Diagnostic Challenges in Sports Cardiology

Diagnostic Challenges in Sports Cardiology

Editors

Lukasz Malek
Marek Postuła

MDPI • Basel • Beijing • Wuhan • Barcelona • Belgrade • Manchester • Tokyo • Cluj • Tianjin

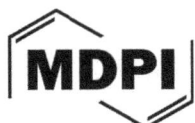

Editors
Lukasz Malek
Department of Epidemiology, Cardiovascular Disease Prevention and Health Promotion
National Institute of Cardiology
Warsaw
Poland

Marek Postuła
Department of Experimental and Clinical Pharmacology
Medical University of Warsaw
Warsaw
Poland

Editorial Office
MDPI
St. Alban-Anlage 66
4052 Basel, Switzerland

This is a reprint of articles from the Special Issue published online in the open access journal *Diagnostics* (ISSN 2075-4418) (available at: www.mdpi.com/journal/diagnostics/special_issues/sports_cardiology).

For citation purposes, cite each article independently as indicated on the article page online and as indicated below:

LastName, A.A.; LastName, B.B.; LastName, C.C. Article Title. *Journal Name* **Year**, *Volume Number*, Page Range.

ISBN 978-3-0365-1203-7 (Hbk)
ISBN 978-3-0365-1202-0 (PDF)

© 2021 by the authors. Articles in this book are Open Access and distributed under the Creative Commons Attribution (CC BY) license, which allows users to download, copy and build upon published articles, as long as the author and publisher are properly credited, which ensures maximum dissemination and a wider impact of our publications.

The book as a whole is distributed by MDPI under the terms and conditions of the Creative Commons license CC BY-NC-ND.

Contents

About the Editors . . . . **vii**

Łukasz A. Małek and Marek Postuła
Can We Provide Safe Training and Competition for All Athletes? From Mobile Heart Monitoring to Side Effects of Performance-Enhancing Drugs and MicroRNA Research
Reprinted from: *Diagnostics* **2021**, *11*, 492, doi:10.3390/diagnostics11030492 . . . . **1**

Małgorzata Stepień-Wojno, Joanna Ponińska, Elżbieta K. Biernacka, Bogna Foss-Nieradko, Tomasz Chwyczko, Paweł Syska, Rafał Płoski and Zofia T. Bilińska
A Recurrent Exertional Syncope and Sudden Cardiac Arrest in a Young Athlete with Known Pathogenic p.Arg420Gln Variant in the *RYR2* Gene
Reprinted from: *Diagnostics* **2020**, *10*, 435, doi:10.3390/diagnostics10070435 . . . . **5**

Tomasz M. Książczyk, Radosław Pietrzak and Bożena Werner
Management of Young Athletes with Asymptomatic Preexcitation—A Review of the Literature
Reprinted from: *Diagnostics* **2020**, *10*, 824, doi:10.3390/diagnostics10100824 . . . . **13**

Wojciech Król, Szymon Price, Daniel Śliż, Damian Parol, Marcin Konopka, Artur Mamcarz, Marcin Wełnicki and Wojciech Braksator
A Vegan Athlete's Heart—Is It Different? Morphology and Function in Echocardiography
Reprinted from: *Diagnostics* **2020**, *10*, 477, doi:10.3390/diagnostics10070477 . . . . **23**

Robert Gajda, Anna Klisiewicz, Vadym Matsibora, Dorota Piotrowska-Kownacka and Elżbieta Katarzyna Biernacka
Heart of the World's Top Ultramarathon Runner—Not Necessarily Much Different from Normal
Reprinted from: *Diagnostics* **2020**, *10*, 73, doi:10.3390/diagnostics10020073 . . . . **33**

Robert Gajda
Is Continuous ECG Recording on Heart Rate Monitors the Most Expected Function by Endurance Athletes, Coaches, and Doctors?
Reprinted from: *Diagnostics* **2020**, *10*, 867, doi:10.3390/diagnostics10110867 . . . . **51**

Robert Gajda
Heart Rate Monitor Instead of Ablation? Atrioventricular Nodal Re-Entrant Tachycardia in a Leisure-Time Triathlete: 6-Year Follow-Up
Reprinted from: *Diagnostics* **2020**, *10*, 391, doi:10.3390/diagnostics10060391 . . . . **63**

Natalia Grzebisz
Cardiovascular Adaptations to Four Months Training in Middle-Aged Amateur Long-Distance Skiers
Reprinted from: *Diagnostics* **2020**, *10*, 442, doi:10.3390/diagnostics10070442 . . . . **77**

Natalia Grzebisz
Determinants of the Cardiovascular Capacity of Amateur Long-Distance Skiers during the Transition Period
Reprinted from: *Diagnostics* **2020**, *10*, 675, doi:10.3390/diagnostics10090675 . . . . **87**

Bartosz Hoffmann, Andrew A. Flatt, Luiz Eduardo Virgilio Silva, Marcel Młyńczak, Rafał Baranowski, Ewelina Dziedzic, Bożena Werner and Jakub S. Gasior
A Pilot Study of the Reliability and Agreement of Heart Rate, Respiratory Rate and Short-Term Heart Rate Variability in Elite Modern Pentathlon Athletes
Reprinted from: *Diagnostics* **2020**, *10*, 833, doi:10.3390/diagnostics10100833 97

Jakub S. Gasior, Bartosz Hoffmann, Luiz Eduardo Virgilio Silva, Łukasz Małek, Andrew A. Flatt, Rafał Baranowski and Bożena Werner
Changes in Short-Term and Ultra-Short Term Heart Rate, Respiratory Rate, and Time-Domain Heart Rate Variability Parameters during Sympathetic Nervous System Activity Stimulation in Elite Modern Pentathlonists—A Pilot Study
Reprinted from: *Diagnostics* **2020**, *10*, 1104, doi:10.3390/diagnostics10121104 119

Łukasz A. Małek, Anna Czajkowska, Anna Mróz, Katarzyna Witek, Dariusz Nowicki and Marek Postuła
Factors Related to Cardiac Troponin T Increase after Participation in a 100 Km Ultra-Marathon
Reprinted from: *Diagnostics* **2020**, *10*, 167, doi:10.3390/diagnostics10030167 135

Sanjay Sivalokanathan, Łukasz A. Małek and Aneil Malhotra
The Cardiac Effects of Performance-Enhancing Medications: Caffeine vs. Anabolic Androgenic Steroids
Reprinted from: *Diagnostics* **2021**, *11*, 324, doi:10.3390/diagnostics11020324 145

Aleksandra Soplinska, Lukasz Zareba, Zofia Wicik, Ceren Eyileten, Daniel Jakubik, Jolanta M. Siller-Matula, Salvatore De Rosa, Lukasz A. Malek and Marek Postula
MicroRNAs as Biomarkers of Systemic Changes in Response to Endurance Exercise—A Comprehensive Review
Reprinted from: *Diagnostics* **2020**, *10*, 813, doi:10.3390/diagnostics10100813 159

About the Editors

Lukasz Malek

Professor Łukasz Małek, M.D., Ph.D., is a preventive cardiologist and a sports cardiologist currently working at the Department of Epidemiology, Cardiovascular Disease Prevention and Health Promotion at the National Institute of Cardiology in Warsaw, Poland, where he leads the Sports Cardiology Unit. He has previously held a position as a professor at the Faculty of Rehabilitation, University of Physical Education, Warsaw. He completed an MSc in Sports Cardiology at St. George's University of London. He specialises in magnetic resonance imaging of the heart for clinical and research purposes. His research focuses on the clinical applications of CMR, sports cardiology, epidemiology, and cardiovascular disease prevention. He has received a number of awards, including the Scopus Young Researcher Award (2009) and the Young Investigator Award—Thrombosis European Society of Cardiology (2007).

Marek Postuła

Professor Marek Postula, M.D., Ph.D., is preventive cardiologist trained both in internal medicine and cardiology. Currently, he holds a full professor position at the Department of Experimental and Clinical Pharmacology, a chief position of the Pharmacogenomic Laboratory. He has previously held the position of Deputy Dean for the English Division at the Medical Faculty, Medical University of Warsaw, Poland. His research focuses on novel biomarkers for cardiovascular diseases, the genetic background of drug responses, and personalized medicine for cardiovascular diseases and diabetes. Importantly, he is also an expert in longevity and ageing research. During his career, he gained experience as a postdoctoral Fulbright fellow in the Laboratory of Perioperative Genomics, Penn State College of Medicine, US.

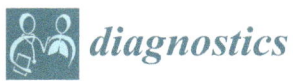

Editorial

Can We Provide Safe Training and Competition for All Athletes? From Mobile Heart Monitoring to Side Effects of Performance-Enhancing Drugs and MicroRNA Research

Łukasz A. Małek [1,*] and Marek Postuła [2]

1. Department of Epidemiology, Cardiovascular Disease Prevention and Health Promotion, National Institute of Cardiology, 04-635 Warsaw, Poland
2. Department of Experimental and Clinical Pharmacology, Medical University of Warsaw, 02-097 Warsaw, Poland; mpostula@wum.edu.pl
* Correspondence: lmalek@ikard.pl

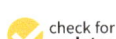

Citation: Małek, Ł.A.; Postuła, M. Can We Provide Safe Training and Competition for All Athletes? From Mobile Heart Monitoring to Side Effects of Performance-Enhancing Drugs and MicroRNA Research. *Diagnostics* **2021**, *11*, 492. https://doi.org/10.3390/diagnostics11030492

Received: 17 February 2021
Accepted: 8 March 2021
Published: 10 March 2021

Publisher's Note: MDPI stays neutral with regard to jurisdictional claims in published maps and institutional affiliations.

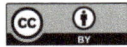

Copyright: © 2021 by the authors. Licensee MDPI, Basel, Switzerland. This article is an open access article distributed under the terms and conditions of the Creative Commons Attribution (CC BY) license (https://creativecommons.org/licenses/by/4.0/).

The foundations of sports cardiology include promoting physical activity and an ability to provide a safe environment for training and competition for all athletes at all levels, from professional to recreational. To combine these two aims, reliable tools to perform pre-participation screening are needed. Moreover, those at high risk of potentially life-threatening events should be advised to limit their training load, while others should be reassured that there is no exercise-related cardiovascular risk. We currently observe an advent of new portable devices for remote and mobile heart monitoring and several new, promising biochemical markers, which can support athletes' diagnostic processes. In this Special Issue of the *Diagnostics* journal entitled "Diagnostic Challenges in Sports Cardiology", we present a series of 13 manuscripts, including eight original works, three reviews, and two case reports, which give a glimpse of the current research topics in the area of sports cardiology.

An excellent example of the balance between the benefits and safety of continued training is a presented case of a 20-year-old athlete with exertional syncope found to harbor a rare genetic disorder causing catecholaminergic polymorphic ventricular tachycardia (CPVT) and predisposing him to severe ventricular arrhythmias and risk of sudden cardiac death [1]. Prompt diagnosis, followed by administration of pharmacological treatment and implantation of a cardiac defibrillator (ICD), permitted the athlete to return to moderate physical activity without clinical events for the time being. This would not have been possible if not for the previous observational reports demonstrating that continued sport participation in such patients might be considered on an individual basis [2]. The current state of knowledge on management and decision-making in several cardiac conditions in athletes should be based on separate algorithms from the non-athletic population and on an individual basis. An example of such an approach concerning the presence of an asymptomatic pre-excitation in junior athletes is demonstrated and discussed in a review of the literature performed by Książczyk et al. [3].

To increase confidence regarding athletes' diagnostic and management decisions, it is crucial to perform differential diagnosis between physiological adaptation to training (namely considering the athlete's heart) and pathological changes. Adaptation to physical activity has been demonstrated in recent decades, mainly in professional athletes, while amateurs, veterans, and other special groups are only now beginning to increasingly enter the scope of research [4]. Interestingly, there may be different athletic pictures of the athlete's heart related to diet, even within the same sports category. Król et al. describe differences between amateur vegan and omnivorous middle-age athletes' hearts. They found a larger left ventricular chamber and signs of better systolic and diastolic function of the left ventricular muscle in the first group, with these changes considered to be positive [5]. Moreover, vegans demonstrated a higher peak oxygen uptake, a marker of physical fitness. On the other hand, an athlete's heart's features may be almost absent in an elite middle-age ultra-marathoner competing at the highest level, as Gajda et al. have demonstrated [6].

Another aspect of sports cardiology is the continuous monitoring of athletes at different time points throughout their careers and during a single season. Doing so may help to detect markers of a new-onset disease, fatigue, and overtraining or predict physical fitness, as described by several articles in this issue. Gajda presents the results of a survey performed on 100 amateur endurance athletes, ten coaches, and ten sports doctors on the importance of heart rate monitoring (HRM) and suggests improvements to make these devices' application more useful [7]. All participants preferred optical rather than strap devices and perceived the possibility of continuous electrocardiogram (ECG) monitoring during training to improve athletes' safety. The manuscript contains a review of new devices used for HRM in athletes and is accompanied by a case report showing how HRM has been applied to detect atrioventricular nodal reentrant tachycardia (AVNRT) over six years in an amateur triathlete unwilling to undergo ablation [8]. Grzebisz looked for determinants of cardiovascular capacity in a group of 16 amateur long-distance skiers before the start of the preparation period. She assessed several morphological and biochemical markers, of which percentage of monocytes, the concentration of sodium, and total calcium were found as predictors of peak oxygen uptake in the regression model [9]. In a series of two articles, Gąsior & Hoffmann et al. focus on the analysis of heart rate (HR), respiratory rate, and heart rate variability (HRV) parameters as potential markers of fatigue and overtraining [10,11]. For that purpose, they studied a group of 12 elite modern pentathlonists and described baseline responses of the studied parameters to sympathetic nervous system activity stimulation, suggesting that the analysis should be individualized [10]. They also found that HRV should be interpreted concerning concomitant differences in HR and respiratory rate and technique of registration [11].

It is still undetermined whether participation in ultra-endurance exercises and competitions leads to acute and prolonged cardiac injury [12]. In this issue, in a group of 18 amateur middle-aged and veteran athletes, we demonstrate that participation in a 100-km running event caused only a mild increase in troponin T, which was not necessarily linked to cardiac injury, as demonstrated by the correlation of troponin T increase with markers of inflammation and lactic acid concentration during the race [13]. This is in line with findings of a detailed cardiac (ECG, echocardiography, cardiac magnetic resonance with resonance spectroscopy) and biochemical panel analysis performed before, 1–2 days after, and ten days after the race in a winner of a 24-h ultra-endurance run [6]. Cardiac imaging did not disclose any alterations, and there were only transient laboratory changes, most likely reflecting muscle damage, liver cell damage, activation of inflammatory processes, effects on the coagulation system, exercise-associated hyponatremia, and cytoprotective or growth-regulatory effects.

Safe sport is dependent on the intended use of legal performance-enhancing medications and the avoidance of illegal substances, which often affect the heart. For that purpose, Sivalokanathan et al. review current data on the cardiac effects of the most commonly used legal and illegal substances (caffeine and anabolic steroids) [14]. A final manuscript of that issue gives a glimpse into the potential future of sports cardiology. Soplińska et al. present a comprehensive review on the role of microRNAs (small particles that regulate the post-transcription gene expression) as biomarkers of systemic changes in response to endurance training [15]. The authors found that miR-1, miR-133, miR-21, and miR-155 are crucial in adaptive response to exercise. It will be interesting to see what the future holds for these markers.

Funding: This research received no external funding.

Conflicts of Interest: The authors declare no conflict of interest.

References

1. Stępień-Wojno, M.; Ponińska, J.; Biernacka, E.K.; Foss-Nieradko, B.; Chwyczko, T.; Syska, P.; Płoski, R.; Bilińska, Z.T. A Recurrent Exertional Syncope and Sudden Cardiac Arrest in a Young Athlete with Known Pathogenic p.Arg420Gln Variant in the *RYR2* Gene. *Diagnostics* **2020**, *10*, 435. [CrossRef]
2. Ostby, S.A.; Bos, J.M.; Owen, H.J.; Wackel, P.L.; Cannon, B.C.; Ackerman, M.J. Competitive Sports Participation in Patients with Catecholaminergic Polymorphic Ventricular Tachycardia: A Single Center's Early Experience. *JACC Clin. Electrophysiol.* **2016**, *2*, 253–262. [CrossRef]
3. Książczyk, T.M.; Pietrzak, R.; Werner, B. Management of Young Athletes with Asymptomatic Preexcitation-A Review of the Literature. *Diagnostics* **2020**, *10*, 824. [CrossRef]
4. Pellicia, A.; Caselli, S. Structural and functional adaptations in the athlete's heart. In *The ESC Textbook of Sports Cardiology*, 1st ed.; Pellicia, A., Heidbuchel, H., Corrado, D., Börjesson, M., Sharma, S., Eds.; Oxford University Press: Oxford, UK, 2019.
5. Król, W.; Price, S.; Śliż, D.; Parol, D.; Konopka, M.; Mamcarz, A.; Wełnicki, M.; Braksator, W. A Vegan Athlete's Heart-Is It Different? Morphology and Function in Echocardiography. *Diagnostics* **2020**, *10*, 477. [CrossRef]
6. Gajda, R.; Klisiewicz, A.; Matsibora, V.; Piotrowska-Kownacka, D.; Biernacka, E.K. Heart of the World's Top Ultramarathon Runner-Not Necessarily Much Different from Normal. *Diagnostics* **2020**, *10*, 73. [CrossRef] [PubMed]
7. Gajda, R. Is Continuous ECG Recording on Heart Rate Monitors the Most Expected Function by Endurance Athletes, Coaches, and Doctors? *Diagnostics* **2020**, *10*, 867. [CrossRef] [PubMed]
8. Gajda, R. Heart Rate Monitor Instead of Ablation? Atrioventricular Nodal Re-Entrant Tachycardia in a Leisure-Time Triathlete: 6-Year Follow-Up. *Diagnostics* **2020**, *10*, 391. [CrossRef] [PubMed]
9. Grzebisz, N. Determinants of the Cardiovascular Capacity of Amateur Long-Distance Skiers during the Transition Period. *Diagnostics* **2020**, *10*, 675. [CrossRef] [PubMed]
10. Hoffmann, B.; Flatt, A.A.; Silva, L.E.V.; Młyńczak, M.; Baranowski, R.; Dziedzic, E.; Werner, B.; Gąsior, J.S. A Pilot Study of the Reliability and Agreement of Heart Rate, Respiratory Rate and Short-Term Heart Rate Variability in Elite Modern Pentathlon Athletes. *Diagnostics* **2020**, *10*, 833. [CrossRef] [PubMed]
11. Gąsior, J.S.; Hoffmann, B.; Silva, L.E.V.; Małek, Ł.; Flatt, A.A.; Baranowski, R.; Werner, B. Changes in Short-Term and Ultra-Short Term Heart Rate, Respiratory Rate, and Time-Domain Heart Rate Variability Parameters during Sympathetic Nervous System Activity Stimulation in Elite Modern Pentathlonists-A Pilot Study. *Diagnostics* **2020**, *10*, 1104. [CrossRef] [PubMed]
12. Merghani, A.; Malhotra, A.; Sharma, S. The U-shaped relationship between exercise and cardiac morbidity. *Trends Cardiovasc. Med.* **2016**, *26*, 232–240. [CrossRef] [PubMed]
13. Małek, Ł.A.; Czajkowska, A.; Mróz, A.; Witek, K.; Nowicki, D.; Postuła, M. Factors Related to Cardiac Troponin T Increase after Participation in a 100 Km Ultra-Marathon. *Diagnostics* **2020**, *10*, 167. [CrossRef] [PubMed]
14. Sivalokanathan, S.; Małek, Ł.A.; Malhotra, A. The Cardiac Effects of Performance-Enhancing Medications: Caffeine vs. Anabolic Steroids. *Diagnostics* **2021**, *11*, 324. [CrossRef] [PubMed]
15. Soplinska, A.; Zareba, L.; Wicik, Z.; Eyileten, C.; Jakubik, D.; Siller-Matula, J.M.; De Rosa, S.; Malek, L.A.; Postula, M. MicroRNAs as Biomarkers of Systemic Changes in Response to Endurance Exercise-A Comprehensive Review. *Diagnostics* **2020**, *10*, 813. [CrossRef] [PubMed]

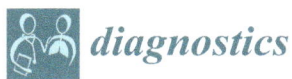

Case Report

A Recurrent Exertional Syncope and Sudden Cardiac Arrest in a Young Athlete with Known Pathogenic p.Arg420Gln Variant in the *RYR2* Gene

Małgorzata Stępień-Wojno [1], Joanna Ponińska [2], Elżbieta K. Biernacka [3], Bogna Foss-Nieradko [1], Tomasz Chwyczko [4], Paweł Syska [5], Rafał Płoski [6] and Zofia T. Bilińska [1,*]

1. Unit for Screening Studies in Inherited Cardiovascular Diseases, National Institute of Cardiology, 04-628 Warsaw, Poland; mstepien@ikard.pl (M.S.-W.); bfn@ikard.pl (B.F.-N.)
2. Department of Medical Biology, National Institute of Cardiology, 04-628 Warsaw, Poland; jponinska@ikard.pl
3. Department of Congenital Heart Diseases, National Institute of Cardiology, 04-628 Warsaw, Poland; kbiernacka@ikard.pl
4. Department of Coronary Artery Disease and Cardiac Rehabilitation, National Institute of Cardiology, 04-628 Warsaw, Poland; tchwyczko@ikard.pl
5. 2nd Department of Arrhythmia, National Institute of Cardiology, 04-628 Warsaw, Poland; psyska@ikard.pl
6. Department of Medical Genetics, Medical University of Warsaw, 02-106 Warsaw, Poland; rploski@ikard.pl
* Correspondence: zbilinska@ikard.pl

Received: 26 May 2020; Accepted: 25 June 2020; Published: 27 June 2020

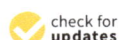

Abstract: Catecholaminergic polymorphic ventricular tachycardia (CPVT) is one of causes of sudden cardiac death in the young, especially in athletes. Diagnosis of CPVT may be difficult since all cardiological examinations performed at rest are usually normal, and exercise stress test-induced ventricular tachycardia is not commonly present. The identification of a pathogenic mutation in *RYR2* or *CASQ2* is diagnostic in CPVT. We report on a 20-year-old athlete who survived two sudden cardiac arrests during swimming. Moreover, he suffered repeated syncopal spells on exercise. The diagnosis was made only following genetic testing using a multi-gene panel, and the p.Arg420Gln *RYR2* variant was identified. We present diagnostic and therapeutic issues in this young athlete with CPVT.

Keywords: sudden cardiac arrest; CPVT; catecholaminergic polymorphic ventricular tachycardia; genetic testing

1. Introduction

Inherited arrhythmia syndromes (e.g., catecholaminergic polymorphic ventricular tachycardia (CPVT)) are common causes of sudden cardiac arrest and cardiac death in the young [1–3], especially in athletes [4]. According to ESC guidelines, CPVT is diagnosed clinically in the presence of a structurally normal heart, normal ECG and exercise- or emotion-induced bidirectional or polymorphic VT, or genetically with the identification of pathogenic mutation(s) in the *RYR2* or *CASQ2* genes [1]. The most common type of the disease is related to mutations in the *RYR2* gene, transmitted in the autosomal dominant way, and *CASQ2* mutations account for the recessive form of the disease. CPVT has an estimated prevalence of 1 in 10,000 [1].

We present diagnostic and therapeutic difficulties with regard to a young athlete who suffered repeated syncopal spells and sudden cardiac arrest twice. The patient provided his written informed consent to participate in the study and to publish his data (Bioethics Committee of National Institute of Cardiology, approval no 1407).

2. Case Description

A 20-year-old male patient, fit and healthy until the age of 17, with a three-year history of exertional syncope (three times within three years), sought medical attention following a swimming-related syncope, followed by sudden cardiac arrest (SCA). The episode was complicated by aspiration pneumonia, and there were no neurological deficits. Structural heart disease was ruled out with routine noninvasive examinations, including ECG, echocardiography, repeated Holter 24-h ECG monitoring, and coronary angiography. Pharmacologic challenges with flecainide and norepinephrine were negative. The patient had two exercise tests: the first without beta-blocker, in which he attained a maximal load of 10.7 METS (85% of the norm for age and sex) with a maximal heart rate (HR) of 171/min (85% of the maximal HR predicted for age and sex); the second one with beta-blocker, in which the attained load was the same, and his maximal HR was 125/min (63% of the maximal HR predicted for age and sex). During both the exercise tests, there was a progressive appearance of premature ventricular contractions at the mean heart rate threshold of 115 bpm, first isolated and monomorphic, and later in bigeminy, as shown in Figure 1.

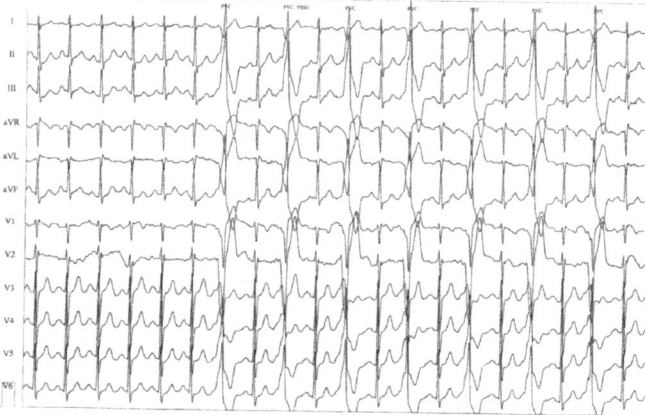

Figure 1. Appearance of ventricular bigeminy during exercise test, which was preceded by isolated premature ventricular contractions.

Premature ventricular contractions disappeared during the recovery period, and the appearance of arrhythmia was asymptomatic. The patient was advised to take beta-blocker. The family history was not informative. An initial diagnosis of unexplained ventricular fibrillation was made.

Despite suffering from SCA, the patient was unwilling to agree to implantable cardioverter-defibrillator (ICD) implantation and, therefore, an implantable loop recorder was implanted and the patient continued to exercise despite being advised against it. One year later, the patient nearly drowned while swimming, was resuscitated, and the loop recorder tracing showed ventricular fibrillation followed by asystole. With a documented mechanism of sudden cardiac arrest, ICD-DR was implanted for secondary prevention, but had to be removed a year later because of the site's infection. Within one month, a subcutaneous (S) S-ICD was implanted, and treatment with beta-blocker was advised again (propranolol at the dose of 120mg/day). At this moment, long QT syndrome was suspected, although the patient has never had long QT in 12-lead ECG.

Despite being fully informed of the nature of the disease, the patient tapered off the medication, continued training in basketball and suffered from SCA in the mechanism of ventricular fibrillation, as shown in Figure 2, while on the basketball court.

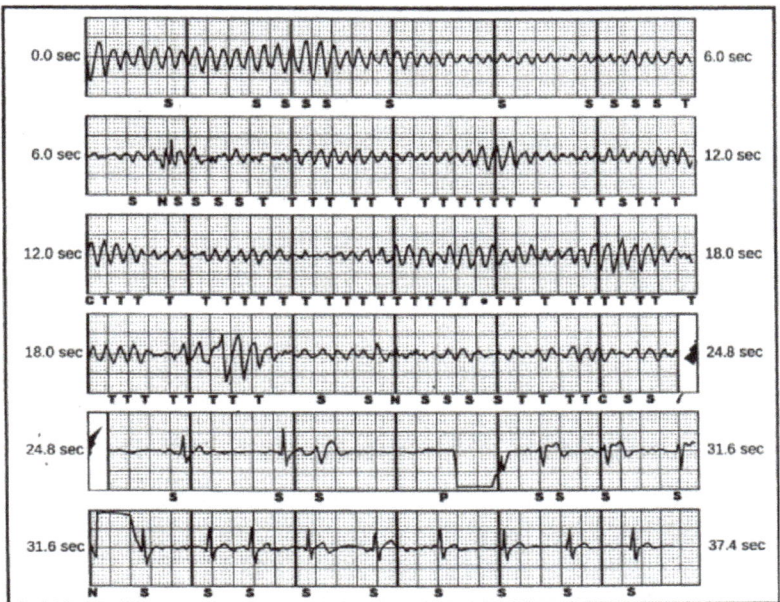

Figure 2. Subcutaneous electrocardiogram showing ventricular fibrillation episode, treated with effective S-ICD shock. Termination of the arrhythmia is followed by sinus beats (S) and, alternately, ventricular extrasystoles of different morphologies (S). One of the beats is a subcutaneously paced beat (P).

Following the adverse event, CPVT was suspected and genetic examination was offered. After obtaining informed consent it was performed with multi-gene panel TruSight Cardio.

A known variant p.Arg420Gln in the N-terminus of *RYR2* gene, as shown in Figure 3, was identified, thus confirming the suspected diagnosis of CPVT.

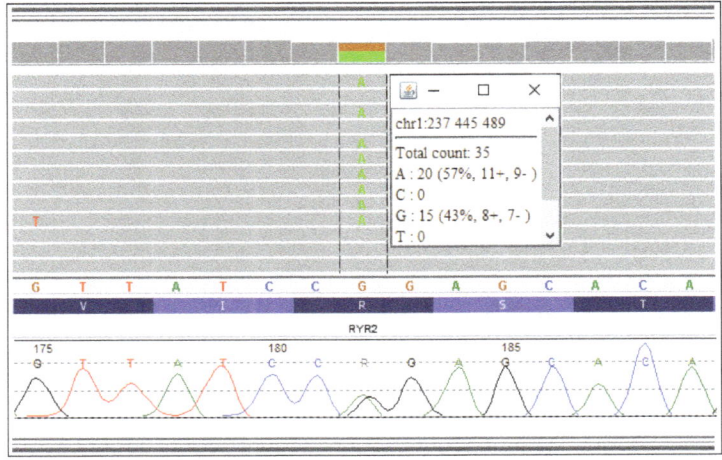

Figure 3. Result of the next generation sequencing and electropherogram showing a variant p.Arg420Gln in the *RYR2* gene.

Following adequate discharge from ICD, the patient agreed to take medication and, with 120 mg of nadolol, he has been free from ICD interventions and syncope for 2 years.

3. Discussion

3.1. Difficulties in Diagnosis—The Role of Genetics

Our patient started being symptomatic rather late, at the age of 17 years with increased physical activity, and first experienced SCA at the age of 20 years. The mean age of onset of symptoms in CPVT is 7–12 years, although onset may be as late as 40 years [5], and the majority of patients with CPVT experience syncope or cardiac arrest by their adulthood. Moreover, the diagnostic hallmark of CPVT [1] is exercise- or emotion-induced bidirectional or polymorphic VT, highly specific for CPVT, but this is also observed in Andersen–Tawil syndrome with *KCNJ2* mutations [6], which were not seen in our patient. The drug challenge was inconclusive. Therefore, the diagnosis in our patient was delayed over three years after onset of symptoms. Only genetic examination helped us to make a proper diagnosis.

The replacement of a positively-charged arginine with a polar glutamine at codon 420 of the RYR2 protein identified in our patient, was first reported in two unrelated individuals from a cohort of patients clinically diagnosed with either CPVT or possible long QT syndrome [7]. Subsequently, it was found in the youths aged 7–14 years diagnosed following syncope [8] or cardiac arrest [9]. Similarly as in our patient, Shigemizu et al. identified the p.Arg420Gln variant in a 12-year-old individual with syncope during swimming who later experienced sudden death at 17 years of age [10]. Additionally, this variant has been identified in a large Spanish family, with nine affected relatives with a clinical diagnosis of CPVT who also had a history of sinus bradycardia, atrial and junctional arrhythmias, and/or giant post-effort U-waves [11]. The functional importance of arginine residue at the 420 position is supported by the identification of a pathogenic variant at the same residue (p.Arg420Trp) in association with polymorphic ventricular tachycardia and experimental studies of mice carrying the variant [12]. Furthermore, the p.Arg420Gln variant resides within the N-terminal domain, one of the three hot-spot regions of the *RYR2* gene, where the majority of pathogenic missense variants have been shown to cluster (e.g., p.Thr415Arg, p.Ile419Phe) [7]. Mutations in *RYR2*, responsible for the autosomal dominant form of CPVT, cause a substantial imbalance in the homeostasis of intracellular calcium, resulting in bidirectional or polymorphic ventricular tachycardia through different mechanisms [13]. Increased diastolic SR Ca^{2+} leaks in ventricular myocytes lead to delayed afterdepolarizations and triggered activity via the Na^+/Ca^{2+} exchanger current, thus promoting ventricular arrhythmia [13]. Another mechanism that seems to be important in triggering arrhythmia is the involvement of Purkinje cells, through increased constitutive intracellular sodium concentration in comparison to ventricular myocytes [13,14].

3.2. Therapeutic Issues

In our patient, several therapeutic problems emerged—first of all, poor compliance to lifestyle modifications. Despite two episodes of SCA the patient continued to perform vigorous physical activity. However, in a recent study on competitive sports participation in patients with CPVT, Ostby et al. [15] analyzed outcome data on 63 patients. In total, 31 (49%) of them were athletes at some point of their life. Compared to non-athletes, they were younger at the time of the diagnosis and more symptomatic. However, following the diagnosis, 21 of 24 (88%) athletes continued competition and, during the follow-up, few adverse events were present both in the athletes and non-athletes (p = NS). Luckily, none of the serious adverse events resulted in death [15]. Of note, the earlier a CPVT is diagnosed, the worse the prognosis [5].

Second problem with our patient was a poor adherence to advised medical treatment protocols, especially treatment with beta-blocker, which is a cornerstone of the therapy in CPVT [1,16]. When left untreated, the mortality rate in CPVT before the age of 40 is 30% [6]. In one third of patients, cardiac arrest is the first symptom of disease [6]. One of the arguments against using beta-blocker therapy presented by the patient was "I am bradycardiac". Indeed, CPVT is associated with bradycardia and aberrant sinus node function may also contribute to atrial tachyarrhythmias [16,17]. Flecainide as monotherapy could be an option, but not applied to our patient due to his reluctant attitude to medical treatment. Hayashi et al. [5] analyzed the outcome in 50 probands and 51 relatives with CPVT. The estimated eight-year cardiac event rate was 32% in the total population, and 27% and 58% in the patients with and without beta-blockers, respectively. The absence of beta-blockers and younger age at diagnosis were independent predictors of major adverse events [5]. Additionally, in the study by Ostby et al., following the experience of any serious adverse event during the follow-up, all patients received an adjustment of their medical therapy [15]. Non-adherence to the prescribed medication was found in 60% of serious cardiac events in the study by Miyake et al. [18] Although beta-blockers remain the mainstay of the therapy, there is some evidence that nadolol is superior to other beta-blockers [19,20]. Only after accepting a high dose of nadolol (120mg/day) is the patient free from arrhythmic episodes. Despite pharmacologic treatment, after numerous syncopes and two episodes of SCA, along with ESC guidelines [1], the avoidance of competitive sports was recommended in our CPVT patient. However, Ostby et al. concluded from their study that the risk of sports participation in CPVT patients may be acceptable for a well-treated and well-informed athlete, although 14% of the athletes experience further events [15]. Nevertheless, recreational activities, not associated with any risk of trauma in case of sudden loss of consciousness/ICD discharge, were advised for our patient.

The third issue that has to be raised relates to ICD therapy in CPVT patients [21]. ICD, in addition to beta-blockers is recommended to patients with a diagnosis of CPVT who experience SCA despite optimal medical therapy [1]. In our patient, ICD was implanted before proper diagnosis and discharged adequately during basketball play, thus saving his life. Since then, he started adhering to medical therapy with no adverse events during the short-term follow-up. Flecainide should be considered in addition to beta-blockers if arrhythmic control in the exercise stress test is incomplete (class IIa) [1]. ESC guidelines also recommend left cardiac sympathetic denervation (LCSD) in CPVT, when recurrent syncope or polymorphic/bidirectional VT/several appropriate ICD shocks occur while patients are on beta-blockers or beta-blockers plus flecainide (class IIb recommendation). There is growing interest in LCSD therapy before ICD implantation, given the increasing evidence of its effectivity [19,22]. Nevertheless, ICDs should be programmed with long delays before discharge since delivered shocks can trigger electrical storms via a vicious circle of adrenergic stimulation in CPVT patients [13,23]. CPVT is characterized by a risk of VF without the need for bradycardia pacing; therefore, when it was possible, S-ICD was implanted in our patient following the removal of the endocardial leads. S-ICD is considered an important option in channelopathies [24,25].

Although beta-blockers extend survival in CPVT and bring relief to patients from life-threatening arrhythmia, there are also reports showing that elevating sinus rates with atropine reduces or eliminates exercise-induced ventricular ectopy in patients with CPVT, suggesting that it may be a novel therapeutic strategy in CPVT [26].

4. Conclusions

In conclusion, the experience that comes from the history of our patient is that CPVT diagnosis may be challenging, and the p.Arg420Gln variant in the *RYR2* gene is inadvertently related to exercise-induced syncope, in particular, related to swimming and playing basketball. Once our patient started following the recommended beta-blocker therapy and adopted lifestyle modifications, no more syncope or ICD discharges were observed during the two-year follow-up.

Author Contributions: Conceptualization, M.S.-W., Z.T.B.; Funding acquisition, M.S.-W.; Investigation, M.S.-W., J.P., E.K.B., T.C., B.F.-N., P.S., R.P., Z.T.B. Supervision, Z.T.B. and R.P.; Writing—Original draft, M.S.-W., Z.T.B.; Writing—Review & editing, M.S.-W., E.K.B, Z.T.B. and R.P. All authors have read and agreed to the published version of the manuscript.

Funding: This study was funded by an internal grant from the National Institute of Cardiology nr 2.19/II/14, M.S.-W. Z.T.B. is supported by a grant from The National Centre for Research and Development, ERA-CVD DETECTIN-HF/2/2017.

Conflicts of Interest: The authors declare no conflict of interest.

References

1. Priori, S.G. 2015 ESC Guidelines for the management of patients with ventricular arrhythmias and the prevention of sudden cardiac death: The Task Force for the Management of Patients with Ventricular Arrhythmias and the Prevention of Sudden Cardiac Death of the European Society of Cardiology (ESC). Endorsed by: Association for European Paediatric and Congenital Cardiology (AEPC). *Eur. Heart J.* **2015**, *36*, 2793–2867. [PubMed]
2. Stepien-Wojno, M. Sudden cardiac arrest in patients without overt heart disease: A limited value of next generation sequencing. *Pol. Arch. Intern. Med.* **2018**, *128*, 721–730. [CrossRef] [PubMed]
3. Stępień-Wojno, M. A different background of arrhythmia in siblings with a positive family history of sudden death at young age. *Ann. Noninvasive Electrocardiol.* **2019**, e12707. [CrossRef]
4. Emery, M.S.; Kovacs, R.J. Sudden Cardiac Death in Athletes. *JACC Heart Fail.* **2018**, *6*, 30–40. [CrossRef]
5. Hayashi, M. Incidence and risk factors of arrhythmic events in catecholaminergic polymorphic ventricular tachycardia. *Circulation* **2009**, *119*, 2426–2434. [CrossRef]
6. Lieve, K.V.; van der Werf, C.; Wilde, A.A. Catecholaminergic Polymorphic Ventricular Tachycardia. *Circ. J.* **2016**, *80*, 1285–1291. [CrossRef]
7. Medeiros-Domingo, A. The RYR2-encoded ryanodine receptor/calcium release channel in patients diagnosed previously with either catecholaminergic polymorphic ventricular tachycardia or genotype negative, exercise-induced long QT syndrome: A comprehensive open reading frame mutational analysis. *J. Am. Coll. Cardiol.* **2009**, *54*, 2065–2074.
8. Van der Werf, C. Flecainide therapy reduces exercise-induced ventricular arrhythmias in patients with catecholaminergic polymorphic ventricular tachycardia. *J. Am. Coll. Cardiol.* **2011**, *57*, 2244–2254. [CrossRef]
9. Ohno, S.; Hasegawa, K.; Horie, M. Gender Differences in the Inheritance Mode of RYR2 Mutations in Catecholaminergic Polymorphic Ventricular Tachycardia Patients. *PLoS ONE* **2015**, *10*, e0131517. [CrossRef]
10. Shigemizu, D. Exome Analyses of Long QT Syndrome Reveal Candidate Pathogenic Mutations in Calmodulin-Interacting Genes. *PLoS ONE* **2015**, *10*, e0130329. [CrossRef]
11. Domingo, D. Non-ventricular, Clinical, and Functional Features of the RyR2(R420Q) Mutation Causing Catecholaminergic Polymorphic Ventricular Tachycardia. *Rev. ESP Cardiol.* **2015**, *68*, 398–407. [CrossRef] [PubMed]
12. Okudaira, N. A knock-in mouse model of N-terminal R420W mutation of cardiac ryanodine receptor exhibits arrhythmogenesis with abnormal calcium dynamics in cardiomyocytes. *Biochem. Biophys. Res. Commun.* **2014**, *452*, 665–668. [CrossRef] [PubMed]
13. Baltogiannis, G.G. CPVT: Arrhythmogenesis, Therapeutic Management, and Future Perspectives. A Brief. Review of the Literature. *Front. Cardiovasc. Med.* **2019**, *6*, 92. [CrossRef] [PubMed]
14. Willis, B.C. Constitutive Intracellular Na^+ Excess in Purkinje Cells Promotes Arrhythmogenesis at Lower Levels of Stress Than Ventricular Myocytes From Mice With Catecholaminergic Polymorphic Ventricular Tachycardia. *Circulation* **2016**, *133*, 2348–2359. [CrossRef]
15. Ostby, S.A. Competitive Sports Participation in Patients with Catecholaminergic Polymorphic Ventricular Tachycardia: A Single Center's Early Experience. *JACC Clin. Electrophysiol.* **2016**, *2*, 253–262. [CrossRef]
16. Postma, A.V. Catecholaminergic polymorphic ventricular tachycardia: RYR2 mutations, bradycardia, and follow up of the patients. *J. Med. Genet.* **2005**, *42*, 863–870. [CrossRef]
17. Sumitomo, N. Association of atrial arrhythmia and sinus node dysfunction in patients with catecholaminergic polymorphic ventricular tachycardia. *Circ. J.* **2007**, *71*, 1606–1609. [CrossRef]
18. Miyake, C.Y. Circadian Variation of Ventricular Arrhythmias in Catecholaminergic Polymorphic Ventricular Tachycardia. *JACC Clin. Electrophysiol.* **2017**, *3*, 1308–1317. [CrossRef]
19. Pflaumer, A. 50 Years of Catecholaminergic Polymorphic Ventricular Tachycardia (CPVT)—Time to Explore the Dark Side of the Moon. *Heart Lung Circ.* **2020**, *29*, 520–528. [CrossRef]

20. Leren, I.S. Nadolol decreases the incidence and severity of ventricular arrhythmias during exercise stress testing compared with β1-selective β-blockers in patients with catecholaminergic polymorphic ventricular tachycardia. *Heart Rhythm* **2016**, *13*, 433–440. [CrossRef]
21. Van der Werf, C. Implantable cardioverter-defibrillators in previously undiagnosed patients with catecholaminergic polymorphic ventricular tachycardia resuscitated from sudden cardiac arrest. *Eur. Heart J.* **2019**, *40*, 2953–2961. [CrossRef] [PubMed]
22. Dusi, V. Cardiac Sympathetic Denervation in Channelopathies. *Front. Cardiovasc. Med.* **2019**, *6*, 27. [CrossRef] [PubMed]
23. Roses-Noguer, F. Outcomes of defibrillator therapy in catecholaminergic polymorphic ventricular tachycardia. *Heart Rhythm* **2014**, *11*, 58–66. [CrossRef] [PubMed]
24. Probst, V. Subcutaneous implantable cardioverter defibrillator indication in prevention of sudden cardiac death in difficult clinical situations: A French expert position paper. *Arch. Cardiovasc. Dis.* **2020**, *113*, 359–366. [CrossRef]
25. Rudic, B. Low Prevalence of Inappropriate Shocks in Patients with Inherited Arrhythmia Syndromes with the Subcutaneous Implantable Defibrillator Single Center Experience and Long-Term Follow-Up. *J. Am. Heart Assoc.* **2017**, *6*, e006265. [CrossRef]
26. Kannankeril, P.J. Atropine-induced sinus tachycardia protects against exercise-induced ventricular arrhythmias in patients with catecholaminergic polymorphic ventricular tachycardia. *Europace* **2020**, *22*, 643–648. [CrossRef]

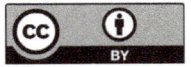

© 2020 by the authors. Licensee MDPI, Basel, Switzerland. This article is an open access article distributed under the terms and conditions of the Creative Commons Attribution (CC BY) license (http://creativecommons.org/licenses/by/4.0/).

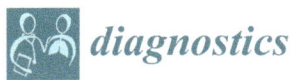

Review

Management of Young Athletes with Asymptomatic Preexcitation—A Review of the Literature

Tomasz M. Książczyk, Radosław Pietrzak and Bożena Werner *

Department of Paediatric Cardiology and General Paediatrics, Medical University of Warsaw, 02–091 Warsaw, Poland; tksiazczyk@wum.edu.pl (T.M.K.); radoslaw.pietrzak@wum.edu.pl (R.P.)
* Correspondence: bozena.werner@wum.edu.pl; Tel./Fax: +48-22-317-95-88

Received: 23 September 2020; Accepted: 12 October 2020; Published: 15 October 2020

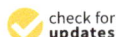

Abstract: Introduction: The management of young athletes with asymptomatic preexcitation remains a challenge, regardless of the progress we have made in understanding the basis of condition and developing catheter ablation procedures. The risk of sudden death, however small, yet definite, being the first symptom is determining our approach. The aim of the study was to establish the current state of knowledge regarding the management of young athletes diagnosed with asymptomatic preexcitation, by conducting a literature review. Material and methods: A comprehensive literature review was completed in accordance to the Preferred Reporting Items for Systematic Reviews and Meta-Analyses (PRISMA) guidelines. The search was limited to English language publications using the following search terms: "asymptomatic" or "incidental" and "pre-excitation" or "Wolff–Parkinson–White" or "delta wave" and "athlete" or "sport". The search was supplemented by hand review of the bibliographies of previous relevant systematic reviews. Results: The search resulted in 85 of abstracts, and the manual search of the bibliographies resulted in 24 additional papers. After careful analysis 10 publications were included in the review. In all but one of the presented papers, the authors used non-invasive methods and then either trans-esophageal or invasive EPS as a way to risk stratify asymptomatic patients. Evidence of rapid conduction through the accessory pathway was considered high risk and prompted sport disqualification. In the analysed reports there were combined: 142 episodes of the life-threatening events (LTE)/sudden death (SCD), of which 56 were reported to occur at rest, 61 during activity and no data were available for 25. Conclusions: athletic activity may impose an increased risk of life-threatening arrhythmias in patients with asymptomatic preexcitation; hence, a separate approach could be considered, especially in patients willing to engage in high-intensity, endurance and competitive sports.

Keywords: asymptomatic preexcitation; athlete; WPW

1. Introduction

Regardless the progress in understanding the electro-pathophysiological basis of the condition, management of asymptomatic young patients with preexcitation remains controversial. We have gone a long way, from the Wolff, Parkinson, and White landmark paper (published in 1930), through description of the mechanisms of atrio-ventricular re-entry tachycardia, linking the episodes of atrial fibrillation with risk of sudden death, to finally developing the modern technique of catheter ablation [1,2]. Further, there are still considerable gaps in our knowledge. Risk of sudden death being the first symptom determines our approach. Preparticipation screening of young athletes is becoming a standard procedure in many countries, leading to increasing numbers of detected asymptomatic patients with ventricular preexcitation (VPE) pattern on the surface electrocardiogram (ECG), who are referred to a cardiologist for risk stratification and treatment or clearance for sport activity [3]. Young athletes are generally at higher risk of arrhythmic events, and the question arises whether they need a separate approach with regard to preexcitation [4,5]. There have been a number of studies published in recent years that tried to estimate the risk of life-threatening events in asymptomatic preexcitation and the usefulness of both invasive and non-invasive tools for its prediction. However, the majority of the major studies on the subject do not address the question of risk related to sport activity. The aim of this study is to establish the risks and management with regard to physical activity and competitive sport in patients with asymptomatic preexcitation.

2. Materials and Methods

2.1. Search Strategy

The authors conducted a comprehensive search for all types of studies in PubMed and EMBASE using the Preferred Reporting Items for Systematic Reviews and Meta-Analyses (PRISMA) checklist [6]. The search was performed through May 2020 and limited to English language publications published between the years 1990 and 2020, using the following search terms: "asymptomatic" or "incidental" and "pre-excitation" or "Wolff–Parkinson–White" or "delta wave" and "athlete" or "sport". The search was supplemented by hand a review of the bibliographies of previous relevant systematic reviews (Figure 1).

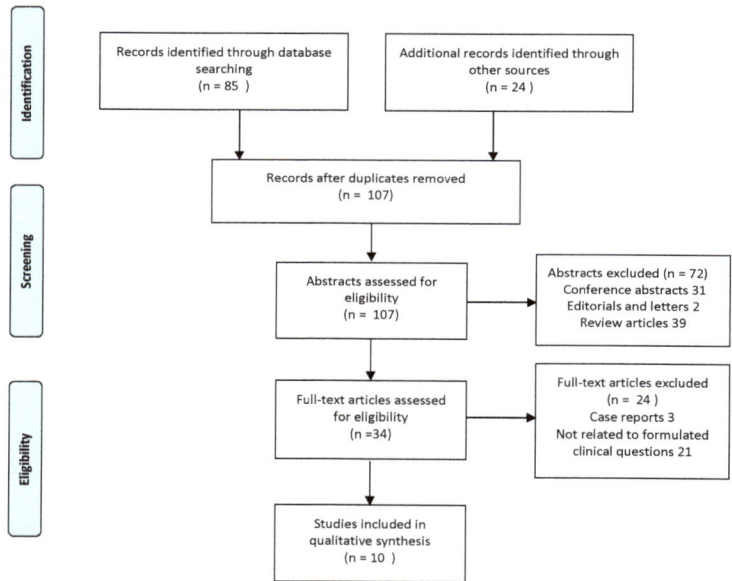

Figure 1. Flowchart detailing the selection of studies for the analysis.

2.2. Selection Criteria

Articles were selected following the title and abstract review on the basis of their relevance to the investigated subject. We formulated following the clinical questions:

1. What was the management of young asymptomatic athletes with VPE in the published studies, and how were they stratified to risk categories?
2. Are the patients with VPE at higher risk of life-threatening arrhythmias while performing physical activity?
3. Should young athletes with VPE be managed differently than other young asymptomatic patients with VPE?

Studies were included if they reflected on the questions formulated above and provided information regarding non-invasive and invasive testing of the properties of the accessory pathway, criteria used for determining high risk patients, and incidence of the life-threatening events (LTE) or sudden death (SCD) including aborted SCD, in the context of the type of activity at the onset of symptoms.

3. Results

The search resulted in 85 abstracts that were reviewed and evaluated by two authors. Manual search of the bibliographies resulted in 24 additional papers. After careful analysis 10 publications were found to provide data relevant to the clinical questions formulated initially.

3.1. Management of Young Athletes with Preexcitation

The details of the analysed studies are summarised in Table 1.

Table 1. Details of the all analysed studies are presented here.

Study	Study Year	Author	Type of Study	Cases	Age of Pts	No of LTE/SCD
1	1993	Munger	Retrospective	53	33 +/− 16	2
2	1993	Brembilla–Perrot	Prospective	40	35 +/− 15	0
3	1995	Timmermans	Retrospective	690	28 +/− 10	15
4	1995	Furlanello	Retrospective	380	20.7	8
5	2003	Sarrubi	Retrospective	57	9.7 +/− 5.4	1
6	2007	Brembilla-Perrot	Prospective	55	14 +/− 3	1
7	2009	Fazio	Retrospective	124	7.8	0
8	2016	Mambro	Prospective	91	11.8 +/− 2.28	0
9	2017	Finocchiaro	Retrospective	19	31 +/− 15	19
10	2018	Ethridge	Retrospective	912	9.7 (+/− 5.3)	96

In 1993 Brembilla-Perrot and Ghawi [7] published a paper that described 40 asymptomatic patients age 35 +/− 15 years, who were followed for a median of 1.8 years. All underwent either invasive electrophysiology study (EPS) or transoesophageal EPS. Patients were considered high risk if the shortest RR interval between pre-excited beats was measured as <250 ms in the control state, or <200 ms during isoproterenol infusion, also in the case of atrial vulnerability or induction of ventricular fibrillation. High-risk features were found in five patients. Two of them underwent ablation procedure, and the other three were discharged and prohibited from participation in competitive sports.

In 2003, Sarubbi et al. [8] followed 98 asymptomatic patients for a mean of 48 months. The mean age at the recruitment was 9.7 years (+/−5.4). Patients were assessed non-invasively at recruitment with clinical examination, ECG, echocardiogram, ECG Holter, and, when possible, exercise testing. Invasive EPS was offered to all the patients. During the follow-up five patients turned symptomatic with supraventricular tachycardia (SVT), and there was one sudden death with no remark about the circumstances. Patients with inducible arrhythmia were offered either medical treatment or RF ablation. In patients with no SVT inducible but with 1:1 conduction over the pathway ≤250 ms in the control state or 220 ms after isoproterenol were discharged without treatment but prohibited from participating in sport activities. The authors comment that this could be seen as controversial but, in their opinion, it was necessary to prevent sudden death.

In 2007, Brembilla-Perrot et al. [9] reported a prospective study of 51 asymptomatic patients, mean age 14 years (+/−3), with average follow-up of five years (+/−1). All patients underwent initial assessment with ECG, 24-h Holter and exercise test, followed by a transoesophageal EPS. High-risk patients were defined if there was a rapid conduction over the pathway ≤250 ms in control and ≤200 after isoproterenol. All high-risk patients were given the recommendation to withdraw from competitive sports. Low-risk and non-inducible patients were allowed to participate. There was one aborted sudden death in a 12-year-old child with high-risk pathway, who did not have an ablation.

At the onset of symptoms, the patient was running with other children. High-risk and inducible patients were offered a catheter ablation.

Fazio et al. in 2009 [10] presented a retrospective analysis of 124 children, median age 7.4 years, followed for a median of 4.2 years. Routine tests (ECG and Holter) were performed. An exercise test was performed in 76 patients. Eight children who wished to participate in competitive sports were offered a transoesophageal EPS. Two of them were found to have pathway of high-risk properties defined as 1:1 conduction over the pathway ≤210 ms or atrio-ventricular refractory period ≤230 ms. There were no LTEs recorded during the follow-up.

In 2016, Mambro et al. [11] published a report on 91 asymptomatic athletes, aged 11.8 +/− 2.28 years, with three years of follow-up. All patients underwent non-invasive assessment including 24-h ECG and exercise test. That was followed by transoesophageal EPS at rest and during exercise test and/or isoproterenol infusion. Based on the result, patients were assigned to three risk categories: low, borderline and high. High-risk was defined as having shortest pre-excited RR interval (SPERRI) ≤250 ms at rest or ≤220 ms during physical stress or sustained atrio-ventricular reentry tachycardia (AVRT) inducibility. Borderline risk was defined as inducibility of non-sustained AVRT and/or an accessory pathway effective refractory period (APERP) of 250 +/− 5 ms at rest, and/or an APERP of 220 +/− 5 ms during physical stress or isoproterenol infusion. Low risk patients were cleared for sport participation. High-risk patients were referred for catheter ablation and were allowed to participate only if the procedure. Patients with unsuccessful attempts or those who refused to have ablation were considered non-eligible for competitive sports. Borderline patients were offered ablation but not as a requirement for sport participation. There were no LTEs recorded during the follow-up period.

3.2. Risk of Life-Threatening Arrhythmia with Sport Activity

The details of the analysed studies are summarised in Table 2

Table 2. Studies that revealed relation of life-threatening events (LTE)/sudden death (SCD) to physical activity are shown here.

Study	Study Year	Author	No of LTE/SCD	LTE/SCD at Rest	LTE/SCD at Physical Activity	No Data
1	1993	Munger	2	0	1	1
2	1995	Timmermans	15	7	6	2
3	1995	Furlanello	8	0	8 (competitive)	
4	2003	Sarrubi	1	no data	no data	1
5	2007	Brembilla–Perrot	1	0	1	
6	2017	Finocchiuro	19	12	2	5
7	2018	Ethridge	96	37	43 (10 competitive)	16

In 1993, Munger et al. [12] attempted to examine the natural history of WPW. In a retrospective manner, they analysed 113 patients included over 36 years of follow-up. Fifty-three of those patients were asymptomatic at the time of diagnosis. There were no sudden deaths in the asymptomatic group over a cumulative period of 537 patient-years. However, 11 patients became symptomatic with tachycardias or palpitations. The patients who became symptomatic were significantly younger at the time of diagnosis than those who remained asymptomatic. Twenty-two patients from the asymptomatic group underwent EPS, and significant arrhythmias were inducible in 18 of them. In the symptomatic group there were two sudden deaths, one during athletic activity.

Important data came from a study by Timmermans et al. in 1995 [13]. A total of 690 patients were retrospectively analysed, 15 of them (mean age 28 +/− 10) suffered from out of-hospital ventricular fibrilliation (VF) and were successfully resuscitated. In eight of them, cardiac arrest was the first manifestation of the condition. At the time of onset of symptoms six patients were exercising, four were under emotional stress, two were at rest, and one was sleeping; data were not available for the two remaining patients. All patients underwent EPS, which showed that in 11 patients, the mean shortest pre-excited RR interval during induced atrial fibrillation was: 206 +/− 42 ms (range 140 to 290).

Furlanello et al. [14] in 1995 performed a retrospective analysis of 1325 competitive athletes (mean age 20.7 years) evaluated at their institution over 19 years. Among them, 380 were diagnosed with WPW. There were six patients with aborted SCD during sport activity as a presenting symptom. There were two more patients diagnosed with VPE, who refused further investigations and that had SCD while playing. Transoesophageal EPS was offered to survivors of the LTE and all patients with WPW.

An interesting analysis was provided by Finocchiaro et al. [15] in 2017. The authors of this report analysed 3684 autopsies performed for SCD and identified a subgroup of 19 patients who had diagnosis of ventricular preexcitation before death. Five of them were asymptomatic. In five cases, additional cardiac pathology was found: hypertrophic cardiomyopathy (HCM), coronary artery disease, cardiac sarcoid. In another four cases autopsy revealed findings of uncertain significance. In two patients, SCD occurred at the time of physical exercise (one in the asymptomatic group); in the remaining patients SCD happened at rest, during sleep, or no data were provided. Five patients had a history of RF ablation for WPW, which was reported to be successful in four of them.

In 2018, a retrospective, multicentre study was published by Ethridge et al. [16], which included 912 patients ≤21 years of age with diagnosed preexcitation, who underwent invasive EPS. Ninety-six patients suffered LTE (case subjects): sudden death, aborted sudden death, or atrial fibrillation with haemodynamic compromise, were compared with the control cases who had no history of LTE. In 62 patients, LTE was a presenting symptom. At the onset of LTE 43 patients were exercising (44%), among them 10 at competitive level (10%), 37 were at rest (39%), and there were no data available for 16 patients—the authors do not distinguish asymptomatic from symptomatic patients here. Accessory pathway characteristics determined during the EPS were compared between the groups. Patients with LTE were more likely to have at least one AP characteristic considered high-risk. SPERRI, APERP, and SPPCL (shortest paced cycle length with preexcitation) were significantly shorter in the case subjects; however, 37% of patients who had at least two characteristics of the AP measured, would be stratified as low-risk patients, and 25% had neither concerning AP parameters nor AVRT inducible.

4. Discussion

Management of young asymptomatic patients with ventricular preexcitation has always been controversial. This is due to problems with risk stratification, which is not straightforward, and, unlike in cardiomyopathies, imaging studies are not very helpful [17]. As we know, there is a small but definite risk of SCD, which is believed to be higher in younger patients and in males [18]. In the analyzed studies the age of the patients was inhomogeneous, however in all of them the mean patient age was below 40 years. The tools traditionally used to assess the risk of SCD are both non-invasive tests and EPS, all of which aim to measure the capability of the accessory pathway to rapidly conduct in antegrade fashion, as well as the inducibility and sustainability of arrhythmias. However, the reliability of those tools has been questioned, as there are problems with general anaesthesia (often used in the paediatric population) affecting the conduction system, and there is no standardisation for the use of isoproterenol [19]. Sudden death and life-threatening arrhythmias can be the first manifestation of the condition, and they have also been reported in patients with intermittent preexcitation and properties of the AP believed to be benign [16,20–22]. In the literature, there are reports with low and high frequency of LTE in asymptomatic children [23,24].

However, when it comes to managing young athletes with asymptomatic pre-excitation, the analyzed studies presented similar approaches. Evidence of the high-risk features of the AP usually prompts disqualification from competitive activities. In all but one of the presented papers the authors used non-invasive methods, but then they used either transoesophageal or invasive EPS as a way to risk stratify asymptomatic patients. The definition of high-risk pathway that has been used by all authors—i.e., evidence of rapid conduction over the pathway with either induced atrial fibrillation or atrial pacing manoeuvres - was proposed for the first time in 1979 by Klein et al. [2]. Shortest pre-excited RR interval (SPERRI) was suggested as marker of high-risk pathway; in later studies other parameters like APERP were proposed as useful [24]. Other recognised risk factors for SCD are younger age, multiple pathways, inducibility of the AVRT during EPS, and septal location of the accessory pathways [25–27].

In the majority of analysed studies, isoproterenol was used to enhance the AP properties and mimic the state of physical activity for risk stratification. Regardless of the small differences in determining the exact threshold for identifying a high-risk pathway, the authors of all the reports share the belief that the presence of the high-risk features of the pathway is enough to prohibit an asymptomatic athletes from participating in sport activities. Importantly, most of them were depending on the either transoesophageal or invasive EPS rather than on non-invasive assessment alone. Some of the authors make the distinction between competitive sport and general physical activity performed in a school environment.

This shows there is a conviction among the researchers that physical activity predisposes to the occurrence of LTE in the presence of the accessory pathway. Sport participation was retained only upon successful ablation of the accessory pathway.

This approach is also reflected in the international guidelines. ESC recommendations for competitive sport participation published in 2005 mandate that risk stratification for asymptomatic athletes is performed with EPS, and RF ablation should be performed in patients with high-risk properties of the AP. Successful ablation or the absence of the risk criteria is a prerequisite for sport eligibility [28].

Published in 2006, ESC Recommendations for leisure-time physical activity suggests that initial assessment could be done with non-invasive tests, reserving EPS for cases with persistent preexcitation. Similarly, to competitive sports recommendations, RF ablation is mandatory if high-risk criteria are present. In the update of those guidelines published in 2020, the same approach is presented, initial non-invasive assessment is suggested for recreational athletes, and EPS should be offered for persistent preexcitation and competitive sports above the age of 12 years [4,26].

In the most recent ESC Guidelines for the Management of Patients with Supraventricular Tachycardia from 2019 [25] and similarly in the ESC Guidelines on Sports Cardiology and Exercise in Patients with Cardiovascular Disease form 2020 it is recommended that all patients with asymptomatic VPE, who are willing to participate in competitive sports undergo invasive EPS for risk stratification and ablation if high-risk properties of the pathway are present. For recreational sport activity, the assessment can be started with non-invasive tests. It is noted that in children younger than 12 years old the risk of a fatal event is small and a conservative approach is suggested [27].

More importance is given to the non-invasive tests in the American guidelines. The PACES/HRS Consensus Statement, published in 2012 makes no distinction between asymptomatic athletes and non-athletes and recommends the same risk stratification protocol regardless of sport activity. Evidence of intermittent pre-excitation or sudden loss of delta wave are considered low risk. EPS and ablation are offered only to asymptomatic patients with high-risk features of the accessory pathway [29].

Similarly, the 2015 AHA/ACC recommendations for competitive sports eligibility conclude that: "in athletes with asymptomatic preexcitation, it is reasonable to attempt risk stratification with stress testing to determine whether the preexcitation abruptly terminates at low heart rates. If low risk is unclear, it is reasonable to recommend invasive electrophysiological evaluation, with ablation of the bypass tract if it is deemed high risk for SCD because of a refractory period ≤250 ms" [30].

Interestingly, the belief that athletic activity should be prohibited in patients with asymptomatic VPE is based on a limited number of cases. Among vast literature on preexcitation and risk of SCD, only a few reports comment on the circumstances and type of activity at the onset of symptoms.

Our review identified only three studies [13,14,16] that provide data on larger groups than single cases, and one post-mortem analysis [15].

Historically, in this regard the greatest influence was made by Timmermans et al. [13], who emphasised the factors that increase the adrenergic tone, like sport activity and emotional stress, as increasing the risk of LTE. However, in this report only six patients out of 15 were exercising at the time of LTE, and the authors interpret them together with the group who suffered VF at the time of emotional stress—four patients, which according to the authors suggests, that the majority of events are provoked by adrenergic stimulation.

In the most recent data provided by Ethridge et al. [16] the total number of events is much greater and a large proportion of them were not related to exercise. Moreover, the authors distinguish between competitive and non-competitive activity, and only 10% of events could be attributed to competitive sports. In view of this, the authors conclude that competitive sport restrictions would not keep the majority of patients safe. At the same time, they would not recommend unrestricted sport participation for athletes with asymptomatic preexcitation. In addition, in this report, the authors suggest that although many of the LTEs were not related to exercise, the time spent performing physical activity is much shorter that the time spent at rest, and in this light the number of LTEs during athletic activity is disproportionally high.

Physical activity, especially on a competitive level, has been linked with increased risk of arrhythmic events in patients with pre-excitation [13,31]. However, it is difficult to establish how many sudden deaths in young athletes occur because of preexcitation, because we do not know the exact number of asymptomatic athletes with WPW pattern, nor how many of them died [32]. Sudden death during exercise is generally more common among the younger population and males [33]. In the long-term registry of SCD among young athletes in the USA, WPW was found to be responsible for about 2% of deaths due to cardiovascular reasons [34].

The rationale behind SCD in pre-excited patients is based on reports mentioned before, with a significant number of patients exercising at the onset of symptoms. At the same time, SCD has been reported in similar numbers to occur at rest and even during sleep. It is also important to consider the mechanism of SCD in pre-excited patients, which is thought to be atrial fibrillation or flutter (occurring either spontaneously or as degeneration of the AVRT) being rapidly conducted to ventricles over the accessory pathway and causing VF [2]. It has been proven that competitive athletes especially in endurance sports are at higher risk of developing atrial fibrillation, even after discontinuation of athletic activity [4,5]. On the other hand intensive training does not seem to affect the properties of the pathway itself [35].

Because of the uncertainty that comes with risk stratification of asymptomatic patients with preexcitation using available methods, and the low complication rate of ablation in the modern era, there is currently a low threshold to offer EPS and ablation to those patients [36,37]. If we agree that physical activity, especially at a competitive level, imposes an increased risk of triggering a potentially life-threatening arrhythmia, then there is even more argument to take this approach in the management of young athletes.

5. Conclusions

Answering the clinical questions formulated initially:

1. In the analyzed studies and in line with recommendations of the major cardiology societies (ESC, AHA/ACC, PACES/HRS), patients should be stratified into risk categories using non-invasive and invasive tests (transoesophageal EPS and invasive EPS) aimed at assessing the properties of the AP. Evidence of the rapid conduction over the pathway either with AF or pacing manoeuvres resulted disqualification from sport until successful ablation could be achieved.
2. Athletic activity may impose an increased risk of life-threatening arrhythmias in patients with asymptomatic preexcitation. However, the data are based on small numbers.

3. Currently there is a low threshold for offering ablation to asymptomatic individuals generally; however, a separate approach to asymptomatic athletes could be considered, especially in patients willing to engage in high-intensity, endurance, and competitive sports.

Author Contributions: Conceptualization, T.M.K. and B.W.; methodology and papers review, T.M.K. and R.P.; data analysis, T.M.K. and B.W.; writing—original draft preparation, T.M.K. and R.P.; writing—review and editing T.M.K. and B.W.; supervision, B.W. All authors have read and agreed to the published version of the manuscript.

Funding: This research received no external funding.

Conflicts of Interest: The authors declare no conflict of interest.

References

1. Yee, R.; Klein, G.J. Syncope in the Wolff-Parkinson-White syndrome: Incidence and electrophysiologic correlates. *Pacing Clin. Electrophysiol.* **1984**, *7*, 381–388. [CrossRef] [PubMed]
2. Klein, G.J.; Bashore, T.M.; Sellers, T.D.; Pritchett, E.L.; Smith, W.M.; Gallagher, J.J. Ventricular fibrillation in the Wolff-Parkinson-White syndrome. *N. Engl. J. Med.* **1979**, *301*, 1080–1085. [CrossRef] [PubMed]
3. Fritsch, P.; Ehringer-Schetitska, D.; Dalla Pozza, R.; Jokinen, E.; Herceg-Cavrak, V.; Hidvegi, E.; Oberhoffer, R.; Petropoulos, A.; European Paediatric Cardiology Working Group Cardiovascular Prevention. Cardiovascular pre-participation screening in young athletes: Recommendations of the Association of European Paediatric Cardiology. *Cardiol. Young* **2017**, *27*, 1655–1660. [CrossRef]
4. Heidbuchel, H.; Panhuyzen-Goedkoop, N.; Corrado, D.; Hoffmann, E.; Biffi, A.; Delise, P.; Blomstrom-Lundqvist, C.; Vanhees, L.; Ivarhoff, P.; Dorwarth, U.; et al. Recommendations for participation in leisure-time physical activity and competitive sports in patients with arrhythmias and potentially arrhythmogenic conditions Part I: Supraventricular arrhythmias and pacemakers. *Eur. J. Cardiovasc. Prev. Rehabil.* **2006**, *13*, 475–484. [CrossRef]
5. Mont, L.; Sambola, A.; Brugada, J.; Vacca, M.; Marrugat, J.; Elosua, R.; Pare, C.; Azqueta, M.; Sanz, G. Long-lasting sport practice and lone atrial fibrillation. *Eur. Heart J.* **2002**, *23*, 477–482. [CrossRef]
6. Moher, D.; Liberati, A.; Tetzlaff, J.; Altman, D.G.; Group, P. Preferred reporting items for systematic reviews and meta-analyses: The PRISMA statement. *BMJ* **2009**, *339*, b2535. [CrossRef] [PubMed]
7. Brembilla-Perrot, B.; Ghawi, R. Electrophysiological characteristics of asymptomatic Wolff-Parkinson-White syndrome. *Eur. Heart J.* **1993**, *14*, 511–515. [CrossRef]
8. Sarubbi, B.; Scognamiglio, G.; Limongelli, G.; Mercurio, B.; Pacileo, G.; Pisacane, C.; Russo, M.G.; Calabro, R. Asymptomatic ventricular pre-excitation in children and adolescents: A 15 year follow up study. *Heart* **2003**, *89*, 215–217. [CrossRef]
9. Brembilla-Perrot, B.; Chometon, F.; Groben, L.; Ammar, S.; Bertrand, J.; Marcha, C.; Cloez, J.L.; Tisserand, A.; Huttin, O.; Tatar, C.; et al. Interest of non-invasive and semi-invasive testings in asymptomatic children with pre-excitation syndrome. *Europace* **2007**, *9*, 837–843. [CrossRef] [PubMed]
10. Fazio, G.; Mossuto, C.; Basile, I.; Gennaro, F.; D'Angelo, L.; Visconti, C.; Ferrara, F.; Novo, G.; Pipitone, S.; Novo, S. Asymptomatic ventricular pre-excitation in children. *J. Cardiovasc. Med. (Hagerstown)* **2009**, *10*, 59–63. [CrossRef] [PubMed]
11. Di Mambro, C.; Drago, F.; Milioni, M.; Russo, M.S.; Righi, D.; Placidi, S.; Remoli, R.; Palmieri, R.; Gimigliano, F.; Santucci, L.M.; et al. Sports Eligibility After Risk Assessment and Treatment in Children with Asymptomatic Ventricular Pre-excitation. *Sports Med.* **2016**, *46*, 1183–1190. [CrossRef] [PubMed]
12. Munger, T.M.; Packer, D.L.; Hammill, S.C.; Feldman, B.J.; Bailey, K.R.; Ballard, D.J.; Holmes, D.R., Jr.; Gersh, B.J. A population study of the natural history of Wolff-Parkinson-White syndrome in Olmsted County, Minnesota, 1953–1989. *Circulation* **1993**, *87*, 866–873. [CrossRef] [PubMed]
13. Timmermans, C.; Smeets, J.L.; Rodriguez, L.M.; Vrouchos, G.; van den Dool, A.; Wellens, H.J. Aborted sudden death in the Wolff-Parkinson-White syndrome. *Am. J. Cardiol.* **1995**, *76*, 492–494. [CrossRef]
14. Furlanello, F.; Bertoldi, A.; Inama, G.; Fernando, F. Catheter ablation in competitive athletes: Indication. *J. Interv. Cardiol.* **1995**, *8*, 837–840. [CrossRef]
15. Finocchiaro, G.; Papadakis, M.; Behr, E.R.; Sharma, S.; Sheppard, M. Sudden Cardiac Death in Pre-Excitation and Wolff-Parkinson-White: Demographic and Clinical Features. *J. Am. Coll. Cardiol.* **2017**, *69*, 1644–1645. [CrossRef] [PubMed]

16. Etheridge, S.P.; Escudero, C.A.; Blaufox, A.D.; Law, I.H.; Dechert-Crooks, B.E.; Stephenson, E.A.; Dubin, A.M.; Ceresnak, S.R.; Motonaga, K.S.; Skinner, J.R.; et al. Life-Threatening Event Risk in Children With Wolff-Parkinson-White Syndrome: A Multicenter International Study. *JACC Clin. Electrophysiol.* **2018**, *4*, 433–444. [CrossRef]
17. Kariki, O.; Antoniou, C.K.; Mavrogeni, S.; Gatzoulis, K.A. Updating the Risk Stratification for Sudden Cardiac Death in Cardiomyopathies: The Evolving Role of Cardiac Magnetic Resonance Imaging. An Approach for the Electrophysiologist. *Diagnostics* **2020**, *10*, 541. [CrossRef]
18. Klein, G.J.; Gula, L.J.; Krahn, A.D.; Skanes, A.C.; Yee, R. WPW pattern in the asymptomatic individual: Has anything changed? *Circ. Arrhythm Electrophysiol.* **2009**, *2*, 97–99. [CrossRef] [PubMed]
19. Shwayder, M.H.; Escudero, C.A.; Etheridge, S.P.; Dechert, B.E.; Law, I.H.; Blaufox, A.D.; Perry, J.C.; Dubin, A.M.; Sanatani, S.; Collins, K.K. Difficulties with invasive risk stratification performed under anesthesia in pediatric Wolff-Parkinson-White Syndrome. *Heart Rhythm.* **2020**, *17*, 282–286. [CrossRef]
20. Di Mambro, C.; Russo, M.S.; Righi, D.; Placidi, S.; Palmieri, R.; Silvetti, M.S.; Gimigliano, F.; Prosperi, M.; Drago, F. Ventricular pre-excitation: Symptomatic and asymptomatic children have the same potential risk of sudden cardiac death. *Europace* **2015**, *17*, 617–621. [CrossRef]
21. Kiger, M.E.; McCanta, A.C.; Tong, S.; Schaffer, M.; Runciman, M.; Collins, K.K. Intermittent versus Persistent Wolff-Parkinson-White Syndrome in Children: Electrophysiologic Properties and Clinical Outcomes. *Pacing Clin. Electrophysiol.* **2016**, *39*, 14–20. [CrossRef] [PubMed]
22. Jastrzębski, M.; Kukla, P.; Pitak, M.; Rudziński, A.; Baranchuk, A.; Czarnecka, D. Intermittent preexcitation indicates "a low-risk" accessory pathway: Time for a paradigm shift? *Ann. Noninvasive Electrocardiol.* **2017**, *22*, e12464. [CrossRef]
23. Inoue, K.; Igarashi, H.; Fukushige, J.; Ohno, T.; Joh, K.; Hara, T. Long-term prospective study on the natural history of Wolff-Parkinson-White syndrome detected during a heart screening program at school. *Acta Paediatr.* **2000**, *89*, 542–545. [CrossRef] [PubMed]
24. Santinelli, V.; Radinovic, A.; Manguso, F.; Vicedomini, G.; Gulletta, S.; Paglino, G.; Mazzone, P.; Ciconte, G.; Sacchi, S.; Sala, S.; et al. The natural history of asymptomatic ventricular pre-excitation a long-term prospective follow-up study of 184 asymptomatic children. *J. Am. Coll. Cardiol.* **2009**, *53*, 275–280. [CrossRef] [PubMed]
25. Calkins, H. The 2019 ESC Guidelines for the Management of Patients with Supraventricular Tachycardia. *Eur. Heart J.* **2019**, *40*, 3812–3813. [CrossRef]
26. Heidbuchel, H.; Adami, P.E.; Antz, M.; Braunschweig, F.; Delise, P.; Scherr, D.; Solberg, E.E.; Wilhelm, M.; Pelliccia, A. Recommendations for participation in leisure-time physical activity and competitive sports in patients with arrhythmias and potentially arrhythmogenic conditions: Part 1: Supraventricular arrhythmias. A position statement of the Section of Sports Cardiology and Exercise from the European Association of Preventive Cardiology (EAPC) and the European Heart Rhythm Association (EHRA), both associations of the European Society of Cardiology. *Eur. J. Prev. Cardiol.* **2020**. [CrossRef]
27. Pelliccia, A.; Sharma, S.; Gati, S.; Back, M.; Borjesson, M.; Caselli, S.; Collet, J.P.; Corrado, D.; Drezner, J.A.; Halle, M.; et al. 2020 ESC Guidelines on sports cardiology and exercise in patients with cardiovascular disease. *Eur. Heart J.* **2020**, *00*, 1–80. [CrossRef]
28. Pelliccia, A.; Fagard, R.; Bjornstad, H.H.; Anastassakis, A.; Arbustini, E.; Assanelli, D.; Biffi, A.; Borjesson, M.; Carre, F.; Corrado, D.; et al. Recommendations for competitive sports participation in athletes with cardiovascular disease: A consensus document from the Study Group of Sports Cardiology of the Working Group of Cardiac Rehabilitation and Exercise Physiology and the Working Group of Myocardial and Pericardial Diseases of the European Society of Cardiology. *Eur. Heart J.* **2005**, *26*, 1422–1445. [CrossRef]
29. Cohen, M.I.; Triedman, J.K.; Cannon, B.C.; Davis, A.M.; Drago, F.; Janousek, J.; Klein, G.J.; Law, I.H.; Morady, F.J.; Paul, T.; et al. PACES/HRS expert consensus statement on the management of the asymptomatic young patient with a Wolff-Parkinson-White (WPW, ventricular preexcitation) electrocardiographic pattern: Developed in partnership between the Pediatric and Congenital Electrophysiology Society (PACES) and the Heart Rhythm Society (HRS). Endorsed by the governing bodies of PACES, HRS, the American College of Cardiology Foundation (ACCF), the American Heart Association (AHA), the American Academy of Pediatrics (AAP), and the Canadian Heart Rhythm Society (CHRS). *Heart Rhythm.* **2012**, *9*, 1006–1024. [CrossRef]

30. Van Hare, G.F.; Ackerman, M.J.; Evangelista, J.A.; Kovacs, R.J.; Myerburg, R.J.; Shafer, K.M.; Warnes, C.A.; Washington, R.L.; American Heart Association Electrocardiography and Arrhythmias Committee of Council on Clinical Cardiology; Council on Cardiovascular Disease in Young; et al. Eligibility and Disqualification Recommendations for Competitive Athletes With Cardiovascular Abnormalities: Task Force 4: Congenital Heart Disease: A Scientific Statement From the American Heart Association and American College of Cardiology. *Circulation* **2015**, *132*, e281–e291. [CrossRef]
31. Wiedermann, C.J.; Becker, A.E.; Hopferwieser, T.; Muhlberger, V.; Knapp, E. Sudden death in a young competitive athlete with Wolff-Parkinson-White syndrome. *Eur. Heart J.* **1987**, *8*, 651–655. [CrossRef] [PubMed]
32. Ceresnak, S.R.; Dubin, A.M. Wolff-Parkinson-White syndrome (WPW) and athletes: Darwin at play? *J. Electrocardiol.* **2015**, *48*, 356–361. [CrossRef]
33. Mellor, G.; Raju, H.; de Noronha, S.V.; Papadakis, M.; Sharma, S.; Behr, E.R.; Sheppard, M.N. Clinical characteristics and circumstances of death in the sudden arrhythmic death syndrome. *Circ. Arrhythm. Electrophysiol.* **2014**, *7*, 1078–1083. [CrossRef]
34. Maron, B.J.; Doerer, J.J.; Haas, T.S.; Tierney, D.M.; Mueller, F.O. Sudden deaths in young competitive athletes: Analysis of 1866 deaths in the United States, 1980–2006. *Circulation* **2009**, *119*, 1085–1092. [CrossRef] [PubMed]
35. Mezzani, A.; Giovannini, T.; Michelucci, A.; Padeletti, L.; Resina, A.; Cupelli, V.; Musante, R. Effects of training on the electrophysiologic properties of atrium and accessory pathway in athletes with Wolff-Parkinson-White syndrome. *Cardiology* **1990**, *77*, 295–302. [CrossRef]
36. Telishevska, M.; Hebe, J.; Paul, T.; Nurnberg, J.H.; Krause, U.; Gebauer, R.; Gass, M.; Balmer, C.; Berger, F.; Molatta, S.; et al. Catheter ablation in ASymptomatic PEDiatric patients with ventricular preexcitation: Results from the multicenter "CASPED" study. *Clin. Res. Cardiol.* **2019**, *108*, 683–690. [CrossRef] [PubMed]
37. Chubb, H.; Campbell, R.M.; Motonaga, K.S.; Ceresnak, S.R.; Dubin, A.M. Management of Asymptomatic Wolff-Parkinson-White Pattern by Pediatric Electrophysiologists. *J. Pediatr.* **2019**, *213*, 88–95.E1. [CrossRef] [PubMed]

Publisher's Note: MDPI stays neutral with regard to jurisdictional claims in published maps and institutional affiliations.

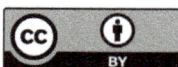

© 2020 by the authors. Licensee MDPI, Basel, Switzerland. This article is an open access article distributed under the terms and conditions of the Creative Commons Attribution (CC BY) license (http://creativecommons.org/licenses/by/4.0/).

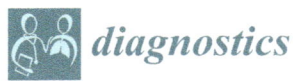

Article

A Vegan Athlete's Heart—Is It Different? Morphology and Function in Echocardiography

Wojciech Król [1], Szymon Price [1], Daniel Śliż [2,*], Damian Parol [2], Marcin Konopka [1], Artur Mamcarz [2], Marcin Wełnicki [2] and Wojciech Braksator [1]

[1] Department of Sports Cardiology and Noninvasive Cardiovascular Imagining, Medical University of Warsaw, 02-091 Warszawa, Poland; wojciech.krol@wum.edu.pl (W.K.); szymonprice@gmail.com (S.P.); marcin.konopka@wum.edu.pl (M.K.); wojciech.braksator@wum.edu.pl (W.B.)

[2] 3rd Department of Internal Medicine and Cardiology, Medical University of Warsaw, 02-091 Warszawa, Poland; damian.parol@wum.edu.pl (D.P.); artur.mamcarz@wum.edu.pl (A.M.); marcin.welnicki@wum.edu.pl (M.W.)

* Correspondence: daniel.sliz@wum.edu.pl

Received: 21 June 2020; Accepted: 10 July 2020; Published: 14 July 2020

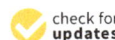

Abstract: Plant-based diets are a growing trend, including among athletes. This study compares the differences in physical performance and heart morphology and function between vegan and omnivorous amateur runners. A study group and a matched control group were recruited comprising $N = 30$ participants each. Eight members of the study group were excluded, leaving $N = 22$ participants. Members of both groups were of similar age and trained with similar frequency and intensity. Vegans displayed a higher VO2max (54.08 vs. 50.10 mL/kg/min, $p < 0.05$), which correlated positively with carbohydrate intake ($\rho = 0.52$) and negatively with MUFA (monounsaturated fatty acids) intake ($\rho = -0.43$). The vegans presented a more eccentric form of remodelling with greater left ventricular end diastolic diameter (LVEDd, 2.93 vs. 2.81 cm/m^2, $p = 0.04$) and a lower relative wall thickness (RWT, 0.39 vs. 0.42, $p = 0.04$) and left ventricular mass (LVM, 190 vs. 210 g, $p = 0.01$). The left ventricular mass index (LVMI) was similar (108 vs. 115 g/m^2, $p = $ NS). Longitudinal strain was higher in the vegan group (−20.5 vs. −19.6%, $p = 0.04$), suggesting better systolic function. Higher E-wave velocities (87 vs. 78 cm/s, $p = 0.001$) and E/e' ratios (6.32 vs. 5.6, $p = 0.03$) may suggest better diastolic function in the vegan group. The results demonstrate that following a plant-based diet does not impair amateur athletes' performance and influences both morphological and functional heart remodelling. The lower RWT and better LV systolic and diastolic function are most likely positive echocardiographic findings.

Keywords: echocardiography; vegan; athletes' hearts; runners; diet

1. Introduction

The vegan diet is one of the fastest-growing trends in nutrition [1]. Between 2014 and 2018, the number of followers of the vegan diet has increased by 600% in the US [2]. This causes both easier access to high-quality vegan products, as well as more research on plant-based diets and better access to knowledge about supplementation and the proper balancing of such diets. This trend can also be observed in the health and fitness industries. Many athletes decide to change their diet and many recent studies focused on the impact this has on their performance.

Regular amateur or professional endurance training induces many morphological and functional adaptations in the cardiovascular system. They include increased dimensions of the heart's chambers and increased wall thickness and muscle mass. Such changes may mimic those observed in pathological conditions and sometimes require monitoring.

In echocardiographic examinations, endurance-trained athletes demonstrate an increased relative wall thickness (RWT), left ventricular mass (LVM), left ventricular end-diastolic internal diameter (LVIDd) and left atrial volume index (LAVI) [3]. The ejection fraction, however, remained similar to untrained control groups. Newer methods using speckle tracking methods to establish global longitudinal strain (GLS) may present more accurate data on the heart's functioning. Recent research shows that GLS may be related to different levels of exercise among athletes and may be different in athletes compared to in healthy controls [4–6].

So far, very little information is available on how a vegan diet affects athletes' hearts. The only research on the impact of a plant-based diet on the cardiovascular system addressed heart failure and other diseases [7,8]. The findings of these studies may suggest that it could potentially be beneficial for athletes. To the best of our knowledge, no study compared the echocardiographic parameters of vegan and non-vegan athletes. The aim of this study was to assess the differences in the athletes' heart morphology and function and the correlation of these with dietary habits.

2. Method

2.1. Subjects

A study and control group were recruited. The participants were recruited from organized amateur running events, such as the Warsaw Marathon, and by online invitation published on social media. Inclusion criteria for the study group (vegan—V) were: having completed at least one organized running event with a distance of at least 10 km, declaring a vegan diet and regular training at least three times a week. The same criteria (excluding the vegan diet) applied to the control group (C), which was age-matched to the study group. The declared vegan diet was then verified by a dietetic survey and nutrition diary. Exclusion criteria for both groups were: age below 18 years, known cardiovascular or respiratory disease and taking any medication on a regular basis. Initially, both groups comprised 30 athletes each. Ultimately, six participants from the study group were excluded due to not following a vegan diet after the dietician's verification and two were excluded due to a suboptimal acoustic window in echocardiography, which did not allow us to perform the required measurements accurately. As a result, the final study group consisted of 22 athletes, and the control group consisted of 30. This study uses the study population from previously published extensive research on plant-based diets in endurance athletes [9].

The study was approved by the Bioethics Committee of the Medical University of Warsaw: No. KB/214/2014 of 4 November 2014 with Annex No. KB/34/A/2015 of 6 May 2015. Written consent was acquired from all participants.

2.2. Tests

The tests carried out among all the participants included: anthropometric measurements (weight, height, skinfold measurement, body composition evaluation using bioimpedance analysis), complex dietetic evaluation based on a 4-day-long nutrition diary, spiroergometric testing on a treadmill and resting echocardiographic tests following current guidelines [10], including global longitudinal strain (GLS) evaluation using speckle tracking methods. In order to accommodate expected differences in height and weight among the participants, the parameters were indexed to the body surface area (BSA) calculated using Mosteller's formula [11].

The echocardiographic measurements were carried out on a GE Vivid 6 echocardiograph using a 4S sector transducer. All the measurements were performed, recorded and evaluated offline using EchoPac (ver. 112 GE, USA) software by one experienced echocardiographer (WK). The chamber size measurements were performed as recommended [10]. The echocardiographer was blinded to the patients' classifications to the V or C group. Segmental strains were calculated using utomated Function imaging (AFI, GE, USA) to obtain GLS measurements. The software automatically divided the left ventricle wall into 17 segments based on manually selected points, two basal and one apical. After the careful assessment of the adequacy of tissue tracing and any necessary adjustments, the software presented the strain curves of all 17 segments and reported peek systolic values. GLS was defined as the average of all examined segments. Following current recommendations, the results concerning LV strain were analysed in absolute values (higher representing better systolic function) [6].

2.3. Statistical Analysis

For the statistical analysis, the commercially available software STATISTICA ver. 13.3 (StatSoft, Tulsa, OK, USA) was used. Continuous variables are presented as mean ± standard deviation (SD), and categorical variables as percentages. The normal distribution of all continuous variables was examined using the Shapiro–Wilk test. The unpaired t-test and the Mann–Whitney U test were used according to data distribution to assess differences between groups in continuous variables and the chi-square test was used for categorical variables. The correlations between continuous variables with normal distributions were assessed using the Pearson correlation coefficient R. The Spearman rank correlation coefficient was used for categorical variables or those with non-normal distributions. Correlations were analysed for all participants together ($N = 52$).

3. Results

3.1. General Characteristics

The general characteristics of the participants are demonstrated in Table 1. The observed insignificant difference in age is a result of excluding eight members of the V group.

Table 1. General characteristics.

Group	V	C
Age (years)	32 ± 5	30 ± 5
Height (cm)	178.5 ± 7	180.5 ± 7
Weight (kg)	68.6 ± 7 *	75.1 ± 6 *
BSA (m^2)	1.75 ± 0.1 *	1.83 ± 0.1 *
BMI (kg/m^2)	21.6 ± 2.1 *	23 ± 1.3 *
Weekly practice time (h)	5.5 ± 4	4.9 ± 2
Weekly distance (km)	48.7 ± 3	48.5 ± 21
Training experience (years)	4.9 ± 4	3.9 ± 3

* $p < 0.05$; BSA—body surface area; BMI—body mass index.

Athletes from the V group weighed significantly less, while being similarly tall. This resulted in lower BMI and BSA. The number of hours spent on training weekly was similar, as was the number of kilometres covered weekly.

3.2. Diet

The daily energy intake for both groups was similar (2647 ± 618 vs. 2408 ± 557 kcal/d, $p = 0.051$). The percentage of energy from protein was significantly lower in the V group (11.8 ± 1.9 vs. 18.1 ± 3.32%, $p < 0.0001$), as was the percentage of energy from fat (25.6 ± 9.8 vs. 31.7 ± 6.6%, $p = 0.0006$). The percentage of energy from carbohydrates was higher in the V group (61.7 ± 11.1 vs. 49.0 ± 7.9%, $p < 0.0001$). Vegans had a lower absolute (g) intake of saturated fatty acids (SFAs, 13.2 ± 7.2 vs. 30.9 ± 11.4 g, $p < 0.0001$), and a higher intake of polyunsaturated fatty acids (PUFAs, 25.7 ± 11.9 vs. 13.8 ± 5.9 g, $p < 0.0001$). The absolute intake of monounsaturated fatty acids (MUFAs) was similar (30.42 ± 15.6 vs. 35.1 ± 12.5 g, $p = 0.11$), however, the percentage of the daily energy intake from MUFAs was significantly higher in the V group (13 ± 3 vs. 11 ± 5%; $p = 0.004$).

3.3. Performance

The peak power output (measured in watts) reached in the treadmill test was similar in both groups. Performance parameters evaluated in the spiroergometry test are presented in Table 2. The absolute exercise capacity, measured as maximal oxygen consumption (VO2max, L/min), was similar in both groups, however the VO2max per kilogram of body mass (mL/min/kg) was higher in the V group. VO2max (mL/min/kg) correlated significantly with the total and per kilogram intake of carbohydrates ($\rho = 0.43$, $\rho = 0.52$, respectively) and correlated negatively with the intake of MUFAs ($\rho = -0.43$).

Table 2. Performance parameters.

Group	V	C
VO2max (L/min)	3.70 ± 0.5	3.75 ± 0.6
VO2 AT (L/min)	2.24 ± 0.7	2.29 ± 0.7
VO2max (mL/kg/min)	54.0 ± 7.0 *	50.1 ± 7.2 *
Power max (W)	309 ± 36	324.2 ± 40.3
Power AT (W)	197 ± 48	216 ± 49
HR max	167 ± 29	168 ± 27
HR AT	144 ± 24	142 ± 19
SBP max (mmHg)	158 ± 30	157 ± 26
DBP max (mmHg)	86.8 ± 10	83 ± 21

* $p < 0.05$; VO2—rate of oxygen consumption; max—measured at peak performance; AT—measured at anaerobic threshold; HR—heart rate; SBP—systolic blood pressure; DBP—diastolic blood pressure.

3.4. Echocardiographic Findings

The morphological findings are demonstrated in Table 3. Vegans presented a more eccentric form of left ventricular remodeling, with greater left ventricular end diastolic diameter (LVEDd) and thinner LV walls (both the intraventricular septum in diastole (IVSd) and the posterior wall in diastole (PWd)). This resulted in a lower relative wall thickness. Both LVM and LVMI correlated negatively with PUFA intake ($\rho = -0.38$, $\rho = -0.37$, respectively). No significant differences were noticed in left atrium (LA) and right atrium (RA) sizes. LA enlargement (>34 mL/m^2) was present in nearly 70% of athletes. Functional systolic and diastolic findings are shown in Table 4. Vegans displayed a higher GLS and higher E-wave velocities of mitral inflow, resulting in a higher E/e'. The GLS correlated positively with SFA and MUFA intakes ($\rho = 0.34$, $r = 0.31$, respectively). The E velocity correlated positively with the intake of plant proteins and carbohydrates ($\rho = 0.32$, $\rho = 0.44$, respectively) and correlated negatively with the intake of SFAs per kilogram of body mass ($\rho = -0.036$).

Table 3. Echocardiographic morphology parameters (with and without BSA indexation).

Group	V	C	p-Value
LVIDd (cm)	5.12 ± 0.2	5.11 ± 0.2	NS
LVIDd/BSA (cm/m^2)	2.93 ± 0.3	2.81 ± 0.2	0.04
IVSd (cm)	1.00 ± 0.10	1.08 ± 0.1	0.01
IVSd/BSA (cm/m^2)	0.58 ± 0.1	0.59 ± 0.1	NS
RVOT	2.92 ± 0.2	2.89 ± 0.3	NS
RVOT/BSA (cm/m^2)	2.3 ± 0.2	2.1 ± 0.2	0.003
LVM (g)	190 ± 34	210 ± 31	0.01
LVMI (g/m^2)	108 ± 17	115 ± 14	NS
RWT	0.39 ± 0.07	0.42 ± 0.06	0.03
LAV (mL)	66.5 ± 19	74.6 ± 16	NS
LAV/BSA (mL/m^2)	38 ± 10	40.3 ± 10	NS
RAA/BSA (cm^2/m^2)	11.9 ± 2.7	11.1 ± 2.2	NS

LVIDd—left ventricular internal dimension at end-diastole; BSA—body surface area indexation; IVSd—interventricular septum thickness at end-diastole; RVOT—right ventricular outflow tract; LVM—left ventricular mass; LVMI—left ventricular mass index; RWT—relative wall thickness; LAV—left atrial volume; RAA—right atrial area.

Table 4. Systolic and diastolic echocardiographic parameters.

Group	V	C	p-Value
E (m/s)	0.87 ± 0.1	0.79 ± 0.1	0.02
A (m/s)	0.44 ± 1.1	0.44 ± 1.4	NS
e' ivs (cm/s)	14.2 ± 2.7	14.3 ± 2.5	NS
e' lat (cm/s)	19.6 ± 3.5	19.1 ± 3.1	NS
E/e'	6.3 ± 1.3	5.60 ± 1	0.03
TVs'	16.1 ± 2.8	15.4 ± 2.8	NS
Peak GLS (%)	20.5 ± 2.2	19.6 ± 1.5	0.04

E—peak velocity of early diastolic transmitral flow; A—peak velocity of late transmitral flow; e'—peak velocity of early diastolic mitral annular motion as determined by pulsed wave Doppler; TVs'—peak velocity of systolic tricuspid annular motion as determined by pulsed wave Doppler; GLS—global longitudinal strain.

4. Discussion

This study presents detailed echocardiographic examination results in a group of vegan athletes and compares them with a well-matched control of athletes on a mixed diet. An additional strength of the study is the wide array of parameters measured in both groups, including detailed dietary data, which allow a more in-depth interpretation of the results.

Overall, the hearts in the V group presented remodelling defined classically as more typical for endurance training—more eccentric, with thinner walls and a larger diameter of the left ventricle [12]. Importantly, despite the ventricle being larger, the LVM was lower in the V group. It has been reported that a higher left ventricular mass in runners is associated with a higher coronary artery calcium (CAC) score, which in the general population is associated with the occurrence of major cardiovascular events. Such a correlation with an increased cardiovascular risk was not confirmed in athletes, although the phenomenon is not yet well described [13–16]. Concentric remodelling and LV hypertrophy are both associated with a higher risk of all-cause mortality [17]. Therefore, the remodelling present in the V group may be more physiologic.

Differences in the diastolic function were also found, measured with tissue Doppler methods (MV E velocity and E/e'). In pathological conditions, such as in patients with hypertension or reduced left ventricular ejection fraction (LVEF), the increased E/e' ratio suggests an elevated filling pressure in the left ventricle [18]. These measurements, however, are not accurate in predicting the filling pressure in normal, healthy subjects [18]. Recent studies confirmed that the athlete's heart is a physiological condition and is not associated with fibrosis or increased filling pressure [19]. In pathologic conditions, decreased E/e' is predominantly caused by lower e' velocities due to the fibrosis of myocardial tissue. Increased E-wave velocity is later present in advanced diastolic dysfunction (restriction). On the contrary, in athletes and in our examined group, high E-wave velocity was concomitant with high e' velocity. In this setting, high E-wave velocity is an indicator of dynamic, efficient inflow during early diastole. It has been demonstrated that better endothelial function and oxidative stress parameters in athletes play an important role in physiological LV remodelling associated with better subendocardial function due to an optimized ventriculo-arterial coupling [19]. The higher E/e' ratio and MV E velocity may therefore be considered a consequence of a more dynamic diastole in a physiological LV. A vegan diet results in lower oxidative stress and may improve endothelial function [8,20,21]. This might be responsible for the better diastolic function in the V group. The correlations of the MV E velocity with plant protein and carbohydrate intakes could suggest a potential influence of these dietary ingredients on a better diastolic function. On the other hand, the higher intake of SFAs may be responsible for the slightly worse diastolic function in non-vegans, based on the negative correlation. A recent pilot study examined the effects of increasing the dietary intake of unsaturated fatty acids in nine individuals with heart failure with preserved ejection fraction (HFpEF) and obesity [22]. The only intervention was to increase the intake of UFA-rich foods (canola, olive oil, tree nuts, peanuts), for 12 weeks without recommendations on energy intake. Aerobic capacity was tested at baseline and at 12 weeks using a treadmill metabolic cart. The authors observed a significant improvement in exercise time and O_2

pulse with a trend toward a significant increase in peak VO$_2$ ($p = 0.069$). Changes in peak VO$_2$ tended to associate with changes in plasma UFAs (R = +0.71; $p = 0.071$). The statistically non-significant result may be due to the small sample size of the pilot study. These results could suggest that the better performance of the vegan group might be due to the higher UFA consumption. Carbone et al. did not perform echocardiography in this pilot study, but their results, together with the results of the present study, may suggest that the improvement in cardiorespiratory fitness is at least partly due to improved cardiac function.

The echocardiographic evaluation of athletes' hearts remains a difficult issue due to the potential overlap of physiological adaptation and pathological conditions [23]. While the LVEF usually remains normal, the echocardiographic diameters of heart chambers may still meet the diagnostic criteria for many serious diseases, such as arrhythmogenic cardiomyopathy and dilated cardiomyopathy [23]. This does not only affect professional athletes, as even moderate training leads to significant changes in the heart and increases the risk of meeting the diagnostic criteria of LV hypertrophy or dilation and RV dilation in cardiac magnetic resonance (CMR) imaging [24]. New techniques, such as GLS evaluation, could give more insight into the function of the athlete's heart [25]. Unfortunately, the results of studies on this parameter are highly controversial. Some evidence suggests that professional athletes have lower GLS compared to controls and recreational athletes [4,6], but another trial yielded opposite results [5]. A recent meta-analysis did not reveal differences in GLS between athletes and controls, but the results were limited by study heterogeneity [26]. Despite these differences, authors generally agree that lower GLS values can be an early marker of LV systolic dysfunction [27]. In this study, the GLS in both groups fell close to the proposed normal value of 19.7% (95% CI, 20.4% to 18.9%) [28]. The strain in the V group was significantly higher, in conjunction with better exercise capability (expressed in VO2max). The correlation between GLS and SFA and MUFA intake could suggest a cause for this difference. This difference could also potentially be related to lower cholesterol levels and better glucose metabolism parameters, which are beneficial for the heart muscle. Such a relationship was demonstrated in type 1 and 2 diabetes patients—GLS was significantly higher with increasing levels of cholesterol remnants and triglycerides [29].

The large proportion of athletes with an enlarged LA in our study is similar to recent studies and is most likely not an indication of pathology, but a physiological adaptation. Even in athletes with advanced atrial remodelling, the left atrial function remains normal, similarly to the left ventricle. Moreover, it has been shown that left atrial volume correlated with exercise capacity in professional athletes [30,31].

The higher VO2max reached by the vegan athletes may imply that they are better trained than the control, thus impacting the echocardiographic findings. However, the weekly training frequency and running distances were similar in both groups, suggesting that other factors may be responsible for the higher VO2max. The moderate correlation of VO2max with the carbohydrate intake and inverse correlation with SFA intake suggests that these dietetic factors may be partly responsible for the difference. It has been found that higher carbohydrate consumption is associated with better performance in an intermittent exercise test [32]. The carbohydrate consumption in the V group in our study (62% of energy) was significantly higher than in the C group, similar to the carbohydrate-enriched diet in the study conducted by Bangsbo et al. (65% of energy) [32]. Our result is also consistent with a recent study which demonstrated that vegetarian athletes had a higher VO2max than omnivorous athletes [33]. Another factor to consider is the similar maximum power output achieved in both groups, despite the higher VO2max in the V group.

5. Conclusions

1. A vegan diet does not result in impaired performance in amateur runners.
2. Following a plant-based diet may influence both morphological and functional heart remodelling.
3. The vegan diet may be associated with certain, most likely positive, characteristics in echocardiography (lower RWT, better LV systolic and diastolic function).

Author Contributions: Conceptualisation, W.K. and D.P.; data curation, W.K., D.Ś. and D.P.; funding acquisition, W.K.; investigation, S.P., D.Ś., M.K. and M.W.; methodology, W.K., D.Ś. and D.P.; project administration, W.K. and D.Ś.; resources, D.P. and M.K.; supervision, A.M. and W.B.; writing—original draft, S.P.; writing—review and editing, W.K. and S.P. All authors have read and agreed to the published version of the manuscript.

Funding: This research did not receive any specific grant from funding agencies in the public, commercial, or not-for-profit sectors.

Conflicts of Interest: The authors have no conflict of interest to declare.

References

1. Parker, J. The Year of the Vegan. *Econ.* 2019. Available online: https://worldin2019.economist.com/theyearofthevegan?utm_source=412&utm_medium=COM (accessed on 5 June 2020).
2. Forgrieve, J. The Growing Acceptance of Veganism. *Forbes* **2018**. Available online: https://www.forbes.com/sites/janetforgrieve/2018/11/02/picturing-a-kindler-gentler-world-vegan-month/#5bdba7b02f2b (accessed on 5 June 2020).
3. Pluim, B.M.; Zwinderman, A.H.; Van Der Laarse, A.; E Van Der Wall, E. The athlete's heart. A meta-analysis of cardiac structure and function. *Circulation* **2000**, *101*, 336–344. [CrossRef] [PubMed]
4. Dores, H.; Mendes, L.; Dinis, P.; Cardim, N.; Monge, J.C.; Santos, J.F. Myocardial deformation and volume of exercise: A new overlap between pathology and athlete's heart? *Int. J. Cardiovasc. Imaging* **2018**, *34*, 1869–1875. [CrossRef] [PubMed]
5. Simsek, Z.; Tas, M.H.; Degirmenci, H.; Yazıcı, A.G.; Duman, H.; Gundogdu, F.; Karakelleoglu, S.; Senocak, H. PP-059 Speckle tracking echocardiographic analysis of left ventricular SYSTOLIC and diastolic functions of young elite athletes with eccentric and concentric type of cardiac remodelling. *Echocardiography* **2013**, *30*, 1202–1208. [CrossRef] [PubMed]
6. Caselli, S.; Montesanti, D.; Autore, C.; Di Paolo, F.M.; Pisicchio, C.; Squeo, M.R.; Musumeci, B.; Spataro, A.; Pandian, N.G.; Pelliccia, A.; et al. Patterns of Left Ventricular Longitudinal Strain and Strain Rate in Olympic Athletes. *J. Am. Soc. Echocardiogr.* **2015**, *28*, 245–253. [CrossRef]
7. Kerley, C.P. A Review of Plant-based Diets to Prevent and Treat Heart Failure. *Card. Fail. Rev.* **2018**, *4*, 54–61. [CrossRef]
8. Tuso, P.; Stoll, S.; Li, W.W. A Plant-Based Diet, Atherogenesis, and Coronary Artery Disease Prevention. *Perm. J.* **2015**, *19*, 62–67. [CrossRef]
9. Parol, D. Ocena wpływu długoterminowego stosowania diety wegańskiej na wydolność fizyczną u osób amatorsko uprawiających biegi długodystansowe. Ph.D. Thesis, Medical University of Warsaw, Warsaw, Poland, 2018.
10. Lang, R.M.; Badano, L.P.; Mor-Avi, V.; Afilalo, J.; Armstrong, A.; Ernande, L.; Flachskampf, F.A.; Foster, E.; Goldstein, S.A.; Kuznetsova, T.; et al. Recommendations for cardiac chamber quantification by echocardiography in adults: An update from the American Society of Echocardiography and the European Association of Cardiovascular Imaging. *Eur. Heart J. Cardiovasc. Imaging* **2015**, *16*, 233–271. [CrossRef]
11. Mosteller, R.D. Simplified Calculation of Body-Surface Area. *N. Engl. J. Med.* **1987**, *317*, 1098.
12. Mihl, C.; Dassen, W.R.M.; Kuipers, H. Cardiac remodelling: Concentric versus eccentric hypertrophy in strength and endurance athletes. *Neth. Hear. J.* **2008**, *16*, 129–133. [CrossRef]
13. Nassenstein, K.; Breuckmann, F.; Lehmann, N.; Schmermund, A.; Hunold, P.; Broecker-Preuss, M.; Sandner, T.A.; Halle, M.; Mann, K.; Jockel, K.-H.; et al. Left ventricular volumes and mass in marathon runners and their association with cardiovascular risk factors. *Int. J. Cardiovasc. Imaging* **2009**, *25*, 71–79. [CrossRef]
14. Neves, P.O.; Andrade, J.; Monção, H. Coronary artery calcium score: Current status. *Radiol. Bras.* **2017**, *50*, 182–189. [CrossRef] [PubMed]

15. Möhlenkamp, P.D.M.S.; Lehmann, N.; Breuckmann, F.; Bröcker-Preuss, M.; Nassenstein, K.; Halle, M.; Budde, T.; Mann, K.; Barkhausen, J.; Heusch, G.; et al. Running: The risk of coronary events: Prevalence and prognostic relevance of coronary atherosclerosis in marathon runners. *Eur. Heart J.* **2008**, *29*, 1903–1910. [CrossRef] [PubMed]
16. Radford, N.; Defina, L.F.; Leonard, D.; E Barlow, C.; Willis, B.L.; Gibbons, L.W.; Gilchrist, S.C.; Khera, A.; Levine, B.D. Cardiorespiratory Fitness, Coronary Artery Calcium, and Cardiovascular Disease Events in a Cohort of Generally Healthy Middle-Age Men. *Circulation* **2018**, *137*, 1888–1895. [CrossRef] [PubMed]
17. Milani, R.V.; Lavie, C.J.; Mehra, M.R.; Ventura, H.O.; Kurtz, J.D.; Messerli, F.H. Left Ventricular Geometry and Survival in Patients With Normal Left Ventricular Ejection Fraction. *Am. J. Cardiol.* **2006**, *97*, 959–963. [CrossRef] [PubMed]
18. Nagueh, S.F.; Smiseth, O.A.; Appleton, C.P.; Byrd, B.F.; Dokainish, H.; Edvardsen, T.; Flachskampf, F.A.; Gillebert, T.C.; Klein, A.L.; Lancellotti, P.; et al. Recommendations for the Evaluation of Left Ventricular Diastolic Function by Echocardiography: An Update from the American Society of Echocardiography and the European Association of Cardiovascular Imaging. *J. Am. Soc. Echocardiogr.* **2016**, *29*, 277–314. [CrossRef] [PubMed]
19. Florescu, M.; Stoicescu, C.; Magda, S.; Petcu, I.; Radu, M.; Palombo, C.; Cinteza, M.; Lichiardopol, R.; Vinereanu, D. "Supranormal" Cardiac Function in Athletes Related to Better Arterial and Endothelial Function. *Echocardiography* **2010**, *27*, 659–667. [CrossRef]
20. Hejazi, K.; Hosseini, S.R.A. Influence of Selected Exercise on Serum Immunoglobulin, Testosterone and Cortisol in Semi-Endurance Elite Runners. *Asian J. Sports Med.* **2012**, *3*, 185–192. Available online: http://www.ncbi.nlm.nih.gov/pubmed/23012638 (accessed on 26 July 2017).
21. Nadimi, H.; Nejad, A.Y.; Djazayery, A.; Hosseini, M.; Hosseini, S. Association of vegan diet with RMR, body composition and oxidative stress. *Acta Sci. Pol. Technol. Aliment.* **2013**, *12*, 311–318.
22. Carbone, S.; Billingsley, H.E.; Canada, J.M.; Kadariya, D.; De Chazal, H.M.; Rotelli, B.; Potere, N.; Paudel, B.; Markley, R.; Dixon, D.L.; et al. Unsaturated Fatty Acids to Improve Cardiorespiratory Fitness in Patients With Obesity and HFpEF: The UFA-Preserved Pilot Study. *JACC Basic Transl. Sci.* **2019**, *4*, 563–565.
23. Dores, H.; Freitas, A.; Malhotra, A.; Mendes, M.; Sharma, S. The hearts of competitive athletes: An up-to-date overview of exercise-induced cardiac adaptations. *Rev. Port. Cardiol.* **2015**, *34*, 51–64. [CrossRef]
24. Dawes, T.J.; Corden, B.; Cotter, S.; De Marvao, A.; Walsh, R.; Ware, J.S.; Cook, S.A.; O Regan, D.P. Moderate Physical Activity in Healthy Adults Is Associated With Cardiac Remodeling. *Circ. Cardiovasc. Imaging* **2016**, *9*, e004712. [CrossRef]
25. Baggish, A.L.; Yared, K.; Wang, F.; Weiner, R.B.; Hutter, A.M.; Picard, M.H.; Wood, M.J. The impact of endurance exercise training on left ventricular systolic mechanics. *Am. J. Physiol. Heart Circ. Physiol.* **2008**, *295*, H1109–H1116. [CrossRef] [PubMed]
26. Beaumont, A.; Grace, F.; Richards, J.; Hough, J.; Oxborough, D.; Sculthorpe, N. Left Ventricular Speckle Tracking-Derived Cardiac Strain and Cardiac Twist Mechanics in Athletes: A Systematic Review and Meta-Analysis of Controlled Studies. *Sports Med.* **2017**, *47*, 1145–1170. [CrossRef] [PubMed]
27. D'Ascenzi, F.; Caselli, S.; Solari, M.; Pelliccia, A.; Cameli, M.; Focardi, M.; Padeletti, M.; Corrado, D.; Bonifazi, M.; Mondillo, S. Novel echocardiographic techniques for the evaluation of athletes' heart: A focus on speckle-tracking echocardiography. *Eur. J. Prev. Cardiol. Engl.* **2016**, *23*, 437–446. [CrossRef]
28. Yingchoncharoen, T.; Agarwal, S.; Popović, Z.B.; Marwick, T.H. Normal Ranges of Left Ventricular Strain: A Meta-Analysis. *J. Am. Soc. Echocardiogr.* **2013**, *26*, 185–191. [CrossRef] [PubMed]
29. Jørgensen, P.G.; Jensen, M.T.; Biering-Sørensen, T.; Møgelvang, R.; Galatius, S.; Fritz-Hansen, T.; Rossing, P.; Vilsbøll, T.; Jensen, J.S. Cholesterol remnants and triglycerides are associated with decreased myocardial function in patients with type 2 diabetes. *Cardiovasc. Diabetol.* **2016**, *15*, 137. [CrossRef]
30. Król, W.; Jędrzejewska, I.; Konopka, M.; Burkhard-Jagodzińska, K.; Klusiewicz, A.; Pokrywka, A.; Chwalbińska, J.; Sitkowski, D.; Dłużniewski, M.; Mamcarz, A.; et al. Left Atrial Enlargement in Young High-Level Endurance Athletes—Another Sign of Athlete's Heart? *J. Hum. Kinet.* **2016**, *53*, 81–90. [CrossRef]
31. D'Ascenzi, F.; Anselmi, F.; Focardi, M.; Mondillo, S. Atrial Enlargement in the Athlete's Heart: Assessment of Atrial Function May Help Distinguish Adaptive from Pathologic Remodeling. *J. Am. Soc. Echocardiogr.* **2018**, *31*, 148–157. [CrossRef] [PubMed]

32. Bangsbo, J.; Nørregaard, L.; Thorsøe, F. The Effect of Carbohydrate Diet on Intermittent Exercise Performance. *Int. J. Sports Med.* **1992**, *13*, 152–157. [CrossRef] [PubMed]
33. Lynch, H.M.; Wharton, C.M.; Johnston, C.S. Cardiorespiratory Fitness and Peak Torque Differences between Vegetarian and Omnivore Endurance Athletes: A Cross-Sectional Study. *Nutrients* **2016**, *8*, 726. [CrossRef] [PubMed]

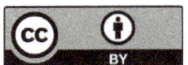

© 2020 by the authors. Licensee MDPI, Basel, Switzerland. This article is an open access article distributed under the terms and conditions of the Creative Commons Attribution (CC BY) license (http://creativecommons.org/licenses/by/4.0/).

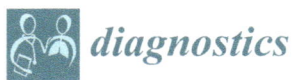

Article

Heart of the World's Top Ultramarathon Runner—Not Necessarily Much Different from Normal

Robert Gajda [1,*], Anna Klisiewicz [2], Vadym Matsibora [3], Dorota Piotrowska-Kownacka [4] and Elżbieta Katarzyna Biernacka [2]

1. Center for Sports Cardiology at the Gajda-Med Medical Center in Pułtusk, ul. Piotra Skargi 23/29, 06-100 Pułtusk, Poland
2. The Cardinal Stefan Wyszyński National Institute of Cardiology, ul. Alpejska 42, 04-628 Warszawa, Poland; aklisiewicz@ikard.pl (A.K.); k.biernacka@ikard.pl (E.K.B.)
3. The 2nd Department of Clinical Radiology, Medical University of Warsaw, ul. Banacha 1A, 02-097 Warsaw, Poland; vadym.matsibora@gmail.com
4. The 1st Department of Radiology, Medical University of Warsaw, ul. Żwirki i Wigury 61, 02-091 Warsaw, Poland; dodo@mrlab.pl
* Correspondence: gajda@gajdamed.pl; Tel.: +48-604286030; Fax: +48-23-6920199

Received: 23 December 2019; Accepted: 25 January 2020; Published: 28 January 2020

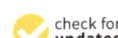

Abstract: The impact of ultramarathon (UM) runs on the organs of competitors, especially elite individuals, is poorly understood. We tested a 36-year-old UM runner before, 1–2 days after, and 10–11 days after winning a 24-h UM as a part of the Polish Championships (258.228 km). During each testing session, we performed an electrocardiogram (ECG), transthoracic echocardiography (TTE), cardiac magnetic resonance imaging (MRI), cardiac ^{31}P magnetic resonance spectroscopy (^{31}P MRS), and blood tests. Initially, increased cholesterol and low-density lipoprotein cholesterol (LDL-C) levels were identified. The day after the UM, increased levels of white blood cells, neutrophils, fibrinogen, alanine aminotransferase, aspartate aminotransferase, creatine kinase, C-reactive protein, and N-terminal type B natriuretic propeptide were observed. Additionally, decreases in hemoglobin, hematocrit, cholesterol, LDL-C, and hyponatremia were observed. On day 10, all measurements returned to normal levels, and cholesterol and LDL-C returned to their baseline abnormal values. ECG, TTE, MRI, and ^{31}P MRS remained within the normal ranges, demonstrating physiological adaptation to exercise. The transient changes in laboratory test results were typical for the extreme efforts of the athlete and most likely reflected transient but massive striated muscle damage, liver cell damage, activation of inflammatory processes, effects on the coagulation system, exercise-associated hyponatremia, and cytoprotective or growth-regulatory effects. These results indicated that many years of intensive endurance training and numerous UMs (including the last 24-h UM) did not have a permanent adverse effect on this world-class UM runner's body and heart. Transient post-competition anomalies in laboratory test results were typical of those commonly observed after UM efforts.

Keywords: professional ultramarathon runner; echocardiography; electrocardiogram; magnetic resonance imaging; Cardiac ^{31}P-MR spectroscopy; blood tests

1. Introduction

Ultramarathon (UM) running is becoming increasingly popular [1,2]. The number of UMs organized worldwide and the number of competitors of both sexes and various ages increase every year [3–6]. Many of these UMs have a long-standing tradition and take place in different weather conditions and on various routes[1]. UMs are considered to be longer the classic marathon (i.e., >42.195 km); there is no upper limit to the distance. Regular events include 100-km and multi-week runs[2] [7]. The longest

UM in history was 5509-km, between New York and Los Angeles, and held in 1928 [8]. Currently, the longest official UM in the world that takes place regularly is the Self-Transcendence 3100-mile race, which covers a total distance of 3100 miles (4989 km)[3]. During the competition, which lasts for many days, competitors must sleep and rest between individual sections of the run, where every section is longer than the marathon (i.e., >42.195 km) [9]. Athletes train for thousands of hours over the course of years [10,11]. Training triggers physiological adaptations, including in the heart and circulatory system [12,13]. The start of the competition is associated with extreme cardiovascular efforts, and the numerous transient changes that are commonly observed in blood test results may indicate damage to the heart or a cytoprotective reaction to long-term stress (e.g., increases in troponin and N-pro brain natriuretic protein [BNP]) [14,15]. Morphological and functional changes to the heart are sometimes observed, but they are not physiological adaptations to extreme endurance efforts. These changes include atrial fibrillation [16,17], bradyarrhythmia, atrioventricular conduction block [18,19], undefined cardiac hypertrophy [20], and non-sustained ventricular tachycardia [21–23], which, in many cases, disappear after training is stopped [24]. Other changes, such as Phidippides cardiomyopathy or presumably exercise-induced arrhythmogenic right ventricular cardiomyopathy, pose significant threats to an athlete's life and do not always disappear after the cessation of training [25,26]. It is not understood why some athletes develop these diseases while others who train in the same way do not. However, there is a relationship between the duration and speed of run and the amount of time spent training and the likelihood of heart disorders [27,28]. One thoroughly tested competitor with elite results who has qualified to compete among the best UM runners in the world has contributed to significantly increasing our knowledge about the potential threats to the body and heart resulting from extreme UM training and competitions. Today, this knowledge is much greater in the case of marathon runs and still scarce in the case of UM runs.

In this study, we tested this 36-year-old athlete (one of the most titled UM runners in the world) before and after the 24-h UM. We hypothesized that many years of intensive UM training as well as competing in a 24-h UM may have adverse effects on the heart and body of this world-class athlete. We assessed him using an electrocardiography (ECG), transthoracic echocardiography (TTE), magnetic resonance imaging (MRI), ^{31}P magnetic resonance spectroscopy (^{31}P MRS), and other laboratory tests.

2. Materials and Methods

2.1. Sports Biography and Main Achievements

The UM runner we tested was 36 years old on the day of the competition (height, 1.73 m; weight, 63 kg; body mass index, 21.05 kg/m^2). He has a sedentary profession and works Monday to Friday from 8:00 h to 16:00 h. He has been running regularly for 20 years and has run approximately 100,000 km in his lifetime. As part of his daily training over the past year, he has run an average of 22 km/day from Monday to Friday; he runs approximately 37 km on Saturdays and Sundays. He also swims, performs gymnastics, and goes to the gym for cross-training. For many years, he has been a Polish representative in UM runs, and his performance over the past several years can be found on his official website[5]. This athlete has participated in approximately 50 UMs, the longest of which was a 48-h run (362-km crown distance, 24-h UM). He has never been injured or seriously ill. The athlete we tested is one of the most successful UM runners in the world. He is a two-time Polish Champion in the 24-h UM (2017, he ran 258.228 km during the UM) and the winner of the Spartathlon in Greece (2016, 246 km). In addition, he holds numerous other honors. In 2014, he set the Polish record for 12-h races (145.572 km). He has participated in the 24-h UM World Championships four times and has won a medal each time. In 2019, he won the 48-h race in Athens (362 km).

2.2. Methods

The athlete tapered his training 2 weeks before the start of the 24-h UM (i.e., gradually reduced exercise over a short period of time and then stopped completely before the competition). The run started at 12:00 h on April 8, 2017 (weather conditions are presented in Figure 1). The competitors ran on a 2-km loop (exact distance, 1.984 km) in a clockwise direction. On one of the straight sections, there was a tent in which the athlete could stop for a meal, a short rest, and basic hygiene. After 12 h, he stopped for 12–15 min for a warm meal, a change of shoes, and other hygiene activities. In addition, he used the toilet three times (2–3 min each). He ate other meals and drank liquids during the run. These competitions comprised the official Polish Championships of the 24-h UM (official website of the competition: https://pzla.pl/aktualnosci/9409-10-mistrzstwa-polski-w-biegu-24-godzinnym).

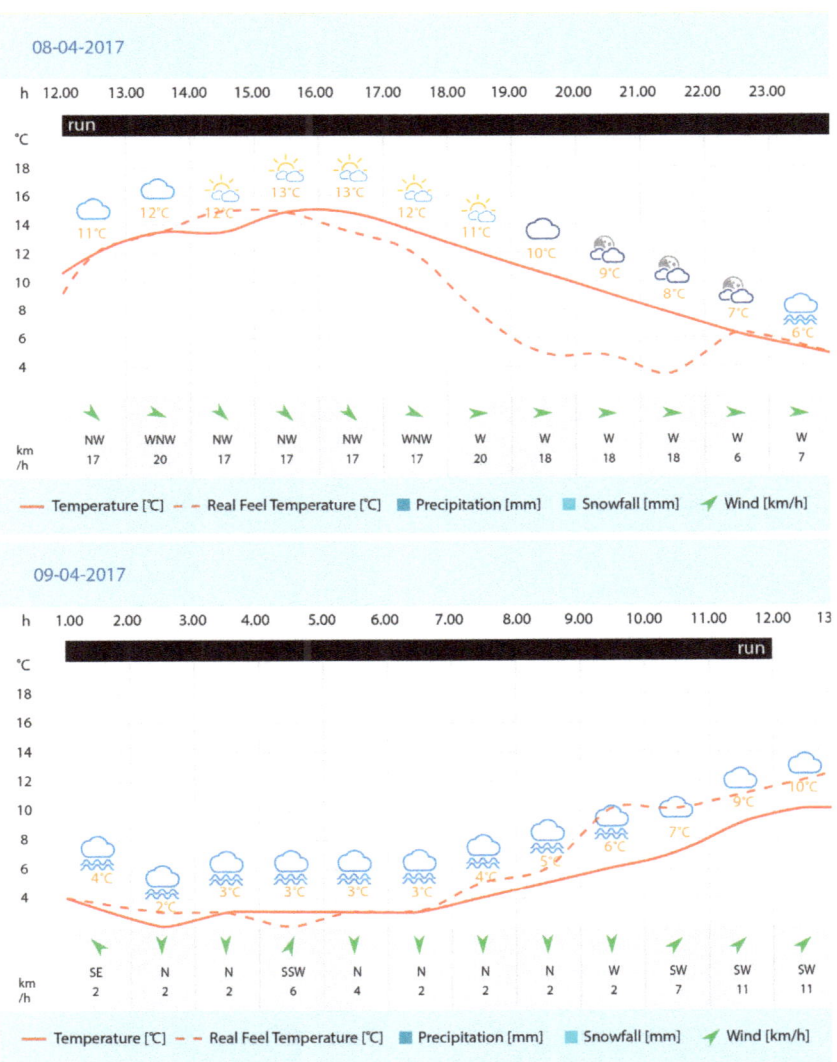

Figure 1. Detailed weather condition in Łódź, Poland, during a 24-h UM competition according to Global Forecast System weather (API by AccuWeather, Inc., State College, Pennsylvania, USA).

2.2.1. Study Protocol

ECG, TTE, MRI, cardiac ^{31}P MRS, and blood tests were performed three times. The dates and types of medical tests are presented in Table 1.

Table 1. Date, place, and type of medical tests.

Days before or after the Run	Before Run	1 Day after the Run	2 Days after the Run	10 Days after the Run	11 Days after the Run
ECG	x	x		x	
TTE	x	x		x	
Blood tests	x	x		x	
MRI	x	x		x	
Cardiac ^{31}P MRS	x		x		x

ECG, electrocardiogram; TTE, transthoracic echocardiography; MRI, magnetic resonance imaging; ^{31}P MRS, cardiac ^{31}P magnetic resonance spectroscopy.

2.2.2. Laboratory Examinations

Blood samples were collected from the median cubital vein with a Kima closed blood collection system. Samples were collected into the following tubes: EDTA K3 (trisodium potassium edetate) tubes for blood morphology testing; 3.2% sodium citrate tubes for coagulation tests; and clotting activator tubes for biochemical and immunochemical tests. Samples for biochemical and coagulation tests were spun in a Nuve NF 800 (Ankara, Turkey) centrifuge for 10 min at 3000 rpm. Blood morphology was analyzed on a SYSMEX XS 1000i analyzer (Kobe, Japan). Biochemical tests were conducted using serum (obtained by centrifugation) and performed using a Roche Integra 400 PLUS (Basel, Switzerland). Immunochemical tests were performed with a Roche Cobas E 411 (Basel, Switzerland). Coagulation tests were conducted using plasma and performed using a Bioksel 6000 (Grudziądz, Poland). The parameters determined were subject to internal and external laboratory controls (COBJ in DL; EQuas of Bio-Rad, Hercules, Kalifornia, USA).

2.2.3. ECG Tests

Standard 12-lead ECG was performed using a Philips PageWriter TC50 apparatus (Eindhoven, Netherlands).

2.2.4. Transthoracic Echocardiography

The patient underwent three complete transthoracic echocardiographic examinations (3 days before, 1 day after, and 10 days after the race) using a GE Medical System Vivid 7 (Chicago, Illinois, USA) with a 2.5-MHz transducer. M-mode, two-dimensional (2D) imaging, and Doppler techniques were used. Left ventricular (LV) end-systolic and LV end-diastolic volume and interventricular septal diastolic diameter and posterior wall thickness diameter were measured. LV systolic function was evaluated by LV ejection fraction (LVEF) and longitudinal strain (global longitudinal strain [GLS]).

LV diastolic function was evaluated using mitral inflow velocities and tissue Doppler imaging (TDI) values. The transmitral early diastolic (E-wave) velocity and atrial (A-wave) velocity were measured. The E/A ratio was calculated. Early diastolic velocity (e′) was measured in addition to E/e′ ratio.

The right ventricular end-diastolic diameter from the parasternal long-axis view and the tricuspid lateral annular systolic velocity wave (S′RV) were measured using TDI. The right atrial area (RAA) and left atrial volume index were calculated using the body surface area

2.2.5. MRI

MRI was performed on a Philips Achieva 3T TX clinical scanner (Philips Medical Systems, Eindhoven, Netherlands) using the multi-coil receive mode. The protocol included B-TFE, s-TFE-GRID,

Q-sFOLW SENSE images, first-pass perfusion module, and delayed enhancement images. Functions of the left and right ventricles were analyzed from short-axis cine images.

2.2.6. P MRS

^{31}P MRS was performed on a 1.5-T scanner (Siemens Avanto SQ T-Class, Tim (76 × 32), multinuclear option, Erlangen, Germany) at three time points: 5 days before the run, 48 h after the run, and 11 days after the run.

An ^{1}H/^{31}P transmit/receive heart/liver coil was used to obtain magnitude proton scout images of the heart and ^{31}P spectra. ECG-gated multiple voxel ^{31}P chemical shift imaging was used for cardiac ^{31}P-MRS. The ratio of phosphocreatine (PCr) to adenosine triphosphate (ATP) was measured from the interventricular septum. The three spectra of the highest quality from each time point were chosen for analysis and the mean results were obtained.

2.2.7. Ethical Approval

This case report was approved by the ethical review board of the Bioethics Committee of the Healthy Lifestyle Foundation in Pułtusk (EC 3/2017/medicine/sports, approval date: 30 March 2017). The runner provided his written informed consent to participate in the analysis and for his data to be published.

3. Results

3.1. Laboratory Examinations (Morphological, Biochemical, Coagulation)

Baseline results were all normal except for cholesterol and LDL-C, which were increased. On the first day after the UM, the following were increased relative to baseline: white blood cells, neutrophils, fibrinogen, alanine aminotransferase, aspartate aminotransferase, creatine kinase (CK), C-reactive protein, and N-terminal type B natriuretic propeptide. In addition, hemoglobin and hematocrit were below normal levels, and cholesterol and LDL-C levels decreased to normal values. Furthermore, the athlete had hyponatremia. On day 10, all results returned to normal and cholesterol and LDL-C returned to their original abnormal values (Table 2).

Table 2. Summary results of blood tests.

Parameters	Units	Before Run	1 Day after the Run	10 Days after the Run	Reference Values
Morphology					
White blood cells	10^9/L	4	↑ 10.87	5.36	4.0–10.0
Neutrophils	10^9/L	↓1.81	↑ 8.46	2.67	2.5–5.0
Neutrophils (%)	%	45.2	↑ 77.8	49.8	45.0–70.0
Lymphocytes	10^9/L	↓ 1.22	↓ 1.18	1.74	1.5–3.5
Lymphocytes (%)	%	30.5	↓ 10.9	32.5	20.0–45.0
Monocytes	10^9/L	0.44	0.72	0.54	0.2–0.8
Monocytes (%)	%	↑ 11.0	6.6	↑10.1	3.0–8.0
Eosinophils	10^9/L	↑ 0.46	↑0.49	0.36	0.04–0.40
Eosinophils (%)	%	↑ 11.5	4.5	↑6.7	1.0–5.0
Basophils	10^9/L	0.07	0.02	0.05	0.020–0.100
Basophils (%)	%	↑ 1.8	0.2	0.9	0.0–1.0
Red blood cells	10^{12}/L	4.96	4.39	5.02	4.1–6.2
Hemoglobin	g/dL	15	↓ 13.4	15.2	14.0–18.0

Table 2. Cont.

Parameters	Units	Before Run	1 Day after the Run	10 Days after the Run	Reference Values
Morphology					
Hematocrit	%	42.8	↓ 38.0	44.2	40.0–54.0
Mean corpuscular volume	fL	86.3	86.6	88	77.0–95.0
Mean corpuscular hemoglobin concentration	g/dL	35	35.3	34.4	32.0–36.0
Biochemistry					
Na	mmol/L	139.28	↓ 135.8	140.02	136.0–145.0
K	mmol/L	4.75	4.13	5.12	3.8–5.2
Cl	mmol/L	99.29	98.89	101.36	98.0–110.0
Protein	g/dL	7	/	6.9	6.0–8.0
Glucose	mg/dL	↑ 105	↑109.0	95	70–99
Creatinine	mg/dL	0.76	0.74	0.64	0.30–1.20
Estimated glomerular filtration rate	mL/min/1.73 m^2	≥60	≥60	≥60	/
Urea	mg/dL	25	35	28	<50
Uric acid	mg/dL	4.2	4.2	4.7	2.7–7.0
Alanine aminotransferase	U/L	12.74	↑73.65	32.96	<40.0
Aspartate amino transferase	U/L	18.42	↑249.18	24.93	<37.0
Gamma-G glutamyl transpeptidase	U/L	25.42	20.64	37	6.00–71.00
Amylase	U/L	51.54	47.21	56.02	10.0–100.0
Creatine kinase	U/L	102.9	↑ 5079.6	91.1	26–174
Cholesterol	mg/dL	↑ 255	177	↑ 240	115–190
HDL-C	mg/dL	67	80	72	>40
Triglycerides	mg/dL	55.04	34.9	82.81	<150.0
Low-density lipoprotein direct measured	mg/dL	185	106	163	<115
Non-HDL-C	mg/dL	188	97	168	40–160
Fe	μg/dL	120	70	134	70–181
Unsaturated iron binding capacity	ug/dL	193.9	179	197.3	150.0–349.0
Transferrin saturation	%	39.75	29.27	40.69	20.00–45.00
Total iron binding capacity	μg/dL	321.85	253.07	332.68	200–400
C-reactive protein	mg/L	0.09	↑144.12	1.52	0.0–5.0
D-Dimers	ng/mL	352.84	398.09	277.3	<113.0
N-terminal-pro hormone BNP	pg/mL	9.9	213.6	16.1	<125.00
Troponin T	pg/mL	3.67	8.11	6.32	<14
BNP	pg/mL	/	29	<2	<35

Table 2. Cont.

Parameters	Units	Before Run	1 Day after the Run	10 Days after the Run	Reference Values
Coagulology					
Activated partial thromboplastin time	sek.	23.9	33	28.7	/
Activated partial thromboplastin time ratio	/	↓0.70	0.97	0.84	0.80–1.20
Prothrombin time	sek.	10.1	10.4	9.5	/
Prothrombin ratio	%	101	98	107	80.0–120.0
International normalized ratio	/	0.99	1.02	0.93	0.80–1.20
Fibrinogen	g/L	3.7	↑8.24	↑4.26	1.80–4.00

BNP, brain natriuretic protein; HDL-C, high-density lipoprotein cholesterol, ↓- under the reference values, ↑ - above the reference values.

3.2. Electrocardiography

During the ECG, we observed sinus rhythm, left atrial enlargement, an incomplete right bundle block, and an increase in QRS amplitude with a normal QRS axis (the QRS voltage criteria for right ventricular hypertrophy were not fulfilled on either side) before, 1 day after, and 10 days after the 24-h UM. Abnormal negative T waves in III and aVF (flat in aVF 1 day after running) together with left atrial enlargement would suggest the need for further evaluation (Table 3, Figure 2A–C).

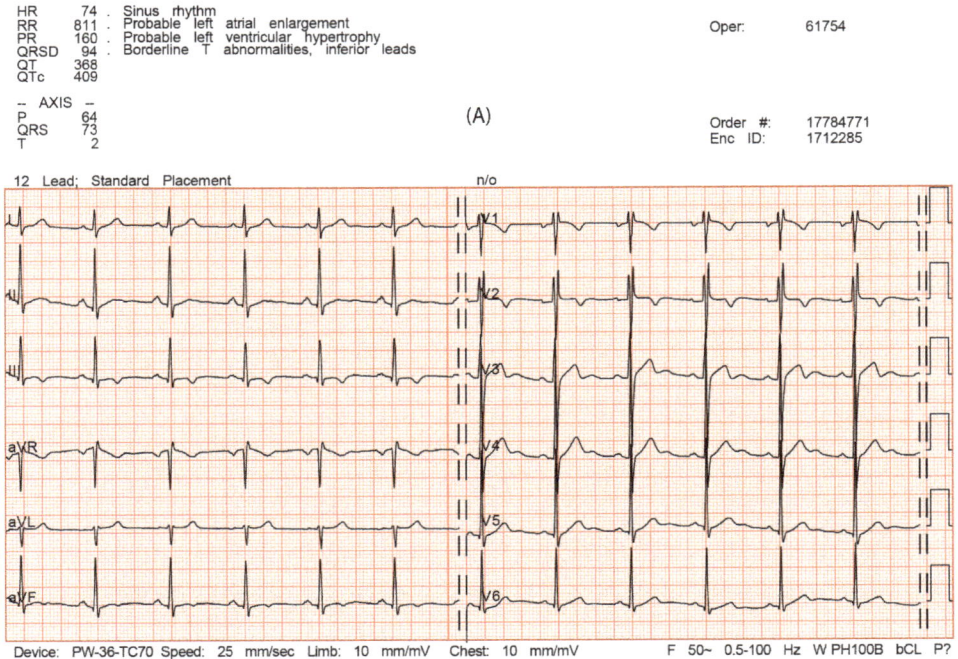

Figure 2. Cont.

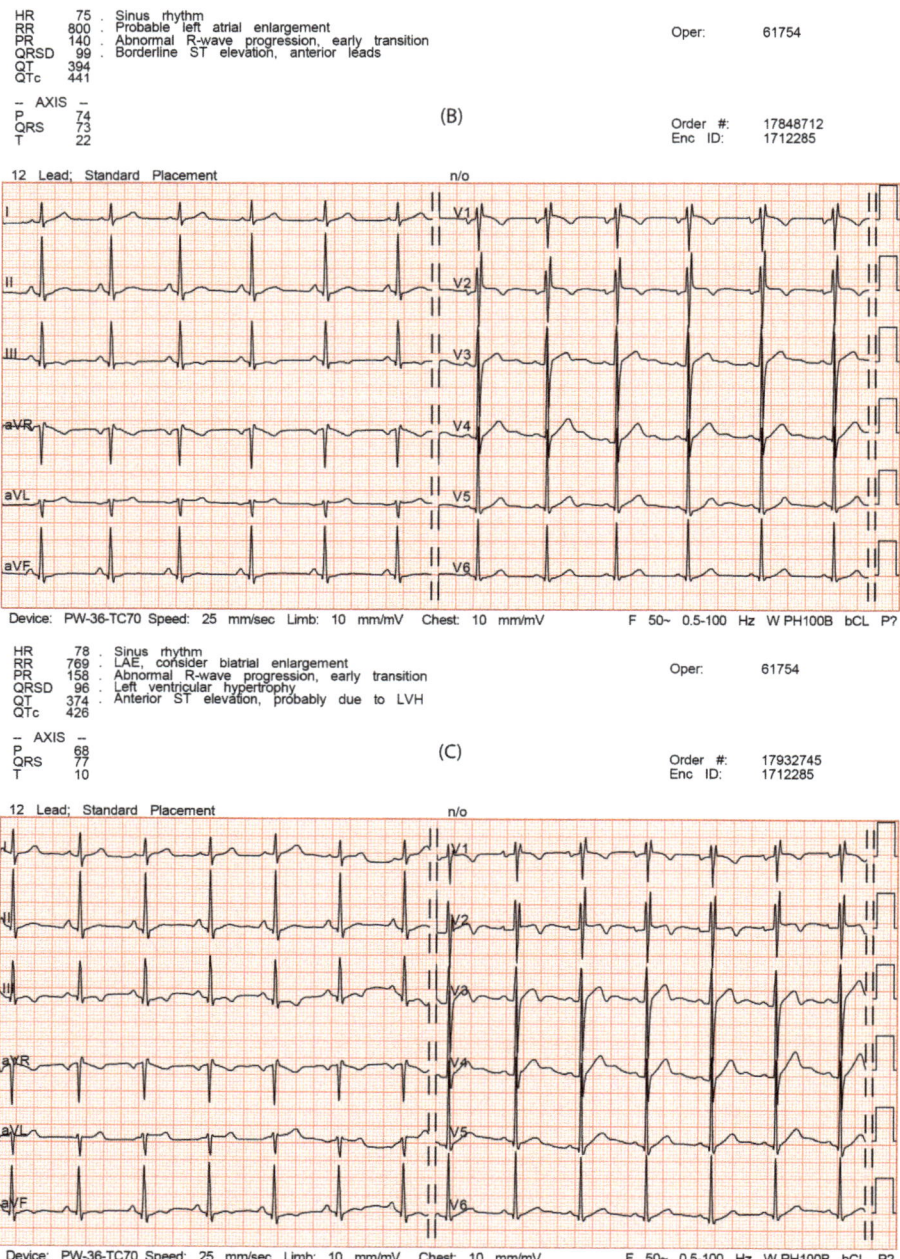

Figure 2. (**A**) ECG: before the run. (**B**). ECG: 1 day after the run. (**C**). ECG: 10 days after the run.

Table 3. Electrocardiography parameters.

Parameters	Units	Before Run	1 Day after the Run	10 Days after the Run
Rhythm	/	Sinus, 74'	Sinus, 75'	Sinus, 78'
PQ duration	ms	160	140	160
The length of PII	ms	120	100	120
P V1 negative deflection amplitude	mm	1	1.5	1
QRS duration	ms	100	100	96
rSr' (leads where present)	/	V1-V2	V1-V2	V1-V2
QRS morphology	/	rSr' V1-V2	rSr' V1-V2	rSr' V1-V2
QRS voltage criteria for left ventricular hypertrophy SV1 + RV5 or RV6 >3.5 mV (35 mm)	mm	32/16?	32/16	32/16
QRS voltage criteria for right ventricular hypertrophy RV1 + SV5 or SV6 >1.1 mV (11 mm)	mm	5.0/1?	4.5/1	4.5/1
QTc duration	ms	410	440	420
T negative (leads when present)	/	III, aVF, V1, V2	III, V1, V2	III, aVF, V1, V2

3.3. Echocardiography

One day after the 24-h UM, we observed an increase in left ventricle volume without a decrease in systolic performance or in EF or GLS assessment results. Indicators of diastolic function (E/e' ratio, e' wave) remained unchanged. An increase in the right ventricle size was noticed with a slight decrease in RV performance (s'RV) and an increase in RAA. All these changes returned to baseline after 10 days of recovery. Despite these differences, all the evaluated parameters remained within the normal ranges and were consistent with the physiology of physical training (Table 4).

Table 4. Heart systolic and diastolic function in echocardiographic parameters.

Parameters	Units (Normal Values)	Before the Run	1 Day after the Run	10 Days after the Run
Left ventricle end-diastolic diameter volume	mL (106 ± 22)	109	126	113
Left ventricle end-systolic diameter volume	mL (41 ± 10)	33	35	33
Ejection fraction 2D (%) bi-plane	% (62 ± 5)	70	72	71
Global longitudinal strain	% (−20)	20.3	21.9	20.3
Interventricular septum diameter	mm (6–10)	9	10	10
Posterior wall diastolic diameter	mm (6–10)	9	9	9
Right ventricular end-diastolic diameter	mm (20–30)	31	34	29
S' right ventricle	cm/s (14.1 ± 2.3)	16	14	17
Left atrium	mm (30–40)	33	36	34
Left atrial volume index	mL/m^2 (16–34)	31.8	32.3	33.5
Right atrial area	cm^2 (16 ± 5)	17.4	20.7	18.7
Mitral valve E-wave	cm/s (73 ± 19)	87	75	75
Mitral valve A-wave	cm/s (69 ± 17)	50	57	46
E' lateral	cm/s (>10)	21	21	20
E' septal	cm/s (>7)	14	12	12
E/e' lateral	ratio (<15)	4.1	3.5	3.8
E/e' septal	ratio (<13)	6.2	6.3	6.2

3.4. MRI

We observed an increase in right ventricle volume after the run, but this was still within the normal range. No myocardial contraction disorders, regional perfusion abnormalities, and late enhancement areas in the myocardium were noted. No presence of myocardial edema on T2-weighted MRI was disclosed (Table 5).

Table 5. Magnetic resonance imaging parameters.

Parameters	Units	Before the Run	1 Day after the Run	10 Days after the Run	Reference Values
Left atrium (4CH)	cm^2	23	24	23	15–29
LV ejection fraction	%	73	73	73	57–75
LV stroke volume	mL	102	107	104	79–135
LV end-diastolic volume index	mL/m^2	79	83	80	66–101
LV end-systolic volume index	mL/m^2	22	23	22	18–39
LV systolic volume index	mL/m^2	57.6	60	58.5	43–67
LV end-diastolic volume	mL	140	148	142	121–204
LV end-systolic volume	mL	38	41	38	33–78
LV mass	g	182	182	182	109–185
Interventricular septal end diastole	mm	10	10	10	6.0–10.4
Cardiac output	L/min	7.1	7.2	7.3	2.8–8.8
Right atrium (4CH)	cm^2	25	28	25	14–30
RV ejection fraction	%	60	63	62	50–76
RV stroke volume	mL	101	107	105	74–142
RV end-diastolic volume index	mL/m^2	96	96.4	95.5	65–111
RV end-systolic volume index	mL/m^2	39	36	36	18–47
RV systolic volume index	mL/m^2	57.5	60.5	59	39–71
RV end-diastolic volume	mL	170	171	170	121–221
RV end-systolic volume	mL	69	64	65	34–94
Heart rate	bpm	70	67	70	60–90
Myocardial contraction disorders	/	no	no	no	/
Perfusion disorders	/	no	no	no	/
Delayed myocardial enhancement	/	no	no	no	/
Tricuspid valve regurgitation	/	+ mild	+ mild	+ mild	/
Myocardial edema on T2-weighted magnetic resonance imaging	/	no	no	no	/

LV, left ventricle/left ventricular; RV, right ventricle/right ventricular.

3.5. P MRS

The mean PCr/ATP values were 1.42 at baseline, 1.26 at 2 days after the run, and 1.65 after 11 days of rest. All results were within normal limits for healthy subjects (2 days after exercise at the lower limit). The ratios of PCr to ATP in the interventricular septum on each day are presented in Table 6.

Table 6. The ratio of phosphocreatine (PCr) to adenosine triphosphate (ATP) in the interventricular septum on particular days.

Parameters	Before Run, Middle Part, IVS	Before Run, Anteromedial Segments, IVS	Before Run, Apical Part, IVS	Before Run, Average Measurements
PCr	5.22	6.27	7.34	6.27
ATP	4.22	4.46	4.89	4.38
PCr/ATP	1.24	1.4	1.5	1.43
Parameters	2 Days after, Middle Part, IVS	2 Days after, Anteromedial Segments, IVS	2 Days after, Apical Part, IVS	2 Days after, Average Measurements
PCr	6.4	4.24	3.99	4.87
ATP	4.42	4.53	2.58	3.84
PCr/ATP	1.45	0.94	1.54	1.26
Parameters	11 Days after, Middle Part, IVS	11 Days after, Anteromedial Segments, IVS	11 Days after, Apical Part, IVS	11 Days after, Average Measurements
PCr	5.06	6.44	5.02	5.49
ATP	3.55	3.36	3.05	3.32
PCr/ATP	1.43	1.91	1.64	1.65

ATP, adenosine triphosphate; IVS, interventricular septum; PCr, phosphocreatine.

4. Discussion

We tested a 36-year-old UM runner before and twice after he won the 24-h UM as part of the Polish Championships. The aim of this study was to assess the impact of this event, as well as many years of training, on the athlete's heart and body via selected laboratory and cardiac tests (ECG, TTE, MRI, and ^{31}P MRS). Initially, only a few lipid parameters were abnormal. On the first day after the UM, we observed changes in some blood test results. On day 10, all the results returned to normal and the blood lipids returned to their original (albeit abnormal) values. Transient changes in laboratory test results are typical of extreme physical effort and represent the reaction of organs to this effort as a result of damage or adaptive mechanisms. Transient changes include massive striated muscle damage, a hepatic cell response, increased inflammation, and coagulation [29]. We found a slight degree of hemolysis (or hyperhydration), as well as minor damage to the cardiomyocytes or a cytoprotective reaction to prolonged stress. The transient minor hyponatremia observed with endurance sports was probably the result of the large amount of fluid consumed by the competitor during the run [30]. The observed ECG changes in athletes are difficult to clearly assess and require a final interpretation in combination with other diagnostic tests [31]. Suspected abnormalities and non-specific changes observed on the ECG were not confirmed by imaging tests, which are crucial in their verification. The TTE, MRI, and ^{31}P MRS changes observed were still in the ranges considered normal for an athlete's heart. The results of this study did not confirm the hypothesis that many years of endurance training and participating in UM competitions have had an adverse effect on this world-class runner.

4.1. How Much Physical Activity Is Too Much or Too Little?

Physical activity dosed individually as part of a healthy lifestyle has reached UM distances in some individuals [32]. Primary prevention and secondary prevention of cardiovascular diseases have established positions [33]. Research has indicated that there is a U-shaped relationship between the amount and intensity of physical activity and health [34,35]. It has been reported that light and moderate-intensity joggers have lower mortality rates than sedentary individuals, whereas the mortality rate of strenuous joggers is not statistically different from that of sedentary individuals [36]. Hypothetically, it can be presumed that excess activity is worse than inactivity. The results of research published thus far do not support this hypothesis. However, exercise-induced arrhythmogenic right ventricular cardiomyopathy and Phidippides cardiomyopathy are both associated with life-threatening ventricular arrhythmias [25,26]. The correlation between endurance sports and FA frequency has also been studied extensively [37]. Often, success in a multi-day UM is associated with resistance to sleep deprivation and ability to run without breaks at a low intensity. The athlete we tested ran at an average pace of 5:34:2 minutes per kilometer[4]. Exercise intensity is well-reflected by heart rate monitors used by many athletes. These monitors accurately determine the heart rate, thus allowing athletes and coaches to determine the intensity of effort throughout the various phases of a run [38–40].

4.2. Lipids

Nutrition is one of the most important elements of preparation for the UM. Extremely long efforts require an adequate energy supply, which is associated with a preferred diet. Ultra-endurance athletes who habitually consumed a very low-carbohydrate/high-fat diet for more than 1 year showed unique cholesterol profiles that were characterized by consistently higher plasma levels of LDL-C and high-density lipoprotein cholesterol (HDL-C). It has been reported that expanding the circulating cholesterol pool helps to meet the heightened demand for lipid transport in highly trained, keto-adapted athletes [41]. In this case study, we observed increased baseline levels of cholesterol and LDL-C, a significant reduction in both lipids immediately after exercise, and a return to baseline on day 10 after the UM. HDL-C was increased at all three timepoints and increased after exercise compared to baseline and during rest. A slightly different change in HDL levels was observed by Chen and others after a 24-h UM [42]. Family history of dyslipidemia is negative in the athlete observed in this study.

4.3. Hemoglobin

In this study, significant decreases in hemoglobin and hematocrit levels were detected 2 days after the run. Anemia due to mechanical hemolysis and oxidative blood cell damage during prolonged physical activity is suggested as the cause of the decreased red blood cell count after long runs [42,43]. However, this may also be associated with excessive fluid intake [44].

4.4. Enzymes and Echocardiography

Increased activity of enzymes released from the muscles (mainly CK) after exercise was first reported in 1958 [45]. CK levels depend on the intensity and duration of prior exercise and peak 24 h after training. Since the duration of exertion is the dominant factor, the highest enzymatic activity of circulating CK after exercise is found after UMs or triathlons [45]. In this case study, we observed a 50-fold increase in CK on the first day after the run. Alanine aminotransferase levels also increased significantly after the race.

Passaglia et al. have obtained different results than those of the current study after blood tests and TTE following a 24-h UM [46]. After the race, they observed a slight increase in troponin levels with decreased LVEF and LV hypertrophy, increased left atrial volume, and decreased E/A ratio in some runners on TTE. Increased troponin levels after the UM without subsequent recognition of permanent myocardial damage is a common phenomenon [47,48]. In the present case, troponin levels were in the normal range, with peak values observed after the run.

Until recently, results of diagnostic analyses of the long-term effects of running on the heart using cardiac biomarkers have been difficult to interpret. The increase in BNP after 100-km trials might show cytoprotective or growth-regulatory effects, but also myocardial insufficiency [49]. In contrast to cardiac patients, it is still unclear whether the appearance of or increase in cardiac biomarkers following exercise in obviously healthy athletes represents a clinically significant cardiac insult or is part of the physiological response to endurance exercise [50]. In this study, the highest BNP level after the run was still within normal limits.

Kosowski et al. reported that marathon running is associated with sharp and significant increases in biomarkers of cardiovascular stress. The profile of these changes, however, along with echocardiographic parameters, did not suggest irreversible myocardial damage [51]. Neilan et al. (2006) screened non-elite Boston Marathon participants using echocardiography and serum biomarkers [47]. Echocardiographic abnormalities after the race were only partly consistent with our results and included altered diastolic filling, increased pulmonary pressures and right ventricular dimensions, and decreased right ventricular systolic function. Unfortunately, no further observations were made.

Myocardial speckle tracking echocardiograms of the right ventricle and left ventricle were obtained before and immediately after a 161-km UM in healthy adults [52]. According to this study, RV size was significantly increased after the race, and there was an increase in LV eccentricity index. The mechanisms responsible for these findings were not clear. Scott et al. (2004) tested UM runners who completed a 160-km race [53]. In contrast to our TTE results, these authors observed post-exercise decreases in LV function after the UM. Similar to our findings, N-terminal type B natriuretic propeptide concentrations increased significantly. Furthermore, transient RV (but not LV) dysfunction during TTE after a 163-km UM at a high altitude has been observed [54]. Some athletes developed marked RV dilation and hypokinesia, paradox septal motion, pulmonary hypertension, and wheezing. In all but one subject, cTnI was undetectable

4.5. MRI

One of the largest UM studies performed using a portable MRI apparatus was conducted during a transcontinental UM (4500 km over the course of 64 days) [9]. According to Klenk et al. [55], LV mass increased significantly over the course of the race, but no other significant changes were observed. It was concluded that the observed structural cardiac change indicated a physiological adaptation to excessive cardiac volume [55]. During our MRI examination, we did not observe these changes or any other abnormalities (nor did we observe gadolinium late enhancement). However, the competition had different characteristics.

4.6. Cardiac ^{31}P MRS

^{31}P MRS is a unique non-invasive imaging modality for probing in vivo high-energy phosphate metabolism in the human heart [56–58]. There are few ^{31}P MRS studies of athletes [59–61]. In our study, all results were within normal limits for healthy subjects.

PCr serves as a cellular energy reservoir; therefore, the observed reduction (average parameters) of the PCr/ATP ratio may have resulted from phosphocreatine depletion after the UM (Table 6, Figure 3). However, these were primary results based on a single-subject study and should be interpreted with caution. In the literature, normal values for the PCr/ATP ratio in healthy volunteers vary widely (range, 0.9 ± 0.3 to 2.5 ± 0.5; mean ± SD, 1.72 ± 0.26) [62,63]. Decreased PCr/ATP has been observed in many cardiac disorders such as cardiomyopathies, ischemic heart diseases, and congenital heart failure; however, significant overlap of normal and abnormal limits has been reported [57,64]. Bakermans et al. [59], investigated whether current ^{31}P MRS methodology would allow for clinical applications to detect exercise-induced changes in (patho-)physiological myocardial energy metabolism and found that this was not the case. Previous studies have not allowed us to identify significant changes in cardiac metabolism during exercise [56,65].

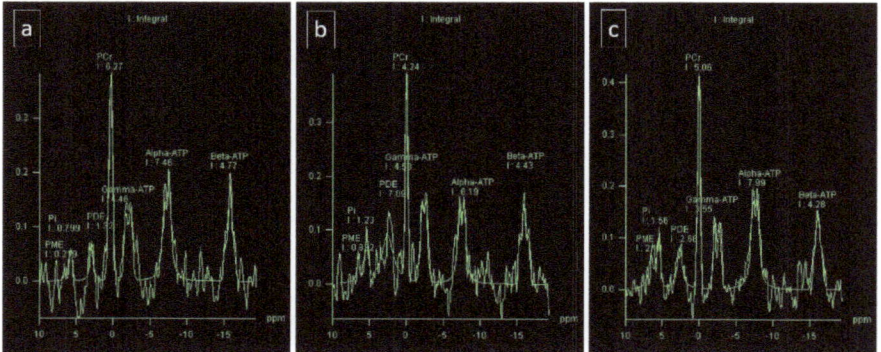

Figure 3. Cardiac-gated 2D CSI ^{31}P spectra from the interventricular septum obtained: (**A**) before the run; (**B**) 2 days after the run; and (**C**) 11 days after the run.

4.7. What Makes Him the Champion of Ultramarathon?

The performed imaging tests did not show typical acute and chronic adaptive features found in many elite endurance athletes neither during the period of normal training nor shortly after the start of a UM. Examples of chronic features such as an eccentric LV hypertrophy in endurance athletes that reflected an increased LV internal dimension and mass, with minor changes in LV wall thickness in echocardiography, or sinus bradycardia, sinus arrhythmia, conduction delays, early repolarization of the ST segment, and isolated voltage criteria for LV hypertrophy in ECG, were not observed. Diastolic dysfunction and atrial dilation typically observed on MRI also did not occur [66]. Contrary to this and other features of Athletes' Heart, the studied athlete has a small heart and very high EF. Even some of the typical acute post-exercise features, such as the increase in troponin levels, were not noticeable in the present case. So, what makes him a champion?

This case study shows that a heart burdened with extreme efforts does not always respond with adaptive features described as Athletes' Heart. It is possible that in the present case, other factors such as mental resistance, pain resistance, and endurance associated with good economics of running at a moderate pace contribute to the athlete's success. With such a "small" heart, it is difficult to run fast. However, it is clearly still possibly be a master of the UM.

4.8. Strength, Limitations, and Perspectives

The main strengths of this work were its performance and ability to allow comparisons of a very wide spectrum of heart imaging results with electrocardiographic and laboratory tests from a UM runner with a history of outstanding sporting achievement. It is difficult to encourage top competitors to undergo multiple tests, especially before the start of a race. Therefore, this spectrum of research has not been performed for any UM runner to date. Undoubtedly, it is extremely rare to perform a ^{31}P MRS to show the energy balance of the heart in response to a 24-h UM. The results of this study are therefore novel.

The major limitation of this study was that it only involved one subject. Another limitation was that the spectroscopic examination was performed on the second day after exercise. Due to the large amount of research performed in different locations, it was not possible to perform all tests immediately after the cessation of the effort. It would be beneficial to examine a larger number of world-class UM runners and to compare their results with those of a control group. However, with such a wide spectrum of medical tests, this would be challenging.

5. Conclusions

Participating in the 24-h UM after many years of professional training as a world-class UM runner did not cause permanent abnormal changes, as assessed by ECG, TTE, MRI, and ^{31}P MRS. The observed changes reflected adaptation to effort. Transient anomalies in laboratory test results at 24 h after the UM were typical of those commonly observed after endurance efforts.

Author Contributions: R.G. conceived of and designed the study. R.G. analyzed the blood tests. E.K.B. conducted and analyzed the E.C.G. A.K. conducted and analyzed the T.T.E. D.P.-K. conducted and analyzed the ^{31}P MRS. V.M. analyzed and interpreted the MRI examinations. R.G. collected the data. R.G. and E.K.B. analyzed and interpreted the collected data. R.G. drafted the manuscript. R.G. and K.B. revised the manuscript and approved the final version. All authors have read and agreed to the published version of the manuscript.

Funding: This research received no external funding.

Acknowledgments: The authors thank Andrzej Radzikowski, a UM runner who consented to the use of his medical data in this study.

Conflicts of Interest: The authors declare no conflict of interest.

References

1. Finn, A. When 26.2 Miles Just Isn't Enough—The Phenomenal Rise of the Ultramarathon. Available online: https://www.theguardian.com/lifeandstyle/2018/apr/02/ultrarunner-ultramarathon-racing-100-miles (accessed on 2 April 2018).
2. Nikolaidis, P.T.; Knechtle, B. Age of peak performance in 50-km ultramarathoners - is it older than in marathoners? *Open. Access. J. Sports. Med.* **2018**, *9*, 37–45. [CrossRef]
3. Hoffman, M.D.; Lebus, D.K.; Ganong, A.C.; Casazza, G.A.; Loan, M.V. Body composition of 161-km ultramarathoners. *Int. J. Sports Med.* **2010**, *31*, 106–109. [CrossRef] [PubMed]
4. Knechtle, B.; Jastrzebski, Z.; Rosemann, T.; Nikolaidis, P.T. Pacing during and physiological response after a 12-hour ultra-marathon in a 95-year-old male runner. *Front. Physiol.* **2019**, *9*, 1875. [CrossRef] [PubMed]
5. Renfree, A.; Crivoi do Carmo, E.; Martin, L. The influence of performance level, age and gender on pacing strategy during a 100-km ultramarathon. *Eur. J. Sport. Sci.* **2016**, *16*, 409–415. [CrossRef] [PubMed]
6. Timms, M. Ultra Pain, Ultra Gain: The Rise of the Ultramarathon. Available online: https://www.businessdestinations.com/relax/health-and-fitness/rise-of-the-ultramarathon-best-events/ (accessed on 19 November 2014).
7. Zaryski, C.; Smith, D.J. Training principles and issues for ultra-endurance athletes. *Curr. Sports. Med. Rep.* **2005**, *4*, 165–170. [CrossRef] [PubMed]
8. Kastner, C.B. *Bunion Derby: The 1928 Footrace across America*; University of New Mexico Press: Albuquerque, NM, USA, 2007.
9. Schütz, U.H.; Schmidt-Trucksäss, A.; Knechtle, B.; Machann, J.; Wiedelbach, H.; Ehrhardt, M.; Freund, W.; Gröninger, S.; Brunner, H.; Schulze, I.; et al. The TransEurope FootRace Project: Longitudinal data acquisition in a cluster randomized mobile MRI observational cohort study on 44 endurance runners at a 64-stage 4,486 km transcontinental ultramarathon. *BMC. Med.* **2012**, *10*, 78. [CrossRef] [PubMed]
10. Badenhausen, K. Ultramarathoner Dean Karnazes on Endurance, Training and Running 350 Miles Straight. Available online: https://www.forbes.com/sites/kurtbadenhausen/2012/05/09/ultramarathoner-dean-karnazes-on-endurance-training-and-running-350-miles-straight/#5400889f43ac (accessed on 9 May 2012).
11. McDougall, C. Born to Run: A Hidden Tribe, Superathletes, and the Greatest Race the World Has Never Seen. Available online: https://en.wikipedia.org/wiki/Born_to_Run:_A_Hidden_Tribe,_Superathletes,_and_the_Greatest_Race_the_World_Has_Never_Seen (accessed on 7 September 2019).
12. Pluim, B.M.; Zwinderman, A.H.; van der Laarse, A.; van der Wall, E.E. The athlete's heart. A meta-analysis of cardiac structure and function. *Circulation.* **2000**, *101*, 336–344. [CrossRef] [PubMed]
13. Riding, N.R.; Salah, O.; Sharma, S.; Carré, F.; O'Hanlon, R.; George, K.P.; Hamilton, B.; Chalabi, H.; Whyte, G.P.; Wilson, M.G. Do big athletes have big hearts? Impact of extreme anthropometry upon cardiac hypertrophy in professional male athletes. *Br. J. Sports. Med.* **2012**, *46*, i90–i97. [CrossRef]

14. Frassl, W.; Kowoll, R.; Katz, N.; Speth, M.; Stangl, A.; Brechtel, L.; Joscht, B.; Boldt, L.H.; Meier-Buttermilch, R.; Schlemmer, M.; et al. Cardiac markers (BNP, NT-pro-BNP, Troponin I, Troponin T, in female amateur runners before and up until three days after a marathon. *Clin. Lab.* **2008**, *54*, 81–87.
15. Kim, Y.J.; Shin, Y.O.; Lee, J.B.; Lee, Y.H.; Shin, K.A.; Kim, A.C.; Goh, C.W.; Kim, C.; Oh, J.K.; Min, Y.K.; et al. The effects of running a 308 km ultra-marathon on cardiac markers. *Eur. J. Sport Sci.* **2014**, *14*, S92–S97. [CrossRef]
16. Biernacka, K. Atrial fibrillation in sportsmen. *Kardiologia po Dyplomie* **2016**, *3*, 32–37.
17. Bosomworth, N.J. Atrial fibrillation and physical activity: Should we exercise caution? *Can. Fam. Physician* **2015**, *61*, 1061–1070. [PubMed]
18. Guasch, E.; Mont, L. Diagnosis, pathophysiology, and management of exercise-induced arrhythmias. *Nat. Rev. Cardiol.* **2016**, *14*, 88–101. [CrossRef] [PubMed]
19. Matelot, D.; Schnell, F.; Khodor, N.; Endjah, N.; Kervio, G.; Carrault, G.; Thillaye du Boullay, N.; Carre, F. Does deep bradycardia increase the risk of arrhythmias and syncope in endurance athletes? *Int. J. Sports Med.* **2016**, *37*, 792–798. [CrossRef]
20. Krysztofiak, H.; Dimitrow, P. Differentiating physiology from pathology in elite athletes. Left ventricular hypertrophy versus hypertrophic cardiomyopathy. *Kardiologia Polska* **2016**, *74*, 705–716. [CrossRef]
21. Baggish, A.L.; Wood, M.J. Athlete's heart and cardiovascular care of the athlete: Scientific and clinical update. *Circulation* **2011**, *123*, 2723–2735. [CrossRef]
22. Biffi, A.; Maron, B.J.; Di Giacinto, B.; Porcacchia, P.; Verdile, L.; Fernando, F.; Spataro, A.; Culasso, F.; Casasco, M.; Pelliccia, A. Relation between training-induced left ventricular hypertrophy and risk for ventricular tachyarrhythmias in elite athletes. *Am. J. Cardiol.* **2008**, *101*, 1792–1795. [CrossRef]
23. Inama, G.; Pedrinazzi, C.; Durin, O.; Nanetti, M.; Donato, G.; Pizzi, R. Ventricular arrhythmias in competitive athletes: Risk stratification with T-wave alternans. *Heart. Int.* **2007**, *3*, 58. [CrossRef]
24. Biffi, A.; Maron, B.J.; Verdile, L.; Fernando, F.; Spataro, A.; Marcello, G.; Ciardo, R.; Ammirati, F.; Colivicchi, F.; Pelliccia, A. Impact of physical deconditioning on ventricular tachyarrhythmias in trained athletes. *J. Am. Coll. Cardiol.* **2004**, *44*, 1053–1058. [CrossRef]
25. Sharma, S.; Zaidi, A. Exercise-induced arrhythmogenic right ventricular cardiomyopathy: Fact or fallacy? *Eur. Heart J.* **2012**, *33*, 938–940. [CrossRef]
26. Trivax, J.E.; McCullough, P.A. Phidippides cardiomyopathy: A review and case illustration. *Clin. Cardiol.* **2012**, *35*, 69–73. [CrossRef] [PubMed]
27. Mont, L.; Sambola, A.; Brugada, J.; Vacca, M.; Marrugat, J.; Elosua, R.; Paré, C.; Azqueta, M.; Sanz, G. Long-lasting sport practice and lone atrial fibrillation. *Eur. Heart J.* **2002**, *23*, 477–482. [CrossRef] [PubMed]
28. Zaidi, A.; Sharma, S. Arrhythmogenic right ventricular remodelling in endurance athletes: Pandora's box or Achilles' heel? *Eur. Heart J.* **2015**, *36*, 1955–1957. [CrossRef] [PubMed]
29. Belli, T.; Macedo, D.V.; de Araújo, G.G.; Nunes, L.A.S.; Brenzikofer, R.; Gobatto, C.A. Mountain Ultramarathon Induces Early Increases of Muscle Damage, Inflammation, and Risk for Acute Renal Injury. *Front. Physiol.* **2018**, *9*, 1368. [CrossRef]
30. Barr, S.I.; Costill, D.L. Water: Can the endurance athlete get too much of a good thing? *J. Am. Diet. Assoc.* **1989**, *89*, 1629–1632, 1635.
31. Sharma, S.; Drezner, J.A.; Baggish, A.; Papadakis, M.; Wilson, M.G.; Prutkin, J.M.; La Gerche, A.; Ackerman, M.J.; Borjesson, M.; Salerno, J.C.; et al. International recommendations for electrocardiographic interpretation in athletes. *Eur. Heart J.* **2018**, *39*, 1466–1480. [CrossRef]
32. Tokudome, S.; Kuriki, K.; Yamada, N.; Ichikawa, H.; Miyata, M.; Shibata, K.; Hoshino, H.; Tsuge, S.; Tokudome, M.; Goto, C.; et al. Anthropometric, lifestyle and biomarker assessment of Japanese non-professional ultra-marathon runners. *J. Epidemiol.* **2004**, *14*, 161–167. [CrossRef]
33. Zachariah, G.; Alex, A.G. Exercise for prevention of cardiovascular disease: Evidence-based recommendations. *J. Clin. Prev. Cardiol.* **2017**, *6*, 109–114.
34. Lee, D.C.; Pate, R.R.; Lavie, C.J.; Sui, X.; Church, T.S.; Blair, S.N. Leisure-time running reduces all-cause and cardiovascular mortality risk. *J. Am. Coll. Cardiol.* **2014**, *64*, 472–481. [CrossRef]
35. Merghani, A.; Malhotra, A.; Sharma, S. The U-shaped relationship between exercise and cardiac morbidity. *Trends Cardiovasc. Med.* **2015**, *26*, 232–240. [CrossRef]
36. Schnohr, P.; O'Keefe, J.H.; Marott, J.L.; Lange, P.; Jensen, G.B. Dose of jogging and long-term mortality: The Copenhagen City Heart Study. *J. Am. Coll. Cardiol.* **2015**, *65*, 411–419. [CrossRef] [PubMed]

37. Stergiou, D.; Duncan, E. Atrial fibrillation (AF) in endurance athletes: A complicated affair. *Curr. Treat. Opt. Cardiovasc. Med.* **2018**, *20*, 98. [CrossRef] [PubMed]
38. Gajda, R.; Biernacka, E.K.; Drygas, W. Are heart rate monitors valuable tools for diagnosing arrhythmias in endurance athletes? *Scand. J. Med. Sci. Sports* **2018**, *28*, 496–516. [CrossRef] [PubMed]
39. Gajda, R.; Biernacka, E.K.; Drygas, W. *The Problem of Arrhythmias in Endurance Athletes: Are Heart Rate Monitors Valuable Tools for Diagnosing Arrhythmias?* Horizons in World Cardiovascular Research; Nova Science Publishers, Inc.: New York, NY, USA, 2018; pp. 1–64.
40. Gajda, R.; Kowalik, E.; Rybka, S.; Rębowska, E.; Śmigielski, W.; Nowak, M.; Kwaśniewska, M.; Hoffman, P.; Drygas, W. Evaluation of the heart function of swimmers subjected to exhaustive repetitive endurance efforts during a 500-km relay. *Front. Physiol.* **2019**, *10*, 296. [CrossRef] [PubMed]
41. Creighton, B.C.; Hyde, P.N.; Maresh, C.M.; Kraemer, W.J.; Phinney, S.D.; Volek, J.S. Paradox of hypercholesterolaemia in highly trained, keto-adapted athletes. *BMJ Open Sport Exerc. Med.* **2018**, *4*, e000429. [CrossRef] [PubMed]
42. Wu, H.J.; Chen, K.T.; Shee, B.W.; Chang, H.C.; Huang, Y.J.; Yang, R.S. Effects of 24 h ultra-marathon on biochemical and hematological parameters. *World J. Gastroenterol.* **2004**, *10*, 2711–2714. [CrossRef] [PubMed]
43. Mairbaurl, H. Red blood cells in sports: Effects of exercise and training on oxygen supply by red blood cells. *Front. Physiol.* **2013**, *4*, 332. [CrossRef]
44. Wirnitzer, K.C.; Faulhaber, M. Hemoglobin and Hematocrit During an 8 Day Mountainbike Race: A Field Study. *J. Sports Sci. Med.* **2007**, *6*, 265–266.
45. Noakes, T.D. Effect of exercise on serum enzyme activities in humans. *Sports Med.* **1987**, *4*, 245–267. [CrossRef]
46. Passaglia, D.G.; Emed, L.G.; Barberato, S.H.; Guerios, S.T.; Moser, A.I.; Silva, M.M.; Ishie, E.; Guarita-Souza, L.C.; Costantini, C.R.; Faria-Neto, J.R. Acute effects of prolonged physical exercise: Evaluation after a twenty-four-hour ultramarathon. *Arq. Bras. Cardiol.* **2013**, *100*, 21–28. [CrossRef]
47. Urhausen, A.; Scharhag, J.; Herrmann, M.; Kindermann, W. Clinical significance of increased cardiac troponins T and I in participants of ultra-endurance events. *Am. J. Cardiol.* **2004**, *94*, 696–698. [CrossRef] [PubMed]
48. Scharhag, J.; Herrmann, M.; Urhausen, A.; Haschke, M.; Herrmann, W.; Kindermann, W. Independent elevations of N-terminal pro-brain natriuretic peptide and cardiac troponins in endurance athletes after prolonged strenuous exercise. *Am. Heart J.* **2005**, *150*, 1128–1134. [CrossRef]
49. Scharhag, J.; George, K.; Shave, R.; Urhausen, A.; Kindermann, W. Exercise-associated increases in cardiac biomarkers. *Med. Sci. Sports Exerc.* **2008**, *40*, 1408–1415. [CrossRef] [PubMed]
50. Kosowski, M.; Młynarska, K.; Chmura, J.; Kustrzycka-Kratochwil, D.; Sukiennik-Kujawa, M.; Todd, J.A.; Jankowska, E.A.; Banasiak, W.; Reczuch, K.; Ponikowski, P. Cardiovascular stress biomarker assessment of middle-aged non-athlete marathon runners. *Eur. J. Prev. Cardiol.* **2019**, *26*, 318–327. [CrossRef] [PubMed]
51. Neilan, T.G.; Januzzi, J.L.; Lee-Lewandrowski, E.; Ton-Nu, T.T.; Yoerger, D.M.; Jassal, D.S.; Lewandrowski, K.B.; Siegel, A.J.; Marshall, J.E.; Douglas, P.S.; et al. Myocardial injury and ventricular dysfunction related to training levels among nonelite participants in the Boston marathon. *Circulation* **2006**, *114*, 2325–2333. [CrossRef] [PubMed]
52. Oxborough, D.; Shave, R.; Warburton, D.; Williams, K.; Oxborough, A.; Charlesworth, S.; Foulds, H.; Hoffman, M.D.; Birch, K.; George, K. Dilatation and dysfunction of the right ventricle immediately after ultraendurance exercise: Exploratory insights from conventional two-dimensional and speckle tracking echocardiography. *Circ. Cardiovasc. Imaging* **2011**, *4*, 253–263. [CrossRef]
53. Scott, J.M.; Esch, B.T.; Shave, R.; Warburton, D.E.; Gaze, D.; George, K. Cardiovascular consequences of completing a 160-km ultramarathon. *Med. Sci. Sports Exerc.* **2004**, *41*, 26–34. [CrossRef]
54. Dávila-Román, V.G.; Guest, T.M.; Tuteur, P.G.; Rowe, W.J.; Ladenson, J.H.; Jaffe, A.S. Transient right but not left ventricular dysfunction after strenuous exercise at high altitude. *J. Am. Coll. Cardiol.* **1997**, *30*, 468–473. [CrossRef]
55. Klenk, C.; Brunner, H.; Nickel, T.; Sagmeister, F.; Infanger, D.; Billich, C.; Beer, M.; Schuetz, U.; Schmidt-Trucksaess, A. P649 Harmonic cardiac adaptation of myocardial structure and mass in the course of a multistage marathon over 4.486 km. *Eur. Heart J.* **2018**, *39*. [CrossRef]
56. Conway, M.A.; Bristow, J.D.; Blackledge, M.J.; Rajagopalan, B.; Radda, G.K. Cardiac metabolism during exercise in healthy volunteers measured by 31P magnetic resonance spectroscopy. *Br. Heart J.* **1991**, *65*, 25–30. [CrossRef]

57. Jung, W.I.; Dietze, G.J. 31P nuclear magnetic resonance spectroscopy: A noninvasive tool to monitor metabolic abnormalities in left ventricular hypertrophy in human. *Am. J. Cardiol.* **1999**, *83*, 19H–24H. [CrossRef]
58. Neubauer, S.; Horn, M.; Hahn, D.; Kochsiek, K. Clinical cardiac magnetic resonance spectroscopy–present state and future directions. *Mol. Cell. Biochem.* **1998**, *184*, 439–443. [CrossRef] [PubMed]
59. Bakermans, A.J.; Bazil, J.N.; Nederveen, A.J.; Strijkers, G.J.; Boekholdt, S.M.; Beard, D.A.; Jeneson, J.A.L. Human cardiac 31P-MR spectroscopy at 3 Tesla cannot detect failing myocardial energy homeostasis during exercise. *Front. Physiol.* **2017**, *8*, 939. [CrossRef] [PubMed]
60. Butterworth, E.J.; Evanochko, W.T.; Pohost, G.M. The 31P-NMR stress test: An approach for detecting myocardial ischemia. *Ann. Biomed. Eng.* **2000**, *28*, 930–933. [CrossRef]
61. Secchi, F.; Di Leo, G.; Petrini, M.; Spairani, R.; Alì, M.; Guazzi, M.; Sardanelli, F. 1H- and 31P-myocardial magnetic resonance spectroscopy in non-obstructive hypertrophic cardiomyopathy patients and competitive athletes. *Radiol. Med.* **2017**, *122*, 265–272. [CrossRef]
62. Bottomley, P.A. NMR Spectroscopy of the human heart. encyclopedia of magnetic resonance. *eMagRes* **2009**. [CrossRef]
63. Neubauer, S.; Horn, M.; Cramer, M.; Harre, K.; Newell, J.B.; Peters, W.; Pabst, T.; Ertl, G.; Hahn, D.; Ingwall, J.S.; et al. Myocardial Phosphocreatine-to-ATP Ratio Is a Predictor of Mortality in Patients with Dilated Cardiomyopathy. *Circulation* **1997**, *96*, 2190–2196. [CrossRef]
64. Mitsunami, K.; Yabe, T.; Kinoshita, M. Diagnosis of myocardial ischemia and viability by 31P nuclear magnetic resonance spectroscopy. *Rinsho Byori* **1998**, *46*, 348–353.
65. Kuno, S.; Ogawa, T.; Katsuta, S.; Itai, Y. In vivo human myocardial metabolism during aerobic exercise by phosphorus-31 nuclear magnetic resonance spectroscopy. *Eur. J. Appl. Physiol. Occup. Physiol.* **1994**, *69*, 488–491. [CrossRef]
66. George, K.; Whyte, G.P.; Green, D.J.; Oxborough, D.; Shave, R.E.; Gaze, D.; Somauroo, J. The endurance athletes heart: Acute stress and chronic adaptation. *Br. J. Sports Med.* **2012**, *46*, i29–i36. [CrossRef]

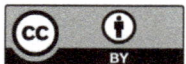

© 2020 by the authors. Licensee MDPI, Basel, Switzerland. This article is an open access article distributed under the terms and conditions of the Creative Commons Attribution (CC BY) license (http://creativecommons.org/licenses/by/4.0/).

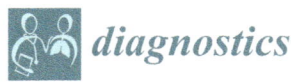

Article

Is Continuous ECG Recording on Heart Rate Monitors the Most Expected Function by Endurance Athletes, Coaches, and Doctors?

Robert Gajda

Center for Sports Cardiology at the Gajda-Med Medical Center in Pułtusk, ul. Piotra Skargi 23/29, 06-100 Pułtusk, Poland; gajda@gajdamed.pl; Tel.: +48-604286030; Fax: +48-23-6920199

Received: 8 September 2020; Accepted: 20 October 2020; Published: 23 October 2020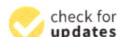

Abstract: Heart rate monitors (HRMs) are important for measuring heart rate, which can be used as a training parameter for healthy athletes. They indicate stress-related heart rhythm disturbances—recognized as an unexpected increase in heart rate (HR)—which can be life-threatening. Most HRMs confuse arrhythmias with artifacts. This study aimed to assess the usefulness of electrocardiogram (ECG) recordings from sport HRMs for endurance athletes, coaches, and physicians, compared with other basic and hypothetical functions. We conducted three surveys among endurance athletes (76 runners, 14 cyclists, and 10 triathletes), 10 coaches, and 10 sports doctors to obtain information on how important ECG recordings are and what HRM functions should be improved to meet their expectations in the future. The respondents were asked questions regarding use and hypothetical functions, as well as their preference for HRM type (optical/strap). Athletes reported distance, pace, instant HR, and oxygen threshold as being the four most important functions. ECG recording ranked eighth and ninth for momentary and continuous recording, respectively. Coaches placed more importance on ECG recording. Doctors ranked ECG recording the highest. All participants preferred optical HRMs to strap HRMs. Research on the improvement and implementation of HRM functions showed slightly different preferences for athletes compared with coaches and doctors. In cases where arrhythmia was suspected, the value of the HRM's ability to record ECGs during training by athletes and coaches increased. For doctors, this is the most desirable feature in any situation. Considering the expectations of all groups, continuous ECG recording during training will significantly improve the safety of athletes.

Keywords: heart rate monitor; ECG; portable/wearable monitoring system; endurance running; cycling; triathlon; long-term assessment; arrhythmia; exertion rhythm disorders; QARDIO MD system

1. Introduction

Heart rate (HR) monitoring during training in endurance sports is a standard method for controlling intensity. It was introduced into training long before heart rate monitors (HRMs). Originally, athletes used a sweep-handed watch and, directly after stopping, the pulse was measured—usually on the radial artery—to assess the intensity range of their training [1]. The appearance of strap HRMs was a revolution. Additional functions related to global positioning systems (GPSs) give information on the length of the route and speed of the athlete's movement, along with many other parameters, such as energy expenditure during training [2]. Originally less perfect and burdened with artifacts, HRMs have shown progressively sophisticated technology related to their used materials, and with it, the precision of the recorded parameters has increased [3,4]. In addition, functions such as determining altitude above sea level, water resistance, and GPS-enabled ease of training in all conditions and scenarios have been added [5]. The ability to measure HR in water was another great step, enabling swimmers and triathletes to monitor their training [6].

Heart rate variability (HRV) is a function that allows indirect evaluation of the cause of arrhythmia indicated by an HRM, thus determining the arrhythmia type [7]. In practice, assessing the distance of the R-R points in an electrocardiogram (ECG)—as indicated by the HRV function—does not allow the cause of the rhythm variability to be determined. The inability to distinguish between supraventricular arrhythmias, ventricular arrhythmias, or an ordinary artifact significantly limits its diagnostic value. The possibility for potentially overlooking a life-threatening ventricular arrhythmia is highly likely [8]. The emergence of ECG recording, which is already offered by some HRMs in conjunction with smartphone applications, was a significant advancement. With its ECG application, the Apple Watch Series 4 can generate an ECG recording similar to that of a single-lead ECG. This was a momentous achievement for a wearable device, allowing it to provide critical data for athletes and their doctors; however, the problem of having to stop training to record the ECG remained [9]. Another important function of HRMs, albeit relatively rarely used, is the measurement of HR at rest and at night. Resting HR is an indicator that is used to observe and analyze the athlete's form—the lower the HR at rest and during sleep, the greater the form [10].

Recently available HRMs can enable continuous ECG recording without training interruption. The QARDIO MD can be described as a typical strap HRM, with the difference being that the information from the transmitter (strap) is transferred to the receiver, which is the Qardio mobile app for the iPhone. After a delay of about 3 min, information from the mobile phone is sent to the "cloud". Downloading information to the Monitoring Center allows us to not only control the ECG recording—which is continuously recorded—but to automatically recognize life-threatening heart rhythm disorders as well. The Monitoring Center offers an ECG recording of three limb leads (modified leads I, II, III) with automated arrhythmia detection, QRS morphology analysis, P-wave detection (for enhanced automated AF detection), and the possibility of manually assessing the PQ, QT, and ST segments. This provides full control of the ECG recording with simultaneous medical supervision, i.e., online data transmission, but the software is currently only available for physicians and hospitals [11].

As HRMs were developed for healthy athletes, the question of their use in ECG recording has become pertinent. The Holter ECG is used to assess arrhythmias and recognizes both the type of arrhythmia and its location with high probability [12]. Many athletes use HRMs daily and have observed unexpected increases in HR during training, suggesting the presence of an arrhythmia, causing them to undergo extensive and unnecessary diagnostic testing, including electrophysiological tests. Ninety-nine percent of anomalies in HR are due to technical problems (artifacts) that mimic an arrhythmia [13]. Therefore, further investigation into the value of ECG monitoring within HRMs for athletes, coaches, and doctors is required.

The aim of this study is to investigate the opinions on the development of HRMs amongst endurance athletes, coaches, and doctors to determine whether the ECG recording function is considered important.

2. Materials and Methods

2.1. Group Characteristics

We conducted three surveys among 100 endurance athletes aged 21–57 years (35.5 ± 4.5 years) who were daily users of sport HRMs and were under the care of our Sports Medicine Clinic. The study group included 76 long-distance runners (50 males, 26 females), 14 cyclists (11 males, 3 females), and 10 triathletes (9 males, 1 female). Most of the athletes were under long-term observation—for up to 10 years—and had participated in previous studies related to the use of HRMs, including their usefulness in the assessment of arrhythmias or exercise intensity [14–16]. The same surveys were conducted amongst 10 coaches aged 26–60 years (47.0 ± 7.5 years), and 10 doctors (33–60 years, 52.0 ± 7.0 years) who were training and examining endurance sportsmen on a daily basis.

Questionnaire One contained 11 questions concerning the usefulness of individual functions, even hypothetical ones, possessed by modern HRMs in a typical situation and the hypothetical assumption of suspicion of arrhythmia in an athlete. The interviewers, assessing the importance of the functions possessed by HRMs, assigned them an importance ranking from 1–11, where 1 point (p.) meant the highest and 11 meant the least important function. The questions concerned functions such as (a) distance; (b) speed/pace; (c) current HR; (d) average training HR; (e) number of calories consumed during training (active kcal); (f) recording of the current ECG "on demand"; (g) continuous ECG recording; (h) the moment of reaching anaerobic threshold (AT) (lactate threshold); (i) altitude (meters above sea level (MASL)); (j) HRV; and (k) 24-h HR measurement.

Athlete inclusion criteria were the use of HRMs, regardless of the brand, for a minimum of 2 years and minimal personal experience with strap and optical HRMs. Some athletes had been using HRMs for more than 10 years. The second questionnaire assessed HRM preferences—optical (OHRM) versus strap (SHRM)—of the athletes, coaches, and doctors in everyday training versus training with the hypothetical assumption of suspicion of heart rhythm disturbances in the athlete (Figure 1). Both types of HRMs are assumed to be valid and resistant to artifacts. Such an assumption was adopted due to common concerns among respondents about artifacts that distort HR values, to a greater extent in OHRMs, and are familiar to their users [13].

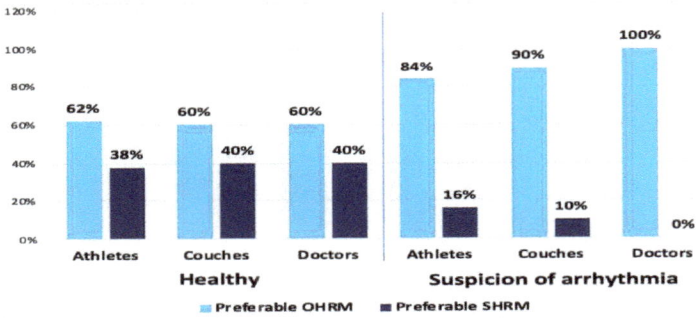

Figure 1. Preferences for the use of HRMs (optical/strap) by athletes, coaches, and doctors in a typical situation and under the hypothetical assumption of suspicion of an arrhythmia in an athlete. Equal and full resistance to artifacts was assumed. Comparison of results of healthy individuals with those of participants with suspected arrhythmia. OHRM, optical heart rate monitor; SHRM, strap heart rate monitor, $p < 0.001$ in every compared pair.

Knowing the results of the preferences in the use of HRMs, all surveyed groups in Questionnaire Three were asked, in detail, about the reasons for their preferences (OHRM versus SHRM selection).

2.2. Statistical Analysis

Normal distributions were analyzed using the Shapiro–Wilk test. As age and experience—both with OHRMs (years) and SHRMs (years)—were characterized by the lack of a normal distribution, descriptive statistics were assessed, namely the median and quarter deviation. Correlations between ranks of HRM functions were measured by Spearman's rank correlation coefficient. Statistical significance in difference in OHRM/SHRM preference depending on the health status of an athlete (healthy vs. suspicion of arrhythmia) was established using chi-squared tests. The average rank of the HRM individual function for every group was set using the mean value. All statistical calculations were performed using STATISTICA 12 (StatSoft, Krakow, Poland). The significance level was set at $p < 0.05$.

2.3. Ethical Approval

This study was approved by the ethical review board of the Bioethics Committee of the Healthy Lifestyle Foundation in Pułtusk (EC 6/2020/medicine/sports, approval date: 1 July 2020). All experiments and procedures were conducted in accordance with the Declaration of Helsinki. The athletes provided their written informed consent prior to participation in the analysis and gave permission for their data to be published.

3. Results

Analyzed answers to Questionnaire One can be found in Figure 2. The data analysis showed that the groups—athletes, coaches, and doctors—had slightly different expectations regarding the importance of the possessed and hypothetical functions and, moreover, the preferred direction of HRM development. There was a strong positive correlation between the ranks of athletes and coaches (r = 0.93); a low negative correlation between the ranks of doctors and athletes (r = −0.27); and an insignificant negative—or even a lack of—correlation between the ranks of coaches and doctors (r = −0.13).

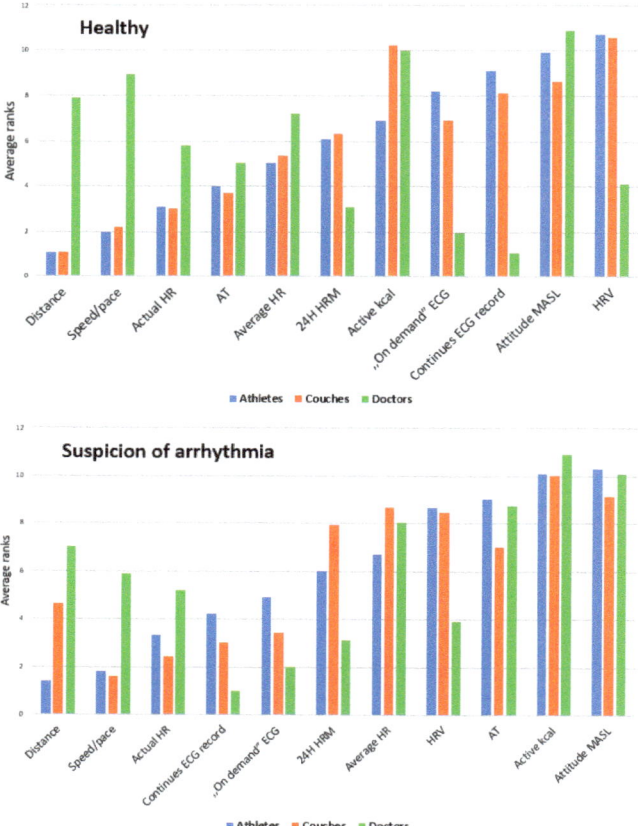

Figure 2. Cumulative results of the survey conducted among athletes, coaches, and doctors regarding the assessment of the importance of individual functions possessed by modern heart rate monitors (HRMs). Two situations are covered: standard use of HRMs and use with the hypothetical assumption of suspected athlete arrhythmia. Data are presented as rankings (mean rankings). Scale rankings 1–11 show decreasing importance of functions. AT: anaerobic threshold; MASL: meters above sea level; HRV: heart rate variability; 24H HRM: 24-h heart rate measurement.

For athletes, the most important functions were the accuracy of the measurements regarding distance, speed/pace, and current HR, and indication of the attainment of anaerobic threshold (first to fourth places, respectively); ECG recording ranked eighth and ninth for on-demand and continuous recording, respectively. Coaches selected the same top four functions as athletes, only differing in terms of the importance of ECG recording (seventh and eighth, respectively). Doctors' assessment of the usefulness of ECG was completely different, placing it in positions 1 (continuous recording) and 2 ("on-demand"). The 24-h HR measurement capability and the HRV function ranked third and fourth, respectively.

The same questions, asked in the case of a hypothetical risk of cardiac arrhythmia, had different levels of relevance, especially among athletes and coaches. For athletes, the fourth most important function was continuous ECG recording, with the first three places remaining unchanged. For coaches, ECG recording (continuous and "on-demand", respectively) was promoted to third and fourth place. Doctors invariably rated the functions describing the work of the heart highly (ECGs, 24-h HR measurement, and HRV). All of the compared groups showed a positive correlation between the given ranks (strong among athletes and coaches, medium among other groups: athletes/coaches, $r = 0.84$; athletes/doctors, $r = 0.55$; doctors/coaches, $r = 0.60$).

The second survey concerned the preferences for the use of HRMs, in terms of OHRM versus SHRM, by athletes, coaches, and doctors in a typical situation and under the hypothetical assumption of suspicion of a cardiac arrhythmia in the athlete (Figure 1). It was hypothetically assumed that both types of HRMs were 100% resistant to artifacts and always correctly indicated assessed parameters. In everyday use, athletes, coaches, and doctors all favored OHRMs (62%, 60%, and 60%, respectively). In the hypothetical heart rhythm disorder situation, the preference of all groups increased in favor of OHRMs (84%, 90%, and 100%, respectively). Observed differences were statistically significant ($p < 0.001$).

Questionnaire Three asked the participants about the reason for their HRM preference (OHRM versus SHRM), assuming that both HRM types had the same functions and level of artifact resistance. The collective results are presented in Table 1.

Table 1. Reasons for preferential use of wrist-worn optical heart rate monitors versus chest strap HRMs by athletes, coaches, and doctors, assuming that the HRMs have the same functions and the same resistance to artifacts.

	Athletes	Coaches	Doctors
Average age (years)	35.5+/−4.5	47.0+/−7.5	52.0+/−7.0
Experience with OHRM (avg. years)	1.3+/−0.5	3.0+/−0.8	2.5+/−1.0
Experience with SHRM (avg. years)	5.3+/−2.0	6.3+/−1.8	5.5+/−1.0
Preferences [OHRM = 1, SHRM = 2]			
Comfort of use during training	1 (88%) *	1 (80%)	1 (80%)
Comfort of use around the clock	1 (95%)	1 (90%)	1 (100%)
Battery life	1 (75%)	1 (60%)	1 (70%)
Skin abrasions from the strap belt	1 (93%)	1 (100%)	1 (100%)
Trend/Fashion	1 (67%)	1 (60%)	1 (60%)
Habit	2 (89%)	2 (90%)	2 (90%)
Confidence in the accuracy of indications	2 (96%)	2 (90%)	2 (90%)
Result: OHRM versus SHRM	5/2	5/2	5/2

* Percentage of votes obtained; 1 = Reason for OHRM preference; 2 = Reason for SHRM preference. OHRM, optical HRM; SHRM, strap HRM.

The survey showed that the two main reasons for selecting optical HRM are related to the all-day comfort of use. Habit and confidence in the indicators were the main reasons for choosing the strap HRM. Most participants (5:2) stated that they would prefer to use an optical HRM in the future. The characteristics of the group and the detailed answers of each respondent to most of the questions asked are found in Table S1 (Supplementary Materials).

4. Discussion

4.1. Analysis of Results

The analysis of information obtained from 120 people (athletes, coaches, and sports doctors) with many years of experience in personal use of HRMs showed different expectations regarding the direction of development for the functions of modern HRMs. Their participation in previous HRM studies on the differentiation of arrhythmias with artifacts was not without significance when answering the questionnaires. The potential health condition of an athlete using an HRM had an impact on the assessment and usefulness of the individual functions of HRMs. While, for athletes, the most important function was to assess the distance, speed, accuracy, and HR during training, the inclusion of potential heart disease with accompanying cardiac arrhythmias "shifted" the continuous ECG recording function quite clearly in the hierarchy of importance (from 9 to 4). This approach seems perfectly justified. Athletes put their training first. Being 'healthy', they do not treat HRMs as medical devices that serve to protect their health. For coaches, the important elements of HRMs were shown to be speed and accuracy in measuring the route, HR during training, and the possibility of determining the oxygen threshold. Regardless of the athlete's health, coaches only appreciated the possibility of continuous ECG recording by HRMs to a slightly higher extent than athletes. This can also be understood by the assumption that trained healthy athletes aim to achieve sports results and are not interested in permanent cardiological control. Doctors, regardless of whether they were dealing with healthy athletes or those suspected of heart rhythm disturbances, ranked the possibility of continuous ECG recording in first place. This is explained by the fact that this is a professional group associated with the training process for whom the athletes' health is more important than results. All three groups stated that they would prefer to use OHRMs (versus SHRMs), provided that they are reliable (resistance to artifacts); however, this is still an area of difficulty. The indicated reason for such a choice was, among others, the ease of use of OHRMs, both in training and in everyday life (Table 1).

4.2. History of Pulse Control from "Fingers on the Radial Artery" to Advanced ECG Recording Technologies

Currently, no HRM in the world has all the functions that respondents were asked about. The indication of oxygen threshold attainment during training by HRMs is a purely theoretical and hypothetical function that is no less desired by athletes and coaches.

The first reports of commercial medical devices for measuring HR came at the beginning of the 18th century [17]. Partially reliable HR control during training appeared with the widespread introduction of sweep hand watches more than two hundred years ago. The athlete had to stop and, most often, count their pulse on the radial artery for ten seconds and then multiply this number by 6 to determine their HR. In this way, they obtained their HR value at the peak of exercise, allowing them to determine the load in the last phase. There was no opportunity to determine the average HR during training; thus, exercise intensity could not be evaluated as a whole.

For doctors, observing the pulse on the radial artery was a factor in making diagnoses long before the advent of classic watches and had nothing to do with competitive sports [18]. Skilled physicians could identify potential arrhythmias and even determine their speed. All HRMs today record HR; however, this is not enough to establish a complete diagnosis of the origin of the rhythm and potential threats to the life and health of the athlete when pathological. There is no ability to determine whether an arrhythmia at a given time is caused by numerous harmless supraventricular beats—or atrial fibrillation—or whether it is a life-threatening ventricular tachycardia [19].

Commonly used SHRMs, which have been commercially available for many years, indicate the correct HR value; however, in the event of an arrhythmia, they are still not a reliable source of information about its type. The introduction of HRV assessment to HRMs has allowed the rhythm "regularity" to be determined; still, it does not define whether a regular or complete arrhythmia is the result of supraventricular/ventricular beats or ordinary artifacts [20]. SHRMs assess the main electric field produced during ventricle contraction. Therefore, they estimate the distance of the R-R points without identifying either P-wave morphology or the QRS complex [21]. This function is completely useless in the case of *commotio cordis*, the mortality rate of which—regardless of the type of HRM or the device controlling the work of the heart (except for the cardioverter-defibrillator)—is very high. However, healthy athletes do not have access to cardioverter-defibrillators [22].

OHRMs have been on the market for about 10 years. The principle of their operation is common, and the accuracy of their measurement is similar to that of the chest SHRM. Optical pulse monitors operate under a completely different principle than SHRMs. While SHRMs work similarly to ECGs, OHRMs use a phenomenon called photoplethysmography (PPG), which constitutes shining light through the skin and measuring the amount of light that is scattered by blood flow. PPG sensors are based on the fact that light entering the body will scatter in a predictable manner as the blood flow dynamics change, such as with changes in the blood pulse rate (HR) or with changes in blood volume (cardiac output). In practice, the optical HR sensor located on the underside of the watch illuminates the blood vessels in the wrist tissue using LEDs, measuring the amount of light dispersed by the blood flow. The advantage of a wrist pulse measurement is convenience, i.e., the ability to measure HR without having to wear a separate strap or other sensors to measure the pulse. Such a watch must be placed directly on the skin with no material in between; occasionally, the watch must be worn higher on the wrist than a normal wristwatch. The sensor detects blood flow through the blood vessels; therefore, the tissue thickness determines the measurement accuracy [14]. OHRMS, as their primary function, can only determine rhythm regularity and, thus, can indirectly be used to make diagnoses, e.g., complete arrhythmia—suspicion of atrial fibrillation [23].

The use of smartphones for arrhythmia monitoring is another advancement for ECG utilization and arrhythmia detection, effectively making the technology available to any smartphone user. Smart wearable technology, while very common, is mostly limited to activity tracking and exercise motivation. Rhythm-strip-generating smartphone products, such as Kardia Mobile by AliveCor and ECG Check by Cardiac Designs, can more accurately detect arrhythmias than wearable monitors. These products, which have been studied in a variety of situations, rely on the use of an external device with metal sensors to create a rhythm strip, which is usually Lead I. A different subset of smartphone products utilize PPG through a phone camera and light to detect atrial fibrillation. Together, these products have created a paradigm shift in rhythm detection and monitoring [9,24].

New electrodes built into the back crystal and digital crown on the Apple Watch Series 4 work together with the ECG app to enable customers to produce an ECG recording similar to a single-lead reading (Figure 3). To take an ECG recording at any time, or following an irregular rhythm notification, users launch the new ECG app on Apple Watch Series 4 and hold their finger on the digital crown. As the user touches the digital crown, the circuit is complete and electrical signals across the heart are measured. After 30 s, the heart rhythm is classified as either AFib, sinus rhythm, or inconclusive. All recordings, their associated classifications, and any noted symptoms are stored securely in the Health application of the iPhone. Users can share a PDF of their results with physicians. Although, similar to the Apple Watch, it is only a record of one limb lead, and it can clearly recognize both the P wave and the QRS complex. This fully corresponds to the classic single Lead 1 ECG recording (Figure 3). The biggest disadvantage of this function is that activity must be paused for recording, contradicting the idea of measurement during training [25].

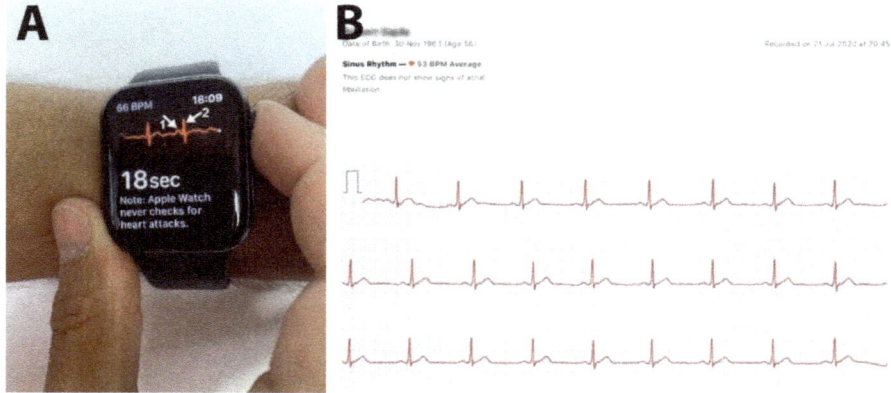

Figure 3. ECG on the Apple Watch, iPhone. (**A**) On the screen, a temporary ECG trace with the morphology of the II limb lead of a classic ECG is shown. Visible: HR 66 bpm. Visible P-waves (arrow 1) and QRS complexes (arrow 2). (**B**) ECG record sent to the iPhone; image taken from the phone screen. Touching the Apple Watch Series 4 Digital Crown completes the circuit and measures electrical signals across the heart.

However, technological advancements brought new solutions including HRMs with applications enabling constant ECG recording during training to the market (Figure 4). The QARDIO MD system (namely, QardioCore ECG with QardioMD remote monitoring cloud based portal) can be described as a typical strap HRM with the difference that the information from the transmitter (strap) is transferred to the Qardio mobile app on the iPhone, i.e., the receiver. After a delay of about 3 min, information from the iPhone is transmitted to the "cloud". The downloading of information to the Monitoring Center (Hospital, Clinic with QardioMD remote monitoring cloud-based portal) allows the control of ECG, which is continuously recorded, and automatic recognition of life-threatening heart rhythm disorders. The inconvenience of carrying a phone during training is a minor difficulty compared to the enormous amount of information stored, which is transferred online to the "cloud" with a slight delay. The Monitoring Center offers an ECG recording with three limb leads (modified leads I, II, III) with automated arrhythmia detection, QRS morphology analysis, P-wave detection (for enhanced automated AF detection), and the possibility of manually assessing PQ, QT, and ST segments. It is a matter of time until automatic diagnosis of stress ischemia with the QardioMD system will become available. Preliminary studies have shown that it is a system with comparable diagnostic value to the standard 3 Lead Holter ECG monitor [26].

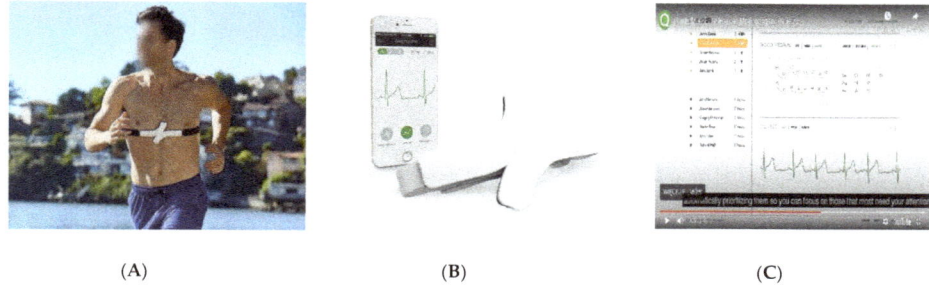

(**A**)   (**B**)   (**C**)

Figure 4. QardioMD ECG solution (QARDIO MD system). (**A**) QardioCore ECG—chest strap with electrode. (**B**) Qardio mobile app (ECG recording on iPhone) and chest strap (QardioCore ECG) with electrode. (**C**) ECG recording on QardioMD remote monitoring web-based portal.

4.3. Strap HRMs or Optical HRM?

The surveyed athletes, coaches, and physicians answered this question unequivocally (Figure 1, Table 1). OHRMs, provided that its indications are reliable, are preferred. Wearing a chest strap is troublesome for athletes for numerous reasons, ranging from battery depletion artifacts, interference in the transmission between the strap and the receiver, to the most important for ultramarathon runners: chafing of the skin during long hours of running by a moving strap [14,15]. It is also common to simply forget to put it on during training, which significantly changes the subsequent evaluation of training. Therefore, OHRMs are preferred on the condition that the accuracy of their indications, which remains a problem, is improved [27]. In the past, an issue was the inability to measure HR by HRMs in the water, which was a significant limitation for triathletes and swimmers; however, this problem has now been resolved [28]. OHRMs usually also have a longer battery life which, in 24- or 48-h ultramarathons, is of great importance [29].

4.4. HRMs Instead of the Holter ECG?

Sports HRMs were introduced to monitor HR values in healthy athletes and were not meant to be, or compete with, medical devices [30]; however, it is impossible to run daily with an ECG Holter to verify periodic indications of incorrect values while training with a HRM. An algorithm has been developed to deal with such cases [14]. Nevertheless, HRMs should be considered as devices with useful and reliable medical functions, such as reliable ECG recording, intended for use by athletes. Today's ECGs recorded by HRMs are single limb lead recordings (Apple Watch) or, as in the case of the QARDIO MD system, a 3-limb lead recording (Figure 3A,B). However, this is an evolutionary advancement, introducing devices "for measuring HR for healthy athletes" as advanced medical diagnostic tools for use in sports cardiology [9].

The trouble-free use of HRMs in everyday life makes them a candidate for use as professional equipment that requires special handling skills and professional knowledge for results interpretation (e.g., Holter ECG). It seems that it will only be a matter of time before HRMs will be able to record a 12-lead ECG with the possibility of assessing any ECG features, including the ST segment, which will be extremely important for the diagnosis of exercise ischemia in a classic exercise test [31]. Other data, such as measuring the QT interval or identifying the origin of ventricular beats, will become automatic information related to these recordings.

Anyone, including potentially healthy top athletes, may experience life-threatening exercise arrhythmias [32]. The registration and early interpretation by the HRMs used today by millions of active people may save lives in the future.

It seems that, in the future, the increasingly perfect ECG data recorded on a typical sports HRM will lead to these devices being treated as medical devices necessary for safe, highly professional, and recreational training. The usefulness of these devices in cardiac rehabilitation is undisputed [33]. Currently, we are starting a long-term observation study of patients with Long QT syndrome type VII, employing modern HRMs for use in ultramarathoners (long "battery life") [34,35].

4.5. Bradyarrhythmia on HRMs—A Lot to Show off in Terms of Observing Athletes

Tachyarrhythmias are mentioned constantly regarding the usefulness of HRMs in the assessment of cardiac arrhythmias; however, the wearing of HRMs—as in the case of OHRMs—may contribute to the registration of not only fast rhythms during training but also night bradyarrhythmias, which are common rhythm disturbances in athletes of endurance disciplines [36]. Undoubtedly, this is a space where HRMs, which are used by many athletes, can contribute both to the diagnosis of arrhythmias—if data are "recorded continuously"—and data collection. All of today's HRM models register a decrease in HR, but they do not all recognize the mechanism by which this decrease occurs (either a conduction block or ordinary bradycardia). In asymptomatic and apparently healthy athletes, either at rest or during sleep, even 15 s pauses in the Holter ECG examination are common. Northcote et al.

examined twenty male veteran endurance runners who underwent resting, exercise, and ambulatory electrocardiography testing. Six athletes had a first degree heart block, four had a Mobitz II second degree block, and three had a complete heart block [37].

The "athlete's heart" and its accompanying bradycardia, or the second-degree A-V block, are physiological adaptations to exercise [38]; however, a break of a few seconds is certainly a pathology that has the potential to be increasingly recognized by athletes using HRMs both in training and at rest and/or sleep. Comfort is also the reason why OHRMs seem to be a more common direction of development.

4.6. Other Expectations from HRMs

The indication of the HR value to diagnose oxygen threshold is nowadays information obtained during the ergospirometric examination [39]. There is an enormous demand for this information by athletes and their coaches and, at the same time, a need for a less complicated measuring method. This function ranked 4th among the surveyed athletes and coaches. There is a need—and it cannot be ruled out—that there will also be a determining method in the future.

4.7. Strength, Limitations, and Perspectives

This study had two main limitations: first, the questionnaire was relatively modest and included few questions and, second, it was conducted on a small sample size.

This study's main strengths were, first, that the group commented on the usefulness of HRMs; second, that most athletes had been under the care of a sports medicine clinic for 5–8 years, constantly using HRMS during their training, and thus had vast experience with different HRMs and could recognize their strengths and weaknesses; and, third, that it included coaches and doctors who were personally acquainted with the athletes and cooperated with the Sports Cardiology Center in which these studies were conducted, rendering them up to date with modern HRM technology.

This study's perspectives included the improvement of the accuracy of already-existing indications in the HRM market and the development of new technology that will allow the widespread use of OHRMs with the function of 24-h ECG recording. Moreover, we are interested in other functions that are not yet available today, such as the expected oxygen threshold indicator. Certainly, there will be new common solutions other than the ones currently available, allowing not only trouble-free ECG recording during training, but also the ability to inform the athlete, coach, and doctor through online means regarding potential threats in the form of heart rhythm disturbances and the emerging features of stress ischemia as well.

The indirect aim of the article was twofold: first, we aimed to investigate and increase the awareness of athletes regarding the need to protect their health during training by controlling heart rhythm and not just heart rate (i.e., ECG recording), and second, we aimed to increase knowledge in this area to protect the lives and health of athletes who sometimes experience tragic cardiac arrhythmias triggered by exercise by encouraging the widespread use of HRM with continuous ECG recording.

5. Conclusions

The conducted analysis indicates the diversity of the expectations of athletes, coaches, and doctors as to the direction of the development of modern HRMs. In the case of suspected heart rhythm disorders, the possibility of ECG recording is a priority feature for sports doctors. Considering all expectations, the paradigm will shift to include continuous ECG recording, especially during training. It seems that users prefer OHRMs over SHRMs as they are more comfortable for use in endurance competitions as well as for non-training use.

Supplementary Materials: The following are available online at http://www.mdpi.com/2075-4418/10/11/867/s1, Table S1.1. Cumulative results of the study groups (athlete, coaches, doctors) including function, sport discipline, gender, age, experience with HRMS, and answers to 11 questions in two situations of healthy athletes or those suspected of arrhythmia., Table S1.2. Number of votes cast for functions by respondents and their percentage share depending on the situation: healthy athlete (A) versus suspected arrhythmia (B), Table S1.2.1. (A) Coaches—Healthy athlete, Table S1.2.1. (B) Coaches—suspected arrhythmia, Table S1.2.2 A. Doctors—healthy athlete, Table S1.2.2. (B) Doctors—suspected arrhythmia, Table S1.2.3. (A) Athletes—healthy athlete, Table S1.2.3. (B) Athletes—Suspicion of arrhythmia, Table S1.3. Reasons for preferential use of wrist-worn optical heart rate monitors (OHRMs) versus chest strap HRMs (SHRMs) by athletes, coaches, and doctors, assuming that both types of HRM have the same functions and the same resistance to artifacts.

Funding: This research received no external funding.

Conflicts of Interest: The author declares no conflict of interest.

References

1. Almeida, M.; Bottino, A.; Ramos, P.; Araujo, C.G. Measuring Heart Rate During Exercise: From Artery Palpation to Monitors and Apps. *Int. J. Cardiovasc. Sci.* **2019**, *32*, 396–407. [CrossRef]
2. De Müllenheim, P.Y.; Chaudru, S.; Emily, M.; Gernigon, M.; Mahé, G.; Bickert, S.; Prioux, J.; Noury-Desvaux, B.; Le Faucheur, A. Using GPS, Accelerometry and Heart Rate to Predict Outdoor Graded Walking Energy Expenditure. *J. Sci. Med. Sport* **2018**, *21*, 166–172. [CrossRef]
3. Xu, X.W.; Liu, Z.F.; He, P.; Yang, J.L. Screen Printed Silver Nanowire and Graphene Oxide Hybrid Transparent Electrodes for Long-Term Electrocardiography Monitoring. *J. Phys. D Appl. Phys.* **2019**, *52*. [CrossRef]
4. Pani, D.; Dessi, A.; Saenz-Cogollo, J.F.; Barabino, G.; Fraboni, B.; Bonfiglio, A. Fully Textile, PEDOT:PSS Based Electrodes for Wearable ECG Monitoring Systems. *IEEE Trans. Biomed. Eng.* **2016**, *63*, 540–549. [CrossRef]
5. Li, R.T.; Kling, S.R.; Salata, M.J.; Cupp, S.A.; Sheehan, J.; Voos, J.E. Wearable Performance Devices in Sports Medicine. *Sports Health* **2016**, *8*, 74–78. [CrossRef]
6. Gajda, R.; Kowalik, E.; Rybka, S.; Rębowska, E.; Śmigielski, W.; Nowak, M.; Kwaśniewska, M.; Hoffman, P.; Drygas, W. Evaluation of the Heart Function of Swimmers Subjected to Exhaustive Repetitive Endurance Efforts During a 500-km Relay. *Front. Physiol.* **2019**, *10*, 296. [CrossRef] [PubMed]
7. Cassirame, J.; Vanhaesebrouck, R.; Chevrolat, S.; Mourot, L. Accuracy of the Garmin 920 XT HRM to perform HRV analysis. *Australas. Phys. Eng. Sci. Med.* **2017**, *40*, 831–839. [CrossRef]
8. Broux, B.; De Clercq, D.; Vera, L.; Ven, S.; Deprez, P.; Decloedt, A.; van Loon, G. Can Heart Rate Variability Parameters Derived by a Heart Rate Monitor Differentiate Between Atrial Fibrillation and Sinus Rhythm? *BMC Vet. Res.* **2018**, *14*, 320. [CrossRef]
9. Garabelli, P.; Stavrakis, S.; Po, S. Smartphone-Based Arrhythmia Monitoring. *Curr. Opin. Cardiol.* **2017**, *32*, 53–57. [CrossRef]
10. Gajda, R. Extreme Bradycardia and Bradyarrhythmias at Athletes. What will Technology Development Bring as a Help to Diagnosis Them? *Res. Inves. Sports Med.* **2019**, *5*. [CrossRef]
11. MindtecStore. QARDIOMD MOBILE ECG VITAL PARAMETERS MONITORING. Available online: https://www.mindtecstore.com/QardioMD-mobile-ECG-vital-parameters-monitoring (accessed on 5 August 2020).
12. Su, L.; Borov, S.; Zrenner, B. 12-lead Holter electrocardiography. Review of the literature and clinical application update. *Herzschrittmacherther Elektrophysiol.* **2013**, *24*, 92–96. [CrossRef]
13. Gajda, R.; Biernacka, E.K.; Drygas, W. Are heart rate monitors valuable tools for diagnosing arrhythmias in endurance athletes? *Scand. J. Med. Sci. Sports* **2018**, *28*, 496–516. [CrossRef]
14. Gajda, R.; Biernacka, E.K.; Drygas, W. The problem of arrhythmias in endurance athletes: Are heart rate monitors valuable tools for diagnosing arrhythmias? In *Horizons in World Cardiovascular Research*; Bennington, H.B., Ed.; Nova Science Publishers: New York, NY, USA, 2009; Volume 15, pp. 1–64.
15. Gajda, R.; Klisiewicz, A.; Matsibora, V.; Piotrowska-Kownacka, D.; Biernacka, E.K. Heart of the World's Top Ultramarathon Runner—Not Necessarily Much Different from Normal. *Diagnostics* **2020**, *10*, 73. [CrossRef]
16. Gajda, R. Heart Rate Monitor Instead of Ablation? Atrioventricular Nodal Re-Entrant Tachycardia in a Leisure-Time Triathlete: 6-Year Follow-Up. *Diagnostics* **2020**, *10*, 391. [CrossRef] [PubMed]
17. Pulse Watch. Available online: https://en.wikipedia.org/wiki/Pulse_watch (accessed on 4 August 2020).
18. de Sá Ferreira, A.; Lopes, A.J. Pulse Waveform Analysis as a Bridge Between Pulse Examination in Chinese Medicine and Cardiology. *Chin. J. Integr. Med.* **2013**, *19*, 307–314. [CrossRef]
19. Müssigbrodt, A.; Richter, S.; Wetzel, U.; Van Belle, Y.; Bollmann, A.; Hindricks, G. Diagnosis of Arrhythmias in Athletes Using Leadless, Ambulatory HR Monitors. *Med. Sci. Sports Exerc.* **2013**, *45*, 1431–1435. [CrossRef]
20. Gajda, R.; Drygas, W. Ventricular Arrhythmias in Endurance Athletes. Are Heart Rate Monitors Suitable Tools for their Diagnostics? *Res. Inves. Sports Med.* **2019**, *5*. [CrossRef]

21. Giles, D.A.; Draper, N. Heart Rate Variability During Exercise: A Comparison of Artefact Correction Methods. *J. Strength Cond. Res.* **2018**, *32*, 726–735. [CrossRef]
22. Gajda, R. Commotio Cordis at Athletes – Under Recognized Problem. *Res. Inves. Sports Med.* **2019**, *5*. [CrossRef]
23. Gajda, R.; Biernacka, E.K.; Drygas, W. Atrial Fibrillation in Athletes—Easier to Recognize Today? *Res. Inves. Sports Med.* **2019**, *5*. [CrossRef]
24. Serhani, M.A.; El Kassabi, H.T.; Ismail, H.; Nujum Navaz, A. ECG Monitoring Systems: Review, Architecture, Processes, and Key Challenges. *Sensors* **2020**, *20*, 1796. [CrossRef]
25. Massoomi, M.R.; Handberg, E.M. Increasing and Evolving Role of Smart Devices in Modern Medicine. *Eur. Cardiol.* **2019**, *14*, 181–186. [CrossRef] [PubMed]
26. Barr, C. Comparison of Accuracy and Diagnostic Validity of a Novel Non-Invasive Electrocardiographic Monitoring Device with a Standard 3 Lead Holter Monitor and an ECG Patch over a 24 h Period. *J. Cardiovasc. Dis. Diagn.* **2019**, *7*, 5.
27. Baek, H.J.; Shin, J. Effect of Missing Inter-Beat Interval Data on Heart Rate Variability Analysis Using Wrist-Worn Wearables. *J. Med. Syst.* **2017**, *41*, 147. [CrossRef]
28. Olstad, B.H.; Bjørlykke, V.; Olstad, D.S. Maximal Heart Rate for Swimmers. *Sports* **2019**, *7*, 235. [CrossRef] [PubMed]
29. Optical HR Armband Shootout: Polar OH1+, Scosche Rhythm 24, Wahoo TICKR FIT. Available online: https://www.dcrainmaker.com/2019/04/optical-heart-rate-sensor-armband-shootout-schosche24-polaroh1-wahoo-tickr-fit.html (accessed on 2 June 2020).
30. Karvonen, J.; Vuorimaa, T. Heart Rate and Exercise Intensity During Sports Activities. Practical Application. *Sports Med.* **1988**, *5*, 303–311. [CrossRef]
31. Marcadet, D.M.; Pavy, B.; Bosser, G.; Claudot, F.; Corone, S.; Douard, H.; Iliou, M.C.; Vergès-Patois, B.; Amedro, P.; Le Tourneau, T.; et al. French Society of Cardiology Guidelines on Exercise Tests (part 1): Methods and Interpretation. *Arch. Cardiovasc. Dis.* **2018**, *111*, 782–790. [CrossRef]
32. Biffi, A.; Maron, B.J.; Di Giacinto, B.; Porcacchia, P.; Verdile, L.; Fernando, F.; Spataro, A.; Culasso, F.; Casasco, M.; Pelliccia, A. Relation Between Training-Induced Left Ventricular Hypertrophy and Risk for Ventricular Tachyarrhythmias in Elite Athletes. *Am. J. Cardiol.* **2008**, *101*, 1792–1795. [CrossRef]
33. Falter, M.; Budts, W.; Goetschalckx, K.; Cornelissen, V.; Buys, R. Accuracy of Apple Watch Measurements for Heart Rate and Energy Expenditure in Patients With Cardiovascular Disease: Cross-Sectional Study. *JMIR mHealth uHealth* **2019**, *7*, e11889. [CrossRef]
34. Krych, M.; Biernacka, E.K.; Ponińska, J.; Kukla, P.; Filipecki, A.; Gajda, R.; Hasdemir, C.; Antzelevitch, C.; Kosiec, A.; Szperl, M.; et al. Andersen-Tawil syndrome: Clinical Presentation and Predictors of Symptomatic Arrhythmias—Possible Role of Polymorphisms K897T in KCNH2 and H558R in SCN5A gene. *J. Cardiol.* **2017**, *70*, 504–510. [CrossRef]
35. Gajda, R.; Walasek, P.; Jarmuszewski, M. Right Knee-The Weakest Point of the Best Ultramarathon Runners of the World? A Case Study. *Int. J. Environ. Res. Public Health* **2020**, *17*, 5955. [CrossRef] [PubMed]
36. Doyen, B.; Matelot, D.; Carré, F. Asymptomatic Bradycardia Amongst Endurance Athletes. *Phys. Sportsmed.* **2019**, *47*, 249–252. [CrossRef]
37. Northcote, R.J.; Canning, G.P.; Ballantyne, D. Electrocardiographic findings in male veteran endurance athletes. *Br. Heart J.* **1989**, *61*, 155–160. [CrossRef] [PubMed]
38. Bessem, B.; De Bruijn, M.C.; Nieuwland, W.; Zwerver, J.; Van Den Berg, M. The Electrocardiographic Manifestations of Athlete's Heart and Their Association with Exercise Exposure. *Eur. J. Sport. Sci.* **2018**, *18*, 587–593. [CrossRef]
39. Tran, D. Cardiopulmonary Exercise Testing. *Methods Mol. Biol.* **2018**, *1735*, 285–295. [CrossRef] [PubMed]

Publisher's Note: MDPI stays neutral with regard to jurisdictional claims in published maps and institutional affiliations.

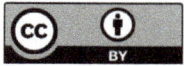

© 2020 by the author. Licensee MDPI, Basel, Switzerland. This article is an open access article distributed under the terms and conditions of the Creative Commons Attribution (CC BY) license (http://creativecommons.org/licenses/by/4.0/).

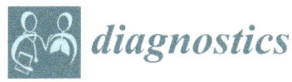

Case Report

Heart Rate Monitor Instead of Ablation? Atrioventricular Nodal Re-Entrant Tachycardia in a Leisure-Time Triathlete: 6-Year Follow-Up

Robert Gajda

Center for Sports Cardiology at the Gajda-Med Medical Centre in Pułtusk, ul. Piotra Skargi 23/29, 06-100 Pułtusk, Poland; gajda@gajdamed.pl; Tel.: +48-604286030

Received: 1 June 2020; Accepted: 8 June 2020; Published: 10 June 2020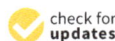

Abstract: This study describes a triathlete with effort-provoked atrioventricular nodal re-entrant tachycardia (AVNRT), diagnosed six years ago, who ineffectively controlled his training load via heart-rate monitors (HRM) to avoid tachyarrhythmia. Of the 1800 workouts recorded for 6 years on HRMs, we found 45 tachyarrhythmias, which forced the athlete to stop exercising. In three of them, AVNRT was simultaneously confirmed by a Holter electrocardiogram (ECG). Tachyarrhythmias occurred in different phases (after the 2nd–131st minutes, median: 29th minute) and frequencies (3–8, average: 6.5 times/year), characterized by different heart rates (HR) (150–227 beats per minute (bpm), median: 187 bpm) and duration (10–186, median: 40 s). Tachyarrhythmia appeared both unexpectedly in the initial stages of training as well as quite predictably during prolonged submaximal exercise—but without rigid rules. Tachyarrhythmias during cycling were more intensive (200 vs. 162 bpm, $p = 0.0004$) and occurred later (41 vs. 10 min, $p = 0.0007$) than those during running (only one noticed but not recorded during swimming). We noticed a tendency ($p = 0.1748$) towards the decreasing duration time of tachycardias (2014–2015: 60 s; 2016–2017: 50 s; 2018–later: 37 s). The amateur athlete tolerated the tachycardic episodes quite well and the ECG test and echocardiography were normal. In the studied case, the HRM was a useful diagnostic tool for detecting symptomatic arrhythmia; however, no change in the amount, phase of training, speed, or duration of exercise-stimulated tachyarrhythmia was observed.

Keywords: AVNRT; endurance training; HRM; triathlon; exertion cardiac arrhythmia; Holter ECG

1. Introduction

Heart-rate monitors (HRMs) are devices designed to control the intensity of training in athletes and are not intended to serve as medical devices to diagnose arrhythmias [1]. However, they can "catch" cardiac arrhythmia during training. While indications of sudden, unexpected heart rate (HR) values on HRMs during training, without clinical symptoms are most often ordinary artifacts, arrhythmias on the HRM which force the athlete to stop training cannot remain undiagnosed [2]. Atrioventricular nodal re-entrant tachycardia (AVNRT) is one of the more common, clinically manifesting arrhythmias in endurance athletes, with and without structural heart disease [3]. Athletes present more frequently with an atypical subform of AVNRT. This is possibly related to cardiac remodeling with dilatation of the cardiac cavities, which leads to changed conduction properties in the septal area [4]. It is dependent on the functional dissociation of atrioventricular nodal conduction over a fast and slow pathway or even over two slow pathways, wherein structural and electrical cardiac remodeling occurs with exercise [5]. The ablation of AVNRT carries the very low, but real risk of inducing conduction tissue damage (0.7%) [6]. Therefore, some athletes decline the procedure. Some choose to stop training altogether, while others increasingly limit the intensity of training. There are no previous long-term observational studies of athletes with heart arrhythmia training with HRMs. We examined a triathlete who, for six years after being diagnosed with exercise-stimulated arrhythmia as AVNRT, consistently participated in amateur triathlon training and competitions, while attempting to limit the number of tachycardic events using HRMs.

2. Materials and Methods

2.1. Sports Biography

A triathlete, 47 years old, 191 cm tall, weighing 91 kg (body mass index, 24.94), performs a free profession by working mentally, has regularly trained as an amateur from 6 years of age, almost every day, treating sports as a factor of a healthy lifestyle and a great adventure.

He was not focused on sports competition, and in the relatively few triathlons or cycling competitions he participated in, he finished more or less in the middle of the competitors, advancing in age groups through the years (currently Master-45). For 8 years of training, he felt violent "heart palpitations", confirmed by high HR values on an HRM, often exceeding 200 bpm, which forced him to stop training until they subsided. Six years ago, he presented to the Center for Sports Cardiology. He reported sudden changes in HR during exercise, from typical for a given phase of training to exceeding the maximum HR. One of the arrhythmias was "caught" on his HRM during cycling training, in which the athlete was also wearing a Holter electrocardiogram (ECG). The arrhythmia registered simultaneously at the 68th min of effort, and HR increased from 167 to 227 bpm, preventing the athlete from continuing (Table A1 pos. 7). The maximum HR of the athlete described, determined empirically (during tests and competitions without arrhythmia, recorded on HRM) was 184 bpm for 6 years and did not change during the observation period. Both devices, i.e., HRM and Holter ECG, noted identical changes in HR values during this symptomatic tachycardia, described as AVNRT in the article by Gajda et al. [7]. Later, AVNRT was recorded on the Holter ECG twice, identical to HR values indicated on the HRM. Clinical studies confirmed the diagnosis of AVNRT with qualification for ablation. However, the triathlete did not report for the proposed treatment. Instead, he trained for the next 6 years with a HRM, collecting data obtained from it on a computer, scrupulously noting all arrhythmia attacks in a training diary. The athlete described tachyarrhythmic attacks as: completely unexpected: mainly at the beginning of training and more often during the running and "predictable" (high probable). The latter appeared most often during long bicycle training in the phases of submaximal effort (and submaximal HR). Sometimes he was able to provoke them with submaximal, interval, long-term training. The start in the competition was a trigger for arrhythmia, which the athlete associated with emotional tension (large adrenergic component) and maximum effort. However, this was not the rule. In adult life, he spent well over 4000 h training and competing in endurance sports (10 years counted), 5–6 times per week. His most preferred triathlon discipline is cycling, and his least is running. He occasionally abstained from physical activity (e.g., during travels). He never got sick and he abstains from alcohol and smoking. During the observation period, he experienced only one arrhythmic attack while swimming, without hemodynamic effects, threatening him with an inability to continue swimming. He never lost consciousness or experienced an arrhythmia while at rest. He did not take any medications (e.g., beta-blockers) that, in the past, occasionally taken gave "discomfort" resulting in abstentions of training. A schematic sport curriculum vitae is presented in Table 1.

2.2. Methods

2.2.1. Study Protocol

In the triathlete, whom we diagnosed with AVNRT six years ago, we analyzed about 1800 training sessions recorded on HRMs during the following 6-year period, some compared with the competitor's notes (training diary). We further analyzed only those trainings in which there were unexpected increases in HR values during training combined with clinical symptoms in the form of a sudden decrease in physical fitness. Sudden "bursts" of HR in training recorded exclusively on HRMs, of which there were about 100 in the analyzed period, without any clinical symptoms, were treated as artifacts, in accordance with previous studies [7]. Finally, we performed 3 simultaneous tests: exercise stress tests, Holter ECGs, and HR measurements using an HRM, to provoke and evaluate exercise arrhythmias and assess the correctness of the HRM indications (Figure 1). We performed ECG and echocardiography directly preceding the exercise stress test. We continued the Holter ECG examination the next day during field training in order to assess HRM indications and record any HR disorders in natural conditions.

Table 1. Involvement in individual sports disciplines of the examined athlete—'sports biography'.

Age (Years)	Discipline	Training—Number of Hours/Week	Number of Years on Training	Hours of Training in Discipline	X- Endurance Sports—Adult Age—Hours at Training
6–8	swimming	4	3	600	
8–11	karate kyokushinkai	4	4	800	
12–14	judo	4	3	600	
15–17	swimming	2	3	300	
15–19	volleyball	7	5	1750	
20–26	kickboxing	6	7	2100	
26–27	sambo sports	6	2	600	
27–32	squash	1	6	300	
27–45	cycling	2	18	1800	X
35–45	swimming	2	10	1000	X
35–45	running	2	10	1000	X
35–45	starts in competitions or tests triathlon/running/cycling/swimming	0.5	10	250	X
17–47	skiing, sailing, waking, other	occasionally	30		
Sport-life in total: 6 to 47 = 41 years	all disciplines	5	40	11,100 (about)	X—about 4050 h in total, on average 6 times/week/10 years

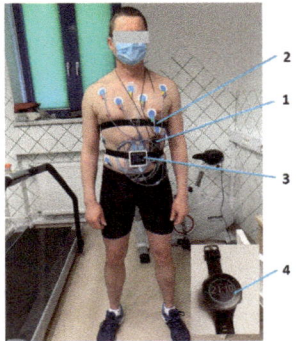

Figure 1. Prepared athlete before exercise stress test on treadmill along with Holter electrocardiogram (ECG) and heart-rate monitor (HRM). 1. Holter ECG, 2. HRM strap, 3. ECG device—from the treadmill exercise stress test set, 4. HRM Polar Vantage V.

2.2.2. Electrocardiogram (ECG) Tests

Standard 12-lead ECG was performed using a BTL Flexi 12 ECG device (BTL Industries Ltd., Hertfordshire, UK).

2.2.3. Transthoracic Echocardiography

The patient underwent complete transthoracic echocardiographic examination using a GE Medical System Vivid 7 with a 2.5-MHz transducer (GE Medical Systems Information Technologies, Inc.,

Wauwatosa, WI, USA). M-mode, two-dimensional (2D) imaging, and Doppler techniques were used. The left ventricular (LV) end-systolic and LV end-diastolic volumes and the interventricular septal diastolic and posterior wall thickness diameters were measured. The LV systolic function was evaluated using the LV ejection fraction (LVEF) and longitudinal strain (global longitudinal strain (GLS)).

LV diastolic function was evaluated using mitral inflow velocities and tissue Doppler imaging (TDI) values. The transmitral early diastolic (E-wave) velocity and atrial (A-wave) velocity were measured and the E/A ratio was calculated. Early diastolic velocity (e') was measured in addition to E/e' ratio.

The right ventricular end-diastolic diameter from the parasternal long-axis view and the tricuspid lateral annular systolic velocity wave (S'RV) were measured using TDI. The left atrial volume index was calculated using the body surface area.

2.2.4. Holter ECG

A 24-h Holter ECG monitoring was performed with the Holter ECG Lifecard CF apparatus and software version: Cardionavigator Plus Impresario 3.07.0158. (Reynolds Medical, Paris, France).

2.2.5. Exercise Stress Test

A treadmill exercise stress test was performed according to the individually modified protocol (by adjusting the speed and incline of the treadmill to lengthen the submaximal exercise phase) using the set: EKG apparatus BTL Flexi 12 ECG (BTL Industries Ltd., Hertfordshire, UK), treadmill BTL-770M (BTL Industries Ltd., Hertfordshire, UK). Software: BTL CardioPoint 6.1.7601.24545 (UK).

2.2.6. Heart-Rate Monitor (HRM) Analyses

HR measurements were obtained over the 6-year period via the following HRMs: Polar Vantage V (POLAR Electro, Kempele, Finland), Polar V800 HR monitors (POLAR Electro, Kempele, Finland), and Forerunner 910 XT GPS, (Garmin® Ltd., Southampton, UK). All HRMs were tested and compared with Holter ECG measurements. The results were analyzed by a cardiologist with extensive experience.

2.2.7. Statistical Analysis

Normal distributions were analyzed using the Shapiro–Wilk test. For variables without a normal distribution, the significance of differences was measured using the Wilcoxon test (by comparing two groups: type of activity; type of tachycardia event) and the Friedman analysis of variance (ANOVA) (by three groups: period). Any significance in changing tachycardia frequencies was established based on trend analysis. All the statistical calculations were performed using the STATISTICA 12 package (StatSoft, Tulsa, OK, USA). The significance level was set at $p < 0.05$.

2.2.8. Ethical Approval

This case report was approved by the ethical review board of the Bioethics Committee of the Healthy Life Style Foundation in Pułtusk (EC 5/2019/medicine/sports, approval date: 29 June 2019). The runner provided his written informed consent to participate in the analysis and for his data to be published.

3. Results

3.1. HRM Data Analysis

Only training sessions in which unexpected increases in HR values recorded on a HRM, resulting in a sudden decrease in physical capacity preventing the continuation of training, were analyzed. Training sessions, for which the quality of data were doubtful, were excluded from the analysis. Taking into consideration over 6 years of training, statistically significant differences in the frequency of tachycardia ($p = 0.6068$), their intensity ($p = 0.2657$) or duration ($p = 0.1748$) were not observed, wherein cycling and running training were analyzed together. Nevertheless, there was a statistically insignificant tendency towards decreasing durations of tachycardia ($p = 0.1748$) (Table 2, Figure 2). Analyzing cycling and running training separately, we observed that the intensity of tachycardia i.e., the rate of ventricular rhythm recognized by HRM as HR, was significantly lower during running activities ($p = 0.0004$) and occurred later ($p = 0.0007$). The rate of tachyarrhythmia (HR) on HRM as well as its duration during cycling training was 165–227 bpm (median: 200 bpm) / 15–186 s (median: 45 s), whereas during running training, it was 150–202 bpm (median: 162 bpm)/10–170 s. (median: 39 s) (Table 2). No other relevant observations have occurred. On three different occasions, tachycardia occurred twice during the same training session (Table A1, position 22a, 28a, 30a); during one training session, the athlete experienced tachycardia three times (Table A1, position 25, 25a, 25b). The episodes of repeated tachycardia were characterized by higher intensity and decreased duration compared to the non-repeated tachycardia, but these characteristics were not statistically significant (respectively $p = 0.2249$ and 0.1380, Table 2). Only three tachycardias (Table A1: no 7, 19, 36, Table 3: no 1, 3, 6) were simultaneously recorded on both the HRM and Holter EEG, wherein AVNRT was confirmed. All of the other episodes of analyzed tachycardia occurred during training sessions, when the participant was not wearing the Holter ECG device. The amateur-triathlete experienced only one tachycardia during swimming training, without good confirmation on HRM. Full data from heart rate monitors obtained during 6 years of observation are in Table A1.

Table 2. Main characteristics of tachycardia events in the analyzed athlete.

Characteristic	Parameters		Start of Tachycardia [min]	HR at Beginning of Tachycardia [bpm]	HR at the end of Tachycardia [bpm]	AVNRT [bpm]	Time of AVNRT [s]
	All N = 40	Median	29	127	119	187	40
		QD	23.7	11.5	8.8	19.0	21.8
		Min-Max	2–131	86–167	90–156	150–227	10–186
Type of activity	Cycling N = 20	Median	41	129	117	200	45
		QD	23.7	14.3	18.5	10.0	17.5
		Min-Max	14–131	86–167	90–156	165–227	15–186
	Running N = 20	Median	10	126	119	162	39
		QD	18.0	8.0	6.3	9.5	22.5
		Min-Max	2–64	100–153	98–132	150–202	10–170
	p-value (Cyc. vs. Run)		0.0007	0.9679	0.681323	0.0004	0.6149
Analyzed years with tachycardia	2014–15 N = 15	Median	23	125	120	180	60
		QD	12.6	13.5	8.5	16.0	40.0
		Min-Max	4–68	90–167	90–156	155–227	15–186
	2016–17 N = 11	Median	33	130	115	190	50
		QD	18.9	13.5	14.0	8.5	19.5
		Min-Max	14–110	86–153	93–139	165–210	20–152
	2018–IV 20 N = 14	Median	32	127	122	173	37
		QD	34.4	8.5	7.5	23.0	10.5
		Min-Max	2–131	100–147	98–140	150–212	10–96
	p-value (comparing periods)		0.1778	0.1778	0.1593	0.2657	0.1748
Features of tachycardia	Primary N = 40	Median	29	127	119	187	40
		QD	23.7	11.5	8.8	19.0	21.8
		Min-Max	2–131	86–167	90–156	150–227	10–186
	Repeated N = 5	Median	180	114	109	201	23
		QD	82.4	5.0	2.0	11.0	13.5
		Min-Max	15–191	93–130	79–118	158–217	7–56
	p-value (primary vs. repeated)		0.2249	0.2249	0.1056	0.2249	0.1380

Legend: Cyc. vs. Run—Cycling versus Running, QD—Quartile Deviation.

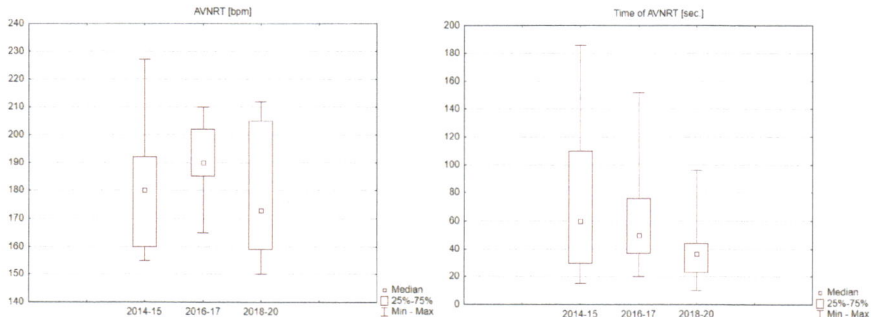

Figure 2. Intensity and time of atrioventricular nodal re-entrant tachycardia (AVNRT) in 2014–2020 of analyzed patient.

3.2. ECG Tests

During the rest ECG, we observed sinus rhythm 63/min. ECG recording normal. (Figure 3).

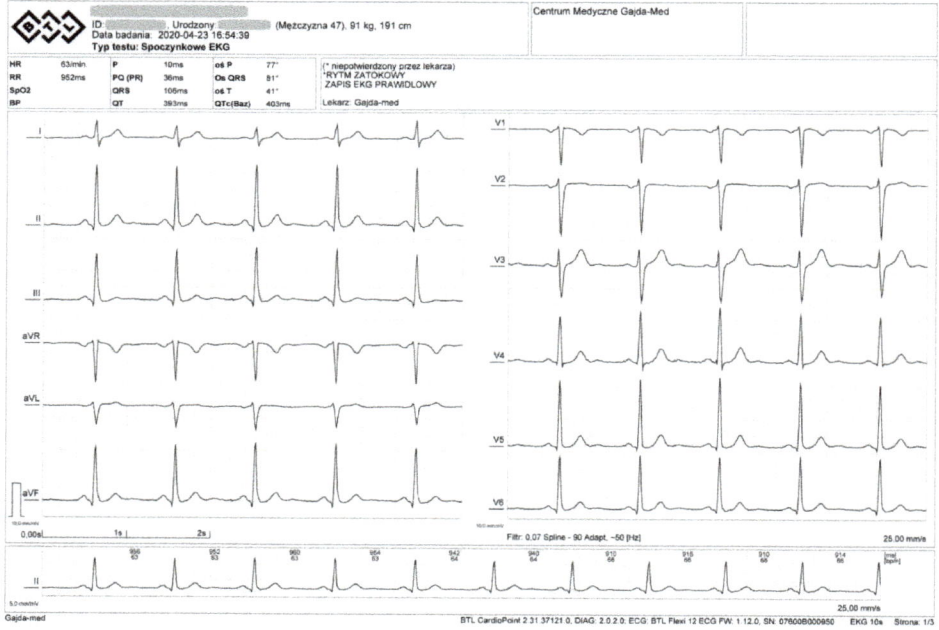

Figure 3. ECG of the examined athlete.

3.3. Echocardiography

All the evaluated parameters remained within the normal ranges (Table 3).

Table 3. Heart systolic and diastolic function in echocardiographic parameters.

Parameters	Units (Normal Values)	Result
Left ventricle end-diastolic diameter volume	mL (106 ± 22)	111
Left ventricle end-systolic diameter volume	mL (41 ± 10)	35
Ejection fraction 2D (%) bi-plane	% (62 ± 5)	65
Global longitudinal strain	% (-20)	20.4
Interventricular septum diameter	mm (6–10)	10
Posterior wall diastolic diameter	mm (6–10)	10
Right ventricular end-diastolic diameter	mm (20–30)	30
S' right ventricle	cm/s (14.1 ± 2.3)	16
Left atrium	mm (30–40)	36
Left atrial volume index	mL/m^2 (16–34)	30.0
Right atrial area	cm^2 16 ± 5	14.4
Mitral valve E-wave	cm/s 73 ± 19	80
Mitral valve A-wave	cm/s (69 ± 17)	50
E' lateral	cm/s (>10)	20
E' septal	cm/s (>7)	12
E/e' lateral	ratio(<15)	4.0
E/e' septal	ratio (<13)	6.6

3.4. Exercise Stress Test

The athlete underwent a treadmill exercise stress test, according to an individual protocol, with the additional goals of provoking an arrhythmia and evaluating the associated HRM indications. The effort ended due to fatigue at the 44th min. The maximum heart rate of 182/min was reached in 35 min. At the same time, the highest metabolic equivalent of task (MET) load of 15.9 was achieved. During the modified test (3× longer when usual), several attempts of interval maximum efforts were made to provoke arrhythmia without success. The athlete exhibited a correct pressure response to effort, without chest pain or ST-segment changes in ECG. Conclusion: negative exercise stress test.

3.5. Heart-Rate Monitor Tests

We tested the correctness of the indications of all 3 HRMs (Polar Vantage V, Polar V800 HR monitors and Forerunner 910 XT GPS) used over the 6-year period several times. Additionally, we simultaneously tested the Polar Vantage V HRM while the athlete was wearing a Holter ECG during an exercise stress test (Figures 1 and 4, Table 4 No. 8). In 2014, we checked the correctness of the HRM then used (Table 4, No. 1) simultaneously with the Holter ECG, when AVNRT was first detected [7]. During the tests, all three HRMs showed the same maximum and average HR values indicated by the Holter ECG. In total, AVNRT on the Holter ECG was recorded 3 times with the same HR as the HRMs' indications. Table 4 indicates the detailed values obtained during HRM tests versus the Holter ECG, showing the highest HR values on HRM and HR values shown simultaneously by the Holter ECG.

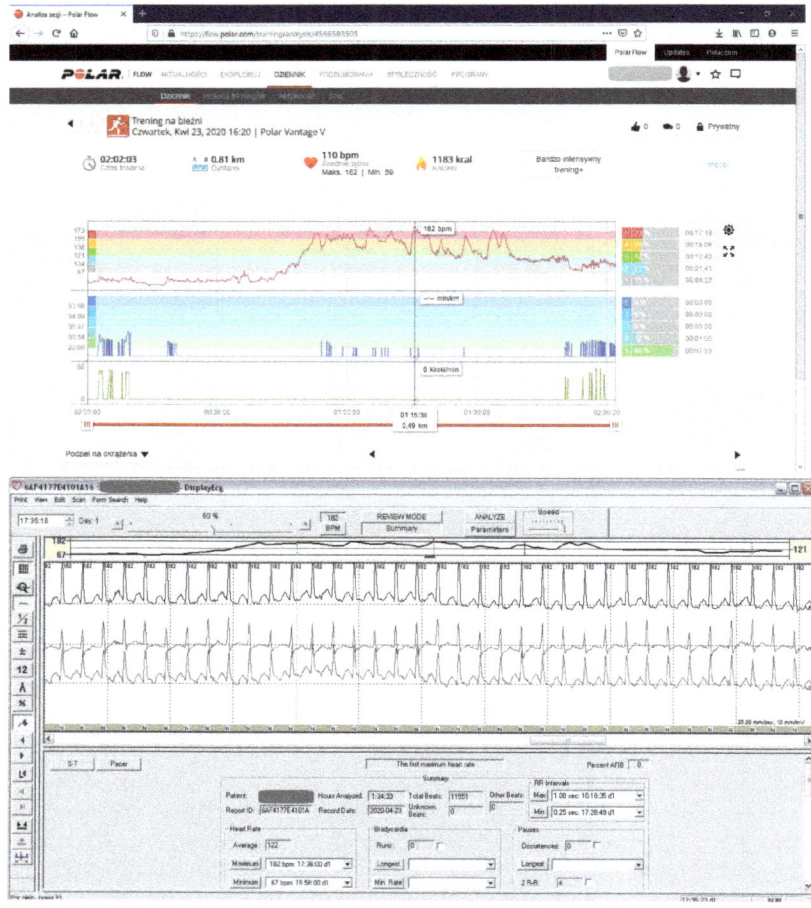

Figure 4. HRM control by comparing heart rate (HR) on HRM and at the same time in Holter ECG. The diagram with HRM indicates max. HR 182/min. At the same time, the Holter ECG indicates a rhythm of 182/min. The test was performed during a modified effort test on a treadmill. (number 8 in Table 4).

Table 4. Tests for the correctness of the HRMs' indications used by the athlete versus Holter ECG.

Measurement Number	Polar Vantage V (Maximum HR Recorded during Training) (bpm)	V800 HR Monitors (Maximum HR Recorded during Training) (bpm)	Forerunner 910 XT GPS Maximum HR Recorded during Training (bpm)	Holter ECG Maximum HR Recorded during Training(bpm)	Difference in bpm Between Devices
1			227	226 AVNRT	1(App.1 No 7)
2			179	179 SHR	0
3		202		203 AVNRT	1(App.1 No 19)
4		178		178 SHR	0
5		177		178 SHR	1
6	205			206 AVNRT	1(App.1 No 36)
7	174			173 SHR	1
8	182			182 SHR	0 (Figure 1, Figure 4)

Legend: SHR—sinus heart rate, AVNRT—atrioventricular nodal re-entrant tachycardia.

4. Discussion

4.1. Discussion of the Results

We analyzed the triathlete's training, recorded on HRMs for 6 years, with recognized effort-stimulated AVNRT. It is a rare and specific situation when an athlete, using HRM, tries to limit the number of symptomatic tachyarrhythmias. During the observation period, we did not notice significant changes: frequency, intensity (speed) and their duration.

Sports HRMs, in which HR is one of several assessed values, are designed to control the intensity of training [8]. Eight years ago, the triathlete described in this study noticed sudden increases in HR on his HRM, which forced him to stop training. Finally, 6 years ago, tachyarrhythmia was simultaneously recorded on the HRM and Holter ECG, and confirmed at the Cardiology Clinic as AVNRT. The analysis of approximately 1800 training sessions recorded on HRM over the past 6 years has allowed us to segregate and analyze 45 tachyarrhythmias, without artifacts, which were also noted in his training diary. Their analysis indicates no significant changes in the frequency of arrhythmias, their speed, length, and the phase of training in which they occurred (Table 2, Figure 2). It is not clear why there is a significant difference in maximal HR during arrhythmia generated during running in relation to cycling. The onset of arrhythmia was also significantly earlier during running (Table 2). The triathlete definitely preferred cycling, which could explain his better adaptation to this type of effort and, thus, the delayed arrhythmia generation. However, this is only speculation. It can be speculated that the fact that there is no arrhythmia during swimming (a one-time episode felt clinically without documentation in the form of a recording from HRMs due to a technical error in recording) is due to the much lower muscular involvement associated with working mainly the upper body during swimming and the decreased stress on the circulatory system. There was an average of 12 AVNRT seizures recorded in the training notebook per year, but the HRM device was only able to reproduce an average of 7/year as "technically well documented". The athlete, refusing ablation, hoped that with time the arrhythmias would subside, slow down, or shorten in duration. Apart from the slight tendency to shorten in duration, this did not happen. It also seems that attempts to reduce the number of seizures by controlling HR and well-being were ineffective, as evidenced by the primary arrhythmias recorded, as well as the three secondary and 1 tertiary tachycardic episodes (Table 2, Table A1). Modified training, aimed at provoking arrhythmias (long-term and submaximal), turned out to be ineffective. No other rules or trends other than those listed were observed. No other factors were found that triggered the, unexpected and anticipated" arrhythmias by analyzing them all together (e.g., the type of the beginning of training, special warm-up, breaks in training, fast start, etc.) Listed by the athlete as provocative for arrhythmias: long, submaximal, interval training, or start in competitions, although often, they were not always triggers of arrhythmias. Judged together with the "unexpected" in the initial phase, they did not allow drawing any additional conclusions or observations. Tachyarrhythmia, each time it occurred, was a very unpleasant feeling for the athlete, which forced him to stop training until it subsided. The echocardiographic examination and exercise stress test did not show any abnormalities. The ECG markers related to sudden cardiac death in the examined athlete, such as P-wave (duration, interatrial block, and deep terminal negativity of the P wave in V1), prolonged QT and Tpeak-Tend intervals, QRS duration and fragmentation, bundle branch block, ST segment depression and elevation, T waves (inverted, T wave axes), premature ventricular contractions, and ECG hypertrophy criteria are missing [9].

4.2. Atrioventricular Nodal Re-Entrant Tachycardia (AVNRT) in Athletes

The development of an athlete's heart is recognized as a risk factor for atrial arrhythmias with AVNRT. Prolonged participation in exercise (moderate to intensive sports for ≥3 h per week for ≥5 years) results in structural and electrical cardiac remodeling. Athletes with AVNRT present more frequently with an atypical forms of AVNRT than non-athletes [4]. Exercise can be implicated as an independent causal factor in the development of AVNRT and is more often involved in the development of atypical subform [4]. Dilatation of the right atrium, as seen in the athletic population, may lead to further stretching of the posteroseptal area, facilitating anisotropy. This in turn forms the basis of dual atrioventricular (AV) nodal conduction pathways and the circuit of AVNRT [10]. In the case of the athlete under study, the right atrium in the echocardiography was normal, which, however, does not exclude changes that could be seen during magnetic resonance imaging (MRI). The effect of the endurance exercise on the atria is more pronounced in men than in women [11]. This could be attributed to the fact that men tend to exercise more intensively than women [12]. The examined leisure-time athlete practiced various physical activities since childhood and spent over 10 years training for endurance activity, practicing almost every day. His goal was never competition and he treated sport as a "healthy lifestyle". However, cumulatively, the amount of activity is impressive and should evoke the adaptation and development of the characteristic "athlete's heart" which, were not observed in ECG and echocardiography.

4.3. The Role of HRMs in Recognizing the Type of Arrhythmia in Athletes

HRMs are devices designed to control training via suitable stimuli, including HR assessments [13]. While constantly measuring HR, they may accidentally "catch" arrhythmias [14]. The use of technology has increased tremendously, by means of more reliable, smaller, more accessible, and, especially, more user-friendly devices, which provide a wider range of features, and promote significant benefits for the population and for health professionals [15]. However, the type of arrhythmia is usually impossible to recognize because of the inability of HRMs to interpret a standard ECG, i.e., the inability to interpret P-waves and QRS complexes [16]. There are smartphone applications on the market that register an incomplete ECG recording (i.e., lead I), with the option of recognizing atrial fibrillation and other arrhythmias [17]. Unfortunately, despite this paradigm shift, ECG recording during activity, e.g., running, is very difficult and constant monitoring is completely impossible. HRMs with the "heart-rate variability" (HRV) function enable differentiation of regular and irregular arrhythmias and provide more information than standard ones. However, we were unable to tell whether this athlete's heart rate variability resulted from premature atrial or ventricular contraction or just irregular sinus rhythm [18]. For some time, HR monitoring under water has also been possible, which allows us to control swim training [19]. Unfortunately, this was not the case with the athlete in this study. Despite the indisputable value for training, many outstanding athletes do not use or stop using HRM, citing an unjustified dispersion of concentration associated with artifacts in the form of false indications of high HR values, which discourages athletes from controlling HR, especially during competitions [20]. However sometimes, HRM can save lives, not only allowing the athlete to determine his location (especially helpful when training in unknown terrain) using Global Positioning System (GPS) functions, but also analyzing HR as a potential cause of loss of consciousness during training [21]. Research conducted by Gajda et al. indicates that the vast majority of sudden unexpected indications of high HR on HRM in asymptomatic patients are mere artifacts, stating that HRMs are not good tools for diagnosing asymptomatic arrhythmias [7]. A single large study confirmed the usefulness of HRMs and smartphone applications used by athletes to recognize symptomatic arrhythmia [22], which was later confirmed only in small groups [23]. These tools mainly confirm arrhythmia (exactly the rate of ventricular rhythm during tachycardia) without the ability to accurately identify its type. This is not resolved by the HRV function mentioned above, which determines the time between R waves (R to R) and thus detects irregularities, indirectly indicative of arrhythmias. Unfortunately, this function in most HRMs works only at rest and cannot be used during training. Two of the three HRMs used in this study (Polar Vantage V and Polar V800 HR) had this function. Only training with the Holter ECG can determine the diagnosis of AVNRT with high probability. For this reason, it is uncertain whether this athlete's arrhythmias were AVNRT, atrial flutter, atrial fibrillation, or another supraventricular or ventricular tachyarrhythmia. Without an electrophysiological examination of the provoked arrhythmia, AVNRT can be mistaken for a different condition (e.g., posteroseptal catecholaminergic atrial tachycardia) [5]. These limitations seem to negate HRMs in the diagnosis of symptomatic arrhythmia. However, they are not medical devices and are not used to diagnose medical conditions. On the other hand, when arrhythmias are accompanied by clinical symptoms, they force athletes to consult a doctor. The examined triathlete, diagnosed with AVNRT in the Cardiology Clinic in 2014, refused the proposed ablation, and continued amateur training, hoping that the symptoms would subside or abate. None of these expectations came true. He never clinically registered or reported a tachyarrhythmia seizure at rest on HRMs. However, it is uncertain whether there was an asymptomatic arrhythmia during the resting periods, which is not uncommon for many athletes [24]. The essence of the observations is that the practical use of 3 types of HRMs (Polar Vantage V, Polar V800 HR, Forerunner 910 XT GPS) recognized symptomatic tachyarrhythmia; thus, HRMs, originally intended for healthy athletes with normal HRs, may act as a "paramedical" device which may have practical, medical significance in cases of symptomatic arrhythmia.

4.4. Limitation

The main limitation of this study is the uncertainty regarding the type of symptomatic arrhythmia that was recorded by the HRMs. Each episode could have been AVNRT, as recognized in 2014, or it could have been any other supraventricular or ventricular tachyarrhythmia. Another limitation is the fact that there is no complete assessment of the tendency of changes in speed, duration, and frequency for this arrhythmia, because about 25% of the clinically noted arrhythmias were not recorded by the HRMs for various technical reasons (battery defect in transmitter, poor adhesion transmitter belt, low battery in the receiver, loss of register due to accidental deletion, not switching on HRM). The athlete "felt" arrhythmias on average 12 times/year, of which 7–8/year were recorded. Another limitation of the study is the fact that there were only three training sessions in which arrhythmia were simultaneously recorded on HRM and Holter ECG (AVNRT each time). Despite numerous tests with HRMs and a parallel Holter ECG test, including effort provocation, arrhythmias could not be provoked "on demand" for accurate analysis. Moreover, the athlete has an additional Holter ECG test confirming AVNRT during bicycle training, wherein he did not turn on HRM, which excludes the examination from evaluation.

4.5. Perspectives

It seems that the most favorable situation would be to encourage athletes to undergo electrophysiological diagnostics and conduct the best type of therapy based on its result, which, in the case of confirmation of AVNRT, is ablation. Regardless, during this time, you can encourage the athlete to use the appropriate smartphone application to control training. Strip-generating smartphone products (Kardia Mobile by AliveCor and ECG Check by Cardiac Designs) are more powerful at arrhythmia detection than wearable monitors. In practice, they record an ECG in the form of one or several leads. The fact that you have to stop training at the moment is not a problem because arrhythmia already forces the athlete to pause until it stops (except QardioMD) [17]. A paradigm shift in this matter has already taken place with the appearance of this function (ECG recording). Improvements, such as the possibility of continuous registration at any time and without time limits and above all during training, will ensure success and start a new era in the meaning of these devices. Originally helpful in training, these devices may become diagnostic arrhythmia medical tools essential for the safety of every athlete or person leading a healthy lifestyle.

5. Conclusions

During the 6-year observation period, this athlete did not experience any significant decrease in the number, frequency, or speed of the exercise-stimulated arrhythmias. However, his HRMs acted as a useful diagnostic tool for detecting and documenting symptomatic arrhythmias. Moreover, in the future, HRMs, originally intended for healthy athletes with normal HRs, may act as a "paramedical" device, which may have practical, medical significance in cases of symptomatic arrhythmia.

Funding: This research received no external funding.

Acknowledgments: The author would like to thank K.J., a triathlete who consented to the use of his medical data in this study.

Conflicts of Interest: The author declares no conflict of interest.

Appendix A

Table A1. Arrhythmias registered on HRM during 6 years of observation. Detailed data.

No.	Date	Type of Training R-Running B-Bicycle	Time from Start of Training to Tachycardia Event [hh:mm:ss]	HR by Beginning of Tachycardia [bpm]	AVNRT	Time From Start of Training to the End of Tachycardia Event [hh:mm:ss]	Duration of AVNRT [s]	HR by the End of Tachycardia [bpm]	Type of Tachycardia
1	02.03.2014	R	00:50:20	155	192	00:52:25	125	143	Primary
2	10.04.2014	B	00:35:16	153	186	00:38:06	170	120	Primary
3	15.06.2014	B	00:59:01	145	180	01:00:06	65	130	Primary
4	29.07.2014	R	00:30:00	145	170	00:31:50	110	140	Primary
5	30.08.2014	R	00:15:40	90	200	00:16:17	37	90	Primary
6	15.09.2014	B	00:10:00	120	169	00:11:12	72	115	Primary
7	10.10.2014	R	01:08:02	167	227	01:11:08	186	156	Primary
8	10.01.2015	B	00:27:32	134	159	00:28:02	30	132	Primary
9	20.02.2015	B	00:05:30	120	160	00:06:10	40	118	Primary
10	30.03.2015	R	00:15:30	100	190	00:15:45	15	100	Primary
11	04.04.2015	B	00:10:00	130	155	00:10:25	25	120	Primary
12	02.07.2015	B	00:04:10	118	160	00:04:37	27	117	Primary
13	27.08.2015	R	00:23:04	120	190	00:24:04	60	115	Primary
14	15.09.2015	R	00:29:30	115	211	00:30:32	62	115	Primary
15	16.10.2015	B	00:08:10	125	160	00:08:40	30	120	Primary
16	18.01.2016	B	01:00:01	130	172	01:01:21	80	126	Primary
17	15.03.2016	R	00:59:53	120	210	01:00:13	20	110	Primary
18	02.04.2016	R	01:50:10	125	200	01:50:50	40	115	Primary
19	14.04.2016	B	00:45:20	137	202	00:46:10	50	130	Primary
20	30.04.2016	R	00:51:27	153	190	00:52:04	37	139	Primary
21	02.05.2016	R	00:31:53	144	165	00:34:25	152	97	Primary
22	23.05.2016	R	00:13:35	86	199	00:14:01	26	103	Primary
22a	23.05.2016	R	00:15:26	93	189	00:15:33	7	109	Secondary
23	23.07.2016	R	00:16:14	135	188	00:16:59	45	130	Primary
24	05.03.2017	R	00:22:04	117	189	00:23:00	56	93	Primary
25	02.04.2017	R	00:27:30	107	210	00:28:27	57	102	Primary
25a	02.04.2017	R	02:59:53	112	211	03:00:15	22	79	Secondary
25b	02.04.2017	R	03:10:14	122	201	03:11:03	49	112	Tertiary
26	20.04.2017	B	00:33:16	149	185	00:34:32	76	116	Primary
27	17.01.2018	B	00:01:35	121	176	00:02:12	37	98	Primary
28	02.02.2018	B	00:04:29	104	164	00:05:05	36	116	Primary
28a	02.02.2018	B	00:25:32	130	158	00:25:55	23	118	Secondary
29	19.02.2018	B	00:03:03	100	159	00:03:36	33	101	Primary
30	08.04.2018	R	02:10:55	128	210	02:11:16	21	119	Primary
30a	08.04.2018	R	03:10:30	114	217	03:11:26	56	108	Secondary
31	19.03.2018	B	00:20:10	135	160	00:20:50	40	130	Primary
32	01.05.2018	R	00:55:55	143	190	00:56:39	44	140	Primary
33	19.11.2018	B	00:02:58	126	150	00:03:19	21	117	Primary
34	19.02.2019	B	00:02:54	118	159	00:03:04	10	130	Primary
35	09.05.2019	B	00:03:05	119	157	00:03:28	23	125	Primary
36	02.07.2019	R	01:30:30	140	205	01:31:50	80	133	Primary
37	18.12.2019	B	01:03:47	124	170	01:05:02	75	115	Primary
38	13.01.2020	B	00:44:07	136	199	00:45:43	96	98	Primary
39	30.03.2020	R	01:11:50	147	207	01:12:27	37	140	Primary
40	10.04.2020	R	02:00:01	130	212	02:00:36	35	128	Primary

References

1. Walsh, J.A., III; Topol, E.J.; Steinhubl, S.R. Novel wireless devices for cardiac monitoring. *Circulation* **2014**, *130*, 573–581. [CrossRef] [PubMed]
2. Gajda, R.; Biernacka, E.K.; Drygas, W. The problem of arrhythmias in endurance athletes: Are heart rate monitors valuable tools for diagnosing arrhythmias? In *Horizons in World Cardiovascular Research*; Nova Science Publishers, Inc.: New York, NY, USA, 2018; Volume 15, pp. 1–64.
3. Josephson, M.E. Supraventricular Tachycardias. In *Clinical Cardiac Electrophysiology Techniques and Interpretations*, 5th ed.; Wolters Kluwer/Lippincott Williams & Wilkins: Philadelphia, PA, USA; Baltimore, MD, USA; New York, NY, USA; London, UK; Buenos Aires, Argentina; Hong Kong, China; Sydney, Australia; Tokyo, Japan, 2008; p. 176.
4. Miljoen, H.; Ector, J.; Garweg, C.; Saenen, J.; Huybrechts, W.; Sarkozy, A.; Willems, R.; Heidbuchel, H. Differential Presentation of Atrioventricular Nodal Re-Entrant Tachycardia in Athletes and Non-Athletes. *Europace* **2019**, *21*, 944–949. [CrossRef] [PubMed]
5. Heidbüchel, H.; Jackman, W.M. Characterization of Subforms of AV Nodal Reentrant Tachycardia. *Europace* **2004**, *6*, 316–329. [CrossRef] [PubMed]
6. Opel, A.; Murray, S.; Kamath, N.; Dhinoja, M.; Abrams, D.; Sporton, S.; Schilling, R.; Earley, M. Cryoablation versus radiofrequency ablation for treatment of atrioventricular nodal reentrant tachycardia: Cryoablation with 6-mm-tip catheters is still less effective than radiofrequency ablation. *Heart Rhythm* **2010**, *7*, 340–343. [CrossRef] [PubMed]
7. Gajda, R.; Biernacka, E.K.; Drygas, W. Are Heart Rate Monitors Valuable Tools for Diagnosing Arrhythmias in Endurance Athletes? *Scand. J. Med. Sci. Sports* **2018**, *28*, 496–516. [CrossRef] [PubMed]
8. Bhavnani, S.P.; Narula, J.; Sengupta, P.P. Mobile technology and the digitization of healthcare. *Eur. Heart J.* **2016**, *37*, 1428–1438. [CrossRef] [PubMed]
9. Mozos, I.; Caraba, A. Electrocardiographic Predictors of Cardiovascular Mortality. *Dis. Markers* **2015**, *2015*, 727401. [CrossRef] [PubMed]
10. Kwaku, K.F.; Josephson, M.E. Typical AVNRT—An Update on Mechanisms and Therapy. *Card Electrophysiol. Rev.* **2002**, *6*, 414–421. [CrossRef] [PubMed]
11. Wilhelm, M.; Roten, L.; Tanner, H.; Wilhelm, I.; Schmid, J.P.; Saner, H. Gender Differences of Atrial and Ventricular Remodeling and Autonomic Tone in Nonelite Athletes. *Am. J. Cardiol.* **2011**, *108*, 1489–1495. [CrossRef] [PubMed]
12. Mohanty, S.; Mohanty, P.; Tamaki, M.; Natale, V.; Gianni, C.; Trivedi, C.; Gokoglan, Y.; Di Biase, L.; Natale, A. Differential Association of Exercise Intensity with Risk of Atrial Fibrillation in Men and Women: Evidence from a Meta-Analysis. *J. Cardiovasc. Electrophysiol.* **2016**, *27*, 1021. [CrossRef] [PubMed]
13. Pesta, D.; Burtscher, M. Importance of Determining Maximal Heart Rate for Providing a Standardized Training Stimulus. *JAMA Intern. Med.* **2016**, *176*, 1883. [CrossRef] [PubMed]
14. Hunt, D.; Tanto, P. Diagnosis of arrhythmias in athletes wearing heart rate monitors. *BMJ Mil. Health* **2017**, *163*, 224. [CrossRef] [PubMed]
15. De Almeida, M.B.; Bottino, A.; Ramos, P.; Araujo, C.G. Measuring Heart Rate During Exercise: From Artery Palpation to Monitors and Apps. *Int. J. Cardiovasc. Sci.* **2019**, *32*, 396–407. [CrossRef]
16. Müssigbrodt, A.; Richter, S.; Wetzel, U.; Van Belle, Y.; Bollmann, A.; Hindricks, G. Diagnosis of Arrhythmias in Athletes Using Leadless, Ambulatory HR Monitors. *Med. Sci. Sports Exerc.* **2013**, *45*, 1431–1435. [CrossRef] [PubMed]
17. Garabelli, P.; Stavrakis, S.; Po, S. Smartphone-based arrhythmia monitoring. *Curr. Opin. Cardiol.* **2017**, *32*, 53–57. [CrossRef] [PubMed]
18. Barbosa, M.P.; da Silva, N.T.; de Azevedo, F.M.; Pastre, C.M.; Vanderlei, L.C. Comparison of Polar® RS800G3™ Heart Rate Monitor with Polar® S810i™ and Electrocardiogram to Obtain the Series of RR Intervals and Analysis of Heart Rate Variability at Rest. *Clin. Physiol. Funct. Imaging* **2016**, *36*, 112–117. [CrossRef] [PubMed]
19. Gajda, R.; Kowalik, E.; Rybka, S.; Rębowska, E.; Śmigielski, W.; Nowak, M.; Kwaśniewska, M.; Hoffman, P.; Drygas, W. Evaluation of the Heart Function of Swimmers Subjected to Exhaustive Repetitive Endurance Efforts During a 500-km Relay. *Front. Physiol.* **2019**, *10*, 296. [CrossRef] [PubMed]

20. Gajda, R.; Klisiewicz, A.; Matsibora, V.; Piotrowska-Kownacka, D.; Biernacka, E.K. Heart of the World's Top Ultramarathon Runner—Not Necessarily Much Different from Normal. *Diagnostics (Basel)* **2020**, *10*, 73. [CrossRef] [PubMed]
21. Thabouillot, O.; Bostanci, K.; Bouvier, F.; Dumitrescu, N.; Stéfuriac, M.; Paule, P.; Roche, N.C. Syncope During Competitive Events: Interrogating Heart Rate Monitor Watches May Be Useful! *Prehosp. Disaster Med.* **2017**, *32*, 691–693. [CrossRef] [PubMed]
22. Turakhia, M.P.; Desai, M.; Hedlin, H.; Rajmane, A.; Talati, N.; Ferris, T.; Desai, S.; Nag, D.; Patel, M.; Kowey, P.; et al. Rationale and design of a large-scale, app-based study to identify cardiac arrhythmias using a smartwatch: The Apple Heart Study. *Am. Heart J.* **2019**, *207*, 66–75. [CrossRef] [PubMed]
23. Hwang, J.; Kim, J.; Choi, K.J.; Cho, M.S.; Nam, G.B.; Kim, Y.H. Assessing Accuracy of Wrist-Worn Wearable Devices in Measurement of Paroxysmal Supraventricular Tachycardia Heart Rate. *Korean Circ. J.* **2019**, *49*, 437–445. [CrossRef] [PubMed]
24. Walker, J.; Calkins, H.; Nazarian, S. Evaluation of Cardiac Arrhythmia Among Athletes. *Am. J. Med.* **2010**, *123*, 1075–1081. [CrossRef] [PubMed]

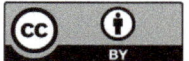

© 2020 by the author. Licensee MDPI, Basel, Switzerland. This article is an open access article distributed under the terms and conditions of the Creative Commons Attribution (CC BY) license (http://creativecommons.org/licenses/by/4.0/).

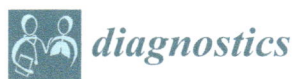 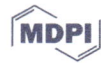

Article

Cardiovascular Adaptations to Four Months Training in Middle-Aged Amateur Long-Distance Skiers

Natalia Grzebisz

Vistula School of Hospitality, Faculty of Dietetics, 02-787 Warsaw, Poland; n.grzebisz@gmail.com; Tel.: +48-22-457-23-00

Received: 16 June 2020; Accepted: 28 June 2020; Published: 30 June 2020

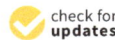

Abstract: Cross-country skiing has a positive effect on health. However, without an individual, thoughtful, and professional plan, it can cause irreversible health problems from overload and injury. The impact of exercise on results is well understood within the group of professional athletes. However, this remains unknown within the group of amateur cross-country skiers and marathon runners—in particular, the impact of the summer preparation period in which training loads performed in the oxygen zone combined with resistance training dominate. The aim of this study was to assess changes in the cardiovascular capacity and body mass composition of male cross-country skiers in the preparation period of their macrocycle. Variables were analyzed using basic descriptive statistics: mean and standard deviation (SD). To compare the results from both measurements (initial and final) the paired Wilcoxon test was used. A statistically significant increase was noted in maximum oxygen uptake and maximum minute ventilation, and a decrease in body fat content, maximum lactate concentration and lactate threshold, and heart rate on anaerobic threshold. Research indicated that in the amateur group increases similar to those in top competitors were achieved in the parameters tested, but the initial level was often significantly lower.

Keywords: cardiovascular capacity; performance; cross-country skiing amateur; heart

1. Introduction

Monitoring of physical effort in competitive sport is a key element in the training process used by trainers, physiologists, and doctors. It also allows to assess the health and capacity of amateurs. In particular, the determination of cardiovascular capacity parameters establishes the initial level before training, allows to assess the progress made and to predict the negative impact of excessive physical exertion. This applies in particular to endurance efforts such as long-distance cross-country skiing. It requires many years of physical activity and the use of periodization of training, for example, to avoid overloading and its negative impact on health.

The parameter used to assess exercise capacity in endurance athletes is the maximum oxygen uptake (VO_{2max}). Its level and change during many years of training is very well described in the literature when it comes to professional athletes. However, there are no reports on the impact of physical effort on the level and change of VO_{2max} in amateur long-distance skiing, which significantly differs in terms of requirements from other sports.

In recent years long-distance skiing (especially the Ski Classics series) has gained the attention of scientists, but the research has been focused on elite skiers [1]. To my knowledge, this paper is the very first on amateur long-distance skiers and their cardiovascular capacity.

The majority of popular long-distance races (30 up to 220 km) are easy in terms of track profile (flat sections and slight climbs, easy downhills), but this type of effort is long-term and characterized by near-threshold intensity. It requires not only efficiency, but also good technique [2].

Cross-country skiing is one of the most demanding sports. In addition to the high energy demand, the specificity of the effort is also important. It involves all body muscles, especially the upper parts [3,4].

This discipline has a positive effect on health. Scientists emphasize the role of systematic physical activity in improving the cardiovascular risk profile and body weight composition in middle-aged men. In the population low body mass index and high body fat percentage are associated with increased mortality. Therefore, qualitative and not quantitative changes in the body are important. In addition, body fat content should be within the reference ranges. This may bring greater cardiovascular benefits than a decrease in body mass index with a decrease in muscle mass [5].

However, without an individual, thoughtful, and professional plan, it can cause irreversible health problems from overload and injury. This is why it is so important to be aware of the body and to control the impact of training. An additional advantage of monitoring is a better adaptation of the training plan and the prevention of fatigue and overtraining. The monitoring process should apply to both athletes and amateurs. Both groups exert submaximal and maximum effort during competition, but professional athletes have a coaching team that checks for negative changes in the body [6].

Amateurs have to take care of this themselves, in terms of physiotherapy, physiological monitoring, biochemistry, diet, supplementation, training loads, as well as monitoring progress. Their work and private lives also have a significant impact on these changes. The impact of exercise on results is well understood within the group of professional athletes. However, it remains unknown within the group of amateur cross-country skiers and marathon runners—in particular, the impact of the summer preparation period, in which training loads performed in the oxygen zone combined with resistance training dominate. The use of roller skis is also unique, as it not only involves almost all muscles in the body but also relieves the joints [7].

The aim of this study was to assess changes in the cardiovascular capacity of cross-country skiers in the preparation period of their macrocycle (the annual cycle of preparations of athletes).

2. Materials and Methods

2.1. Subjects

The study was conducted in accordance with the guidelines of Good Clinical Practice and the Helsinki Declaration. The study was approved by the Bioethics Committee at the Faculty of Human Nutrition and Consumption at Warsaw University of Life Sciences (SGGW) (Nr. 38p/2018, approved on 22 January 2019). All subjects and parents gave their written consent before any testing. The research group consisted of 16 well-trained amateur skiers (mean age 37.5 +/− SD years, and 37.9 in the second test). The competitors worked professionally in a big city and could spend up to 90 min daily for physical training. There were no data on cardiovascular risk factors and changes in response to training for this group.

The research was carried out at the end of the transitional period in May and after the preparation period in September. The criteria for inclusion in the study were: consent to participate in the study, possession of current medical approval, and completion of at least three long-distance races in the last season. Exclusion criteria were: lack of consent for participation in the study, poor health (any disease occurrence), or lack of medical consent.

2.2. Anthropometric Measurements

Body weight was measured on the Tanita MC-980 MA Plus Body Composition Analyzer, consisting of an eight-point touch electrode system. The test was carried out just before the incremental exercise tests began. The following were determined: body weight, water content, minerals, vitamins, fat content in the body (% and kg) and slim mass muscle (muscle mass in % and kg), WHR (waist-to-hip ratio), and BMI (body mass index). All measurements were carried out at Sportslab Sports Diagnostics Center in Warsaw, Poland.

2.3. Measurement of Aerobic Capacity (VO_{2max} Test)

To assess the aerobic capacity expressed by the level of maximum oxygen uptake (VO_{2max}) a time trial test was used with gradually increasing intensity. This test was performed on a treadmill using HP Cosmos CPET equipment and Cosmed Quark/k4B2. The test started at a speed of 6 km/h and a 0% treadmill inclination. Then every 3 min, the speed was increased by 1 km/h, and the inclination by 1%. The test was continued until the subjective feeling of exhaustion by the competitor (to refuse). The frequency of heart contractions at rest and during exercise was recorded using the Garmin ANT+ heart rate monitor. The paper presents the maximum results of the test below. Dr. Müller Super GL Analyser was used to measure lactate concentrations. All measurements were carried out at Sportslab Sports Diagnostics Center in Warsaw, Poland.

2.4. Training Loads

For four months, the skiers performed a systematic endurance and strength effort. It consisted of running, resistance training in the gym, cycling, and, above all, targeted training, which was on roller skis. Individual exercise zones were designated for each person during the first exercise studies.

Figures 1–3 summarize the comprehensive efforts (running, cycling, swimming, general development exercises) and targeted training (ski imitation, roller skis, Ercolina, which is the machine for strengthening the arms and upper body, and special exercises). These data contain information about the intensity and volume of hourly training during the test period. The intensity was pre-rated in five exercise zones: I, II-aerobic, AT (anaerobic threshold)-mixed, anaerobic-Submaximal (Submax), and maximal (Max).

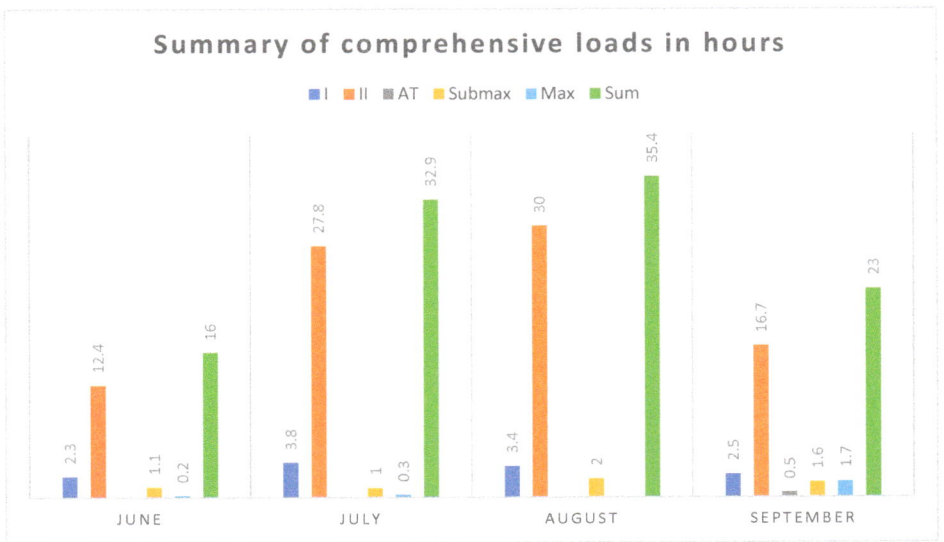

Figure 1. Monthly summary of comprehensive loads in hours.

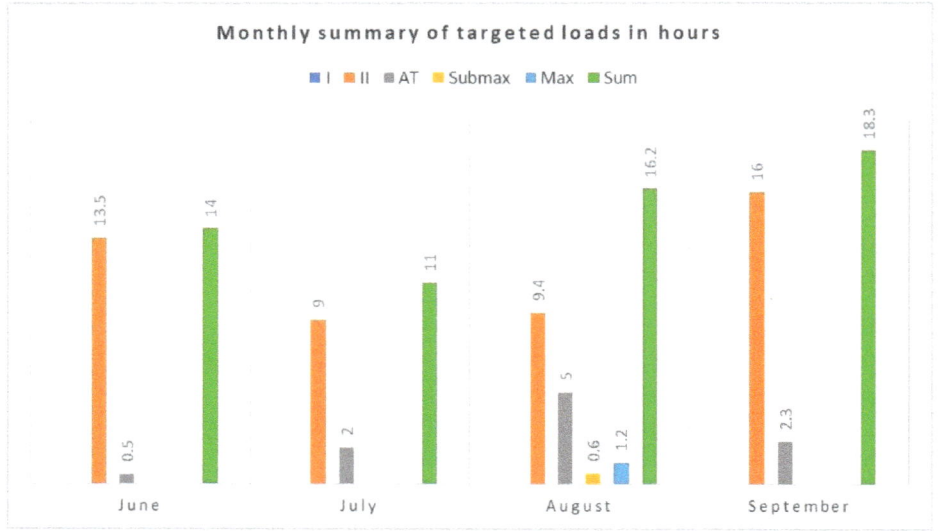

Figure 2. Monthly summary of targeted loads in hours.

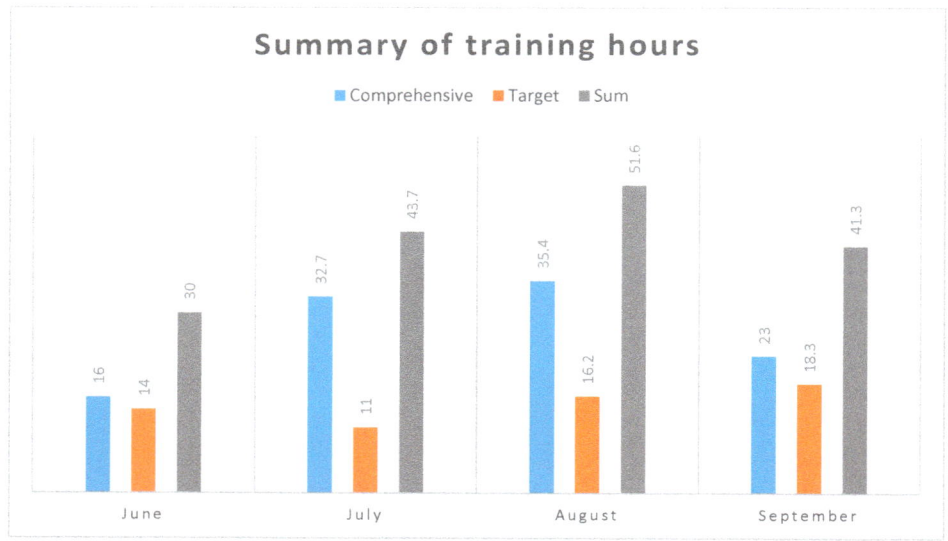

Figure 3. Summary of training hours.

2.5. Statistics

Variables were analyzed using basic descriptive statistics: arithmetic mean and standard deviation (SD). To compare the results from both measurements (initial and final) the paired Wilcoxon test was used, taking a materiality level of 0.05. The value of 0.05 was assumed as the significance level (denoted by * $p < 0.05$, * $p < 0.01$, *** $p < 0.001$).

3. Results

A comparison of the results of the body weight and exercise parameters of the first and second tests is presented in Table 1. Statistically significant changes were recorded in the: percentages of body fat mass, body fat mass (kg), VO_{2max} (relative) (mL/kg/min), maximum lactate concentration (mmol/L), maximum ventilation (L/min), lactate concentration (on the threshold) AT (mmol/L), and breathing rate on AT (bpm). The other parameters did not show statistically significant changes (see Table 1).

Table 1. Comparison of the results of the first and second tests.

Parameter Mean (Standard Deviation)	Result 1	Result 2	p–Value
Height (cm)	182.2 (6.0)	182.2 (5.8)	1.000
Body weight (kg)	78.8 (6.3)	78.4 (6.0)	0.333
BMI (kg/height^2)	23.7 (1.3)	23.6 (1.2)	0.191
% body fat mass	15.3 (2.6)	14.6 (3.0)	0.038
Body fat mass (kg)	12.1 (2.6)	11.4 (2.7)	0.023
Test duration (s)	1566.7 (130.4)	1592.7 (133.5)	0.267
Running speed (maximum km/h)	14.0 (0.7)	14.2 (0.8)	0.181
VO_{2max} (relative) (mL/kg/min)	49.0 (4.5)	51.1 (4.6)	0.008
VO_{2max} (absolute) (L/min)	3.9 (0.4)	4.0 (0.5)	0.054
Maximum heart rate (heartbeats per minute)	183.9 (9.8)	182.3 (10.1)	0.195
Maximum lactate concentration (mmol/L)	12.5 (2.8)	10.8 (2.5)	0.013
Maximum ventilation (L/min)	147.3 (20.5)	151.2 (22.2)	0.038
The frequency of maximum breathing (number of breaths/min)	59.7 (12.4)	60.4 (10.6)	0.410
Running speed anaerobic threshold (AT) (km/h)	11.1 (0.7)	11.2 (0.7)	0.575
Oxygen uptake–VO_2 (relative) on AT (mL/kg/min)	44.8 (3.8)	44.9 (3.6)	0.934
Oxygen uptake–VO_2 (absolute) on AT (L/min)	3.6 (0.4)	3.5 (0.4)	0.609
Heart rate on AT (number of breaths per min)	170.4 (7.7)	168.1 (10.4)	0.073
Lactate concentration (on the threshold) AT (mmol/L)	4.9 (1.3)	4.0 (0.9)	0.017
AT ventilation (L/min)	108.9 (17.9)	112.2 (18.6)	0.229
Heart rate on AT (bpm)	40.09 (6.2)	43.4 (7.1)	0.024

4. Discussion

The main findings of this study are: (1) a statistically significant change in relative VO_{2max} ($p = 0.008$), similar to that in elite cross-country skiing; (2) a change in body fat mass (in absolute terms as well as in %); (3) a change in maximum ventilation.

In the study, the largest statistically significant change was recorded in relative VO_{2max} ($p = 0.008$). This corresponded to an increase of 2.1 mL/kg/min, which was 4.3% on a percentage basis. There are a lack of publications on the impact of a training program (especially roller ski training) on performance parameters in amateur long-distance skiing that could be used to compare these changes. However, we can compare the results to research on other endurance disciplines, e.g., triathlon. A group of 32 participants followed a training program lasting five months with the goal to finish the Half-Ironman competition (which is a long-distance event, similar in hours of effort to 90 km of skiing) [8]. The program significantly increased the maximal oxygen consumption of participants (45.9 ± 8.2 to 48.6 ± 7.5 mL/kg/min, $p = 0.002$) and the difference between tests was 5.9%. In elite cross-country skiing the change in relative VO_{2max} was slightly lower (3.1 ± 4.5%) in response to loads in the preparation mesocycle [9].

These results confirm that regular physical activity increases the values of VO_{2max}, which is the main indicator of the fitness level. Many other studies have also confirmed the positive effects of regular training on VO_{2max} for people over 30 years of age. These effects were greater in the cases of people who led sedentary lifestyles, as well as in cases of introducing HIIT (high intensity interval training) to the training program [10]. Furthermore, high-intensity exercise may reduce by up to 50% the decline in VO_{2max} in young and middle-aged men if the activity is maintained long term. It is worth noting that age-related loss of VO_{2max} is 10% [11]. Researchers indicated that in the elite the changes occurred between the early, middle, and late preparation phases of the macrocycle with minor changes in the competitive season [12]. It can be assumed that this period of preparation in amateurs also significantly affects health-related changes in the body.

It is worth emphasizing that studies did not show significant differences between the results of the time-to-exhaustion test in running and roller skiing. Elite cross-country skiers did not elicit higher VO_{2max} during roller ski skating than during running, and this relationship did not change during the pre-season training period. This may be a monitoring tip for trainers and physiologists, for whom the use of roller skis on a treadmill is limited or impossible.

Several studies have demonstrated that male and female world-class skiers are among the endurance athletes with the highest VO_{2max}. Accordingly, world-class performance has been associated with maximal values above 70 and 80 mL/kg/min, or 4.0 and 6.0 L/min, in female and male skiers, respectively [13]. Values of VO_{2max} [14] in a group of athletes (55.46 mL/kg/min) were significantly greater than in a group of nonathletes (37.78 mL/kg/min), and, in particular, aerobic athletes (like runners, cyclists, and skiers, excluding sprinters) showed higher values than anaerobic athletes (like sprinters and heavy weightlifters) (58.88 mL/kg/min vs. 52.04 mL/kg/min).

Increasing the VO_{2max}, lowering the fat content, and increasing the ventilation are evidences of good adaptation to the effort and an increase in the cardiovascular efficiency [15]. Minute ventilation and lung diffusion capacity are factors related to the functioning of the respiratory system affecting the value of VO_{2max}. In people with good physical fitness it is about 110–130 L/min, in sportsmen 150–160 L/min, and in some cases up to 200–210 L/min [16]. Its increase, as in these studies, indicates an improvement in exercise capacity and better oxygenation of the body during maximum effort.

Higher maximum values have been recorded [17]. The winners of Marcialonga, Vasaloppet, and Birkebeinerrennet (which are the three most prestigious long-distance ski races) also presented higher values [18]. Of course, it is not surprising, if we take into consideration the generally higher sports level of subjects and professional training. Elite skiers train mostly around 20–25 h per week during the preparation period from May to October [3]. In this study amateur skiers trained a mean of 41.7 h per month, which is 10.4 h per week.

As a result, amateurs show lower maximum values for minute ventilation. Therefore, the tendency and increase in response to training should be evaluated. It also indicates a positive adaptation of the cardiovascular system to effort.

Statistically significant differences were also shown in cases of the percentage and kilogram reductions of body fat. Studies have shown that this factor significantly affects VO_{2max} [19]. In other studies it was noted that skiers should aim to achieve a body composition with a high percentage of lean mass and a low percentage of fat mass. A focus on trunk mass through increased muscle mass appears to be important, especially for amateur and long-distance skiing, where double-poling is the most common technique [20,21]. Another research suggested that large amounts of lean body mass, especially in the arms, seem to be of great importance for cross-country skiing performance [22]. Elite male cross-country skiers have approximately 10.5% body fat [23]. In this research the level was higher: 15.3 ± 2.6 in the first test, and 14.6 ± 3.0 in the second. The level was similar to young non-athletes [24] but BMI was similar to athletes. Interestingly, the parameters were much better than those obtained in [8], where body fat mass in % was 23.4 ± 7.5 in the first test (before the training program) and 23.6 ± 7.0 in the second, after a six-month triathlon training program. BMI was 25.0 ± 2.7 and 24.7 ± 2.4, respectively.

In this study, a statistically significant decrease in body fat mass was recorded. Similar trends were also seen in pilot studies [25]. It was proven that a decrease in body fat mass can improve exercise capacity and results [26]. Optimal body fat for men in endurance disciplines is around 8–10% (during the competitive period) [27]. In [28] it was recommended that cross-country skiers should have 7% to 12% fat mass in the body. A reduction of body fat below 4%, however, can affect the body's regenerative capacity and adversely affect the immune system. A value of >10% of body fat translates into poorer sports results because of, among other factors, higher than optimal body weight. By lowering body weight accordingly, by reducing body fat, we increase the level of oxygen intake per kilogram of body weight. Higher oxygen availability translates into better exercise options [27].

In addition, researchers highlighted the link between high body fat content and mortality. Reducing body fat instead of total weight seems to benefit the cardiovascular system more than a decrease in body mass index [29]. The results of these studies indicated the health impact of physical activity on the health of amateurs. A further decline may positively affect the effort and health of these amateurs but should not fall below 8%. Researchers suggested that a low lean mass index can be a strong indicator of mortality in men [30,31]. Reducing body fat and engaging in physical activity are important factors in improving the cardiovascular risk profile in middle-aged men. Achieving the correct body fat content can bring many health benefits for male amateur cross-country skiers.

The mean race intensity in the Vassaloppet race was 82% of maximal heart rate (HR) and did not differ between performance groups, even though elite skiers skied ~15% faster than amateurs. The research showed that the amateur group contributed a longer effort in zones two and three, in comparison with elite cross-country skiers [32]. This emphasizes the role of aerobic and mixed possibilities in amateur efforts.

An increase in heart rate on lactate threshold (HR AT) was recorded in these studies. This indicates a positive adaptation to effort in response to a four-month workout. Delaying the transition from exercise in an aerobic to an anaerobic zone has a positive effect on exercise capacity. Shifting the lactate curve to the right results in a greater use of fat stores than of muscle glycogen, of which reserves in the body are limited.

During endurance training, the exercise load at the anaerobic threshold level is considered to be the most effective in relatively long exercises. Subsequent crossing of the lactate threshold during increasing work load allows you to extend your effort. When lactate increases, hydrogen ions are also released, which is the main cause of fatigue. A decrease in lactate concentration at the anaerobic threshold and in the maximum concentration will indicate correct adaptation to exercise. The optimal training of a long-distance skier should mainly approach the maximum oxygen consumption–VO_{2max} with the least accumulation of lactic acid in the blood [33]. Lowering the concentration of lactic acid and minimizing the effects of its secretion at higher speeds are important matters of training for long-distance runners. It is also worth noting that lactate shows a high correlation with other indicators, e.g., VO_{2max} [34].

The correct response to exercise was recorded in these studies. This was indicated by a decrease in lactate concentration at the threshold and in maximum values. However, it should be emphasized that a decrease in lactate concentration may also be an indicator of fatigue. A low-carbohydrate diet may be another factor affecting its lower values. Both of these factors will reduce the body's exercise capacity.

5. Conclusions

The study indicates that a four-month comprehensive training for amateur long-distance skiers with the use of roller skis has a positive effect on the cardiovascular system. In addition, reducing body fat can be an important factor in protecting against heart disease in middle-aged men. A statistically significant increase was noted in maximum oxygen uptake and maximum minute ventilation, and a decrease in body fat content, maximum lactate concentration and lactate threshold, and heart rate on AT. Research indicated that in the amateur group increases similar to those in top competitors were achieved in the parameters tested, but the initial level was often significantly lower. Future research may focus on the analysis of a larger research group, include control groups, and focus especially on upper body training.

Funding: This research received financial support by the Ministry of Science and Higher Education (grant No. 217906/E-716 /M/2018) for young scientists.

Conflicts of Interest: The author declare that there is no conflict of interests regarding the publication of this article.

References

1. Sagelv, E.H.; Engseth, T.P.; Pedersen, S.; Pettersen, S.A.; Mathisen, G.; Heitmann, K.A.; Welde, B.; Thomassen, T.O.; Stöggl, T.L. Physiological Comparisons of Elite Male Visma Ski Classics and National Level Cross-Country Skiers During Uphill Treadmill Roller Skiing. *Front. Physiol.* **2018**, *9*, 1523. [CrossRef] [PubMed]
2. Carlsson, M.; Assarsson, H.; Carlsson, T. The influence of sex, age, and race experience on pacing profiles during the 90 km Vasaloppet ski race. *J. Sports Med.* **2016**, *7*, 11–19. [CrossRef] [PubMed]
3. Sandbakk, Ø.; Hegge, A.M.; Losnegard, T.; Skattebo, Ø.; Tønnessen, E.; Holmberg, H.C. The Physiological Capacity of the World's Highest Ranked Female Cross-country Skiers. *Med. Sci. Sports Exerc.* **2016**, *48*, 1091–1100. [CrossRef] [PubMed]
4. Sandbakk, Ø.; Holmberg, H.C. Physiological Capacity and Training Routines of Elite Cross-Country Skiers: Approaching the Upper Limits of Human Endurance. *Int. J. Sports Physiol. Perform.* **2017**, *12*, 1003–1011. [CrossRef] [PubMed]
5. Padwal, R.; Leslie, W.; Lix, L.; Majumdar, S. Relationship Among Body Fat Percentage, Body Mass Index, and All-Cause Mortality: A Cohort Study. *Ann. Intern. Med.* **2016**, *164*, 532–541. [CrossRef] [PubMed]
6. Holmberg, H.C. The elite cross-country skier provides unique insights into human exercise physiology. *Scand. J. Med. Sci. Sports* **2015**, *25*, 100–109. [CrossRef] [PubMed]
7. Bolger, C.M.; Bessone, V.; Federolf, P.; Ettema, G.; Sandbakk, Ø. The influence of increased distal loading on metabolic cost, efficiency, and kinematics of roller ski skating. *PLoS ONE* **2018**, *13*, e0197592. [CrossRef]
8. Lalond, F.; Martin, S.M.; Boucher, V.G. Preparation for an Half-Ironmantm Triathlon amongst Amateur Athletes: Finishing Rate and Physiological Adaptation. *Int. J. Exerc. Sci.* **2020**, *13*, 766–777.
9. Losengard, T.; Hallén, J. Elite cross-country skiers do not reach their running VO2max during roller ski skating. *J. Sports Med. Phys. Fitness.* **2014**, *54*, 389–393.
10. Bacon, A.P.; Carter, R.E.; Ogle, E.A.; Joyner, M.J. VO2max trainability and high intensity interval training in humans: A meta-analysis. *PLoS ONE* **2013**, *8*, e73182. [CrossRef]
11. Hawkins, S.; Wiswell, R. Rate and Mechanism of Maximal Oxygen Consumption Decline with Aging. *Sports Med.* **2003**, *33*, 877–888. [CrossRef] [PubMed]
12. Losnegard, T.; Myklebust, H.; Spencer, M.; Hallén, J. Seasonal variations in VO2max, O2-cost, O2-deficit, and performance in elite cross-country skiers. *J. Strength Cond. Res.* **2013**, *27*, 1780–1790. [CrossRef] [PubMed]
13. Losnegard, T. Energy system contribution during competitive cross-country skiing. *Eur. J. Appl. Physiol.* **2019**, *119*, 1675–1690. [CrossRef] [PubMed]
14. Kostić, V. Differences in aerobic capacity and spirometric parameters between athletes and nonathletes. *Porto. Biom. J.* **2017**, *2*, 184. [CrossRef]
15. Grzebisz, N.; Piejko, L.; Sulich, A. Determinants of cardiorespiratory fitness in amateur male cross-country skiers. *Russian J. Cardiol.* **2019**, 109–113. [CrossRef]
16. Ehrman, J.K.; Gordon, P.M.; Visich, P.S.; Keteyian, S.J. *Clinical Exercise Physiology*, 2nd ed.; Human Kinetics: Champaign, IL, USA, 2009.
17. Fabre, N.; Passelergue, P.; Bouvard, M.; Perrey, S. Comparison of heart rate deflection and ventilatory threshold during a field cross-country roller-skiing test. *J. Strength Cond. Res.* **2008**, *22*, 1977–1984. [CrossRef]
18. Skattebo, Ø.; Losnegard, T.; Stadheim, H.K. Double-Poling Physiology and Kinematics of Elite Cross-Country Skiers: Specialized Long-Distance Versus All-Round Skiers. *Int. J. Sports Physiol. Perform.* **2019**, *14*, 1190–1199. [CrossRef]
19. Calbet, J.A.; Joyner, M.J. Disparity in regional and systemic circulatory capacities: Do they affect the regulation of the circulation? *Acta Physiol. (Oxf.)* **2010**, *199*, 393–406. [CrossRef]
20. Stöggl, T.; Enqvist, J.; Muller, E.; Holmberg, H.C. Relationships between body composition, body dimensions, and peak speed in cross-country sprint skiing. *J. Sports Sci.* **2010**, *28*, 161–169. [CrossRef] [PubMed]
21. Øfsteng, S.; Sandbakk, Ø.; van Beekvelt, M.; Hammarström, D.; Kristoffersen, R.; Hansen, J.; Paulsen, G.; Rønnestad, B.R. Strength training improves double-poling performance after prolonged submaximal exercise in cross-country skiers. *Scand. J. Med. Sci. Sport.* **2018**, *28*, 893–904. [CrossRef] [PubMed]
22. Larsson, P.; Henriksson-Larsén, K. Body composition and performance in cross-country skiing. *Int. J. Sports Med.* **2008**, *29*, 971–975. [CrossRef] [PubMed]

23. Udebake, V.; Berg, J.; Tjonna, A.; Sandbakk, Ø. Comparison of Physiological and Perceptual Responses to Upper-, Lower-, and Whole-Body Exercise in Elite Cross-Country Skiers. *J. Strength Cond. Res.* **2019**, *33*, 1086–1094. [CrossRef] [PubMed]
24. Rakovac, A.; Andric, L.; Karan, V.; Bogdan, M.; Slavić, D.; Klasnja, A. Evaluation of spirometric parameters and maximum oxygen consumption in athletes and non-athletes. *Medicinski. Pregled.* **2018**, *71*, 157–161. [CrossRef]
25. Grzebisz, N.; Piejko, L. The impact of endurance exercise on the cardiovascular capacity of a male amateur cross country skier. Pilot study. *World Sci. News* **2018**, *110*, 72–83.
26. Carlsson, M.; Carlsson, T.; Hammarstroem, D.; Malm, C.; Tonkonogi, M. Prediction of race performance of elite cross-country skiers by lean mass. *Int. J. Sports Physiol. Perform.* **2014**, *9*, 1040–1045. [CrossRef] [PubMed]
27. Ettema, G.; Holmberg, H.C.; Sandbakk, Ø. Analysis of a sprint ski race and associated laboratory determinants of world-class performance. *Eur. J. Appl. Physiol.* **2011**, *1*, 947–957.
28. Jeukendrup, A.; Gleeson, M. *Sport Nutrition*, 3rd ed.; Human Kinetics Publishers: Champaign, IL, USA, 2019.
29. Dong, B.; Peng, Y.; Wang, Z.; Adegbija, O.; Hu, J.; Ma, J.; Ying-Hua, M. Joint association between body fat and its distribution with all-cause mortality: A data linkage cohort study based on NHANES (1988–2011). *PLoS ONE* **2018**, *23*, e0193368. [CrossRef]
30. McGee, D.; Reed, D.; Stemmerman, G.; Rhoads, G.; Yano, K.; Feinleib, M. The relationship of dietary fat and cholesterol to mortality in 10 years: The Honolulu Heart Program. *Int. J. Epidemiol.* **1985**, *14*, 97–105. [CrossRef]
31. Graf, C.; Karsegard, V.; Spoerri, A. Body composition and all-cause mortality in subjects older than 65 y. *Am. J. Clin. Nutr.* **2015**, *101*, 760–767. [CrossRef]
32. Stöggl, T.L.; Hertlein, M.; Brunauer, R.; Welde, B.; Andersson, E.P.; Swarén, M. Pacing Exercise Intensity, and Technique by Performance Level in Long-Distance Cross-Country Skiing. *Front. Physiol.* **2020**, *11*, 17. [CrossRef]
33. Moxnes, J.F.; Sandbakk, Ø. The kinetics of lactate production and removal during whole-body exercise. *Theor. Biol. Med. Model.* **2012**, *9*, 7. [CrossRef] [PubMed]
34. Brooks, G.A. Lactate: Link beetwen glycolytic and oxidative metabolism. *Sports Med.* **2007**, *37*, 341–343. [CrossRef] [PubMed]

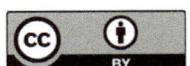

© 2020 by the author. Licensee MDPI, Basel, Switzerland. This article is an open access article distributed under the terms and conditions of the Creative Commons Attribution (CC BY) license (http://creativecommons.org/licenses/by/4.0/).

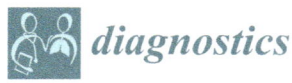

Article

Determinants of the Cardiovascular Capacity of Amateur Long-Distance Skiers during the Transition Period

Natalia Grzebisz

Faculty of Dietetics, Vistula School of Hospitality, 02-787 Warsaw, Poland; n.grzebisz@gmail.com

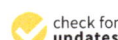

Received: 30 July 2020; Accepted: 4 September 2020; Published: 5 September 2020

Abstract: The aim of this study was to identify determinants of the cardiovascular capacity of 16 male amateur long-distance skiers during the transition period. These factors can vary from amateur marathon skiers, who represent a sort of midpoint between inactive people and professional athletes. Cardiovascular capacity depends mainly on the volume and intensity of the training, which are different between these groups. Finding the factors affecting heart condition of amateur athletes can be an important element in their health care and can help the athletes to achieve their full performance potential. Therefore, ergospirometric and hematological tests were performed. As a result, predictors for volume oxygen uptake were determined using a regression model, which included the following variables: the percentage of monocytes ($p = 0.031$), the concentration of sodium ($p = 0.004$), and total calcium ($p = 0.03$). All these parameters negatively affected VO2 max. Biochemical and physiological monitoring of amateur athletes can help to protect their health and prepare them properly for their training. The growing popularity of long-distance competitions among middle-aged amateur athletes and the lack of guidance on how to assess their health indicate the need for further research.

Keywords: biomarkers; amateur; sports cardiology

1. Introduction

Physical activity provokes adaptive changes in the body, which allow for a fuller use of physiological reserves. These changes are monitored, for example, in the circulatory-respiratory, nervous, and endocrine systems or body weight and composition. The maximum oxygen uptake (VO2 max) is known as the main determining factor for high performance potential (aerobic fitness). Research indicates that this is the main determinant of success in many disciplines, especially in endurance sports (e.g., cross-country skiing). VO2 max is genetically conditioned, and also influenced by body weight and composition, age, gender, diet and supplementation, and biochemical parameters of blood. Monitoring of these factors and the use of this knowledge can have a significant impact on endurance exercise capabilities and can help provide protection against overloading of the body and overtraining. This is particularly important in terms of participation in long-term endurance and strength efforts, such as long-distance races (40 km and more), and in the administration of effective training processes [1].

Adaptation changes also apply to amateur athletes, who are increasingly involved in sports competition. An example is the famous Vasaloppet race, with an attendance of more than 15,000 people. The Worldloppet series (20 races around the globe) attracted 64,000 skiers in the 2019/2020 season [2]. In addition to raising the capabilities of the amateur athletes, it is important to protect their health during long and demanding training sessions and races. This can be particularly relevant to men struggling with stress and around 40 years of age. They participate in sports competition often without prior, long-term, and adapted fitness preparation. This group is significantly vulnerable to the possibility of adverse health outcomes, such as early heart attacks. Above-average effort, like a ski marathon, contributes to this risk. However, the risk can be reduced by regular, fitted exercise that improves body composition and lipogram results and increases cardiovascular capacity and adaptation. Factors affecting the VO2 max level in professional athletes are well understood. Among amateur cross-country skiers, there is still a lack of information about the level of performance they present and the factors that significantly affect it [3]. This knowledge is essential for coaches to create an appropriate training plan for amateur athletes to not only improve their cardiovascular capacity but also support their health and protect against overtraining and its consequences. The aim of this research was to identify biochemical determinants for maximum oxygen uptake in amateur cross-country skiers. It is known that biochemical profiles are different between individuals who are characterized by inactive lifestyles and individuals who are professional athletes, however, the potential differences and similarities are poorly understood in individuals with distinctly elevated physical activity levels (e.g., long distance skiers), but who are not training professionally. In addition, the immune, endocrine, and hormonal systems' responses to demanding physical exertion are poorly understood in this group. This knowledge can be important for doctors, trainers, and nutritionists to assess baseline levels

2. Materials and Methods

2.1. Subjects

The study was conducted in accordance with the guidelines of Good Clinical Practice and the Helsinki Declaration. The study was approved by the Bioethics Committee at the Faculty of Human Nutrition and Consumption at Warsaw University of Life Sciences (SGGW) (No. 38p/2018, approved on 22 January 2019). All subjects gave their written consent before any testing. The study group consisted of 16 well-trained (but working full-time and living in a big city) male amateur cross-country skiers who had participated at least three times in long distance races (40 km or more) in the previous season. They had to give written consent before the test and were required to have a current medical certificate. The test was conducted in May at the end of transition period (i.e., the period after the last race and before the start of the preparation period). The goal of the research was to determine and evaluate the parameters of circulatory-respiratory fitness and predictors of maximum oxygen uptake.

2.2. Anthropometric Measurements

During the test, the weight and body composition of the participants were measured (using Tanita Body Composition Analyzer BODY IN MC-980 MA (Tokyo, Japan) consisting of an eight-point touch electrode system) just before the ergospirometry stress test began. The following were determined: body weight, water content, minerals, vitamins, fat content in the body (% and kg), lean muscle mass (muscle mass in % and kg), WHR (waist to hip ratio), and BMI (body mass index).

2.3. Measurement of Aerobic Capacity (VO2 max Test)

The ergospirometry stress test (time-to-exhaustion test) was conducted to assess the aerobic capacity of the participants and to determine their VO2 max (the level of maximum oxygen uptake). The treadmill HP Cosmos CPET equipment (Nussdorf-Traunstein, Germany) and Cosmed Quark/k4B2 (Rome, Italy) were used. The test started at a speed of 6 km/h and 0% inclination. Then, every 3 min the speed was increased by 1 km/h and the inclination by 1% until the subject reported the feeling of exhaustion. The heart rate of each participant was monitored using a Garmin ANT+ heart rate monitor (Olathe, KS, USA). This paper presents the maximum results of the test.

2.4. Venous Blood Sampling and Analysis

Venous blood was sampled from the subjects in the morning (7:00–10:00 AM), before the first meal, on the day of the exercise test. Alifax (Polverara, Italy) and the automatic methodology were set to measure ESR (erythrocyte sedimentation rate). Cobas 8000 (Basel, Switzerland) and spectrophotometric methods were used to measure creatinine, uric acid, urea, iron, magnesium, total calcium, amylase, alanine amino transferase (ALT), aspartate amino transferase (AST), gamma-glutamyl transpeptidase (GGTP, alkaline phosphatase (ALP), total bilirubin, and glucose. The spectrophotometric method was used to measure sodium and potassium, and the electrochemiluminescence immunoassay (ECLIA) method for the following hormone determinations: thyroid stimulating hormone (TSH), cortisol, and testosterone. The spectrophotometric method also measured lipid profile indicators (total cholesterol, high density lipoprotein-cholesterol (HDL-C), low density lipoprotein-cholesterol (LDL-C), and triglycerides), and C-reactive protein (CRP) was determined by immunoturbidimetric method.

2.5. Statistics

Variables were analyzed using the following basic descriptive statistics: number of persons (N), arithmetic mean, median, minimum (Min), maximum (Max), and standard deviation (SD). The Shapiro–Wilk's test was used to evaluate the normality of the data. The Pearson correlation coefficients were used, whose values—in the case of statistical significance—can be interpreted as follows in Table 1. Regressive models were also developed for dependent variables, among which those with the highest determination factor R^2 were selected. The value of 0.05 was assumed as the significance level (denoted by * $p < 0.05$, ** $p < 0.01$, *** $p < 0.001$).

Table 1. The Pearson correlation coefficients used in the case of statistical significance [1].

Coefficient (r)	Interpretation
$0.0 \leq |r| \leq 0.2$	no correlation
$0.2 < |r| \leq 0.4$	weak correlation
$0.4 < |r| \leq 0.7$	average correlation
$0.7 < |r| \leq 0.9$	strong correlation
$0.9 < |r| \leq 1.0$	very strong correlation

[1] The calculations were made in statistical software (ver. 3.6.0). (Chicaco, IL, USA).

3. Results

Detailed data characteristics of the study group and VO2 max are shown in Table 2.

Table 2. Anthropometric measurements and VO2 max level.

Variable	Arithmetic Average ($N = 16$) Means ± SD (Difference Δ—Delta)
Age (years)	38.69 ± 7.95 (28.00–56.00)
Body height (cm)	181.44 ± 6.53 (169.00–197.00)
Body mass (kg)	78.52 ± 6.18 (68.10–91.50)
Fat mass (kg)	12.22 ± 2.53 (7.90–16.00)
Fat mass (%)	15.51 ± 2.59 (10.00–19.30)
BMI (kg/m^2)	23.84 ± 1.35 (21.00–25.70)
VO2 max (mL/kg/min)	48.37 ± 5.06 (38.54–55.81)

BMI: body mass index; N: number of patients; VO2 max: maximal oxygen uptake; SD: standard deviation. All data are presented as means ± standard deviation and the difference (Δ—delta).

3.1. Hematological Parameters of Participants

Hematological parameters of participants are shown in Table 3. All measured parameters, except bilirubin, were within the norm.

Table 3. Hematological parameters of participants.

Morphology	Mean	Standard Deviation	Min	Max
Leukocytes (thou/μL)	5.4	0.88	4.2	9.1
Erythrocytes (M/μL)	5.06	0.29	4.2	6
Hemoglobin (g/dL)	15.19	0.5	14	18
Hematocrit %	43.86	1.53	40	51
Mean corpuscular value (MCV) (fL)	88.03	3.41	80	99
Mean corpuscular hemoglobin (MCH) (pg)	30.49	1.01	27	35
Mean corpuscular hemoglobin concentration (MCHC) (g/dL)	34.66	0.93	32	37
Platelets (thou/μL)	214.06	35.74	140	440
Red blood cell distribution width-standard deviation (RDW-SD) (fL)	40.77	2.97	35.1	43.9
Red blood cell distribution width-coefficient of variation (RDW-CV) %	12.98	0.79	11.6	14.4
Platelet distribution width (PDW) (fL)	13.45	2.14	9.8	16.1
Mean platelet volume (MPV) (fL)	10.64	1.06	9	13
Platelet-large cell ratio (P-LCR) %	31.83	8.69	13	43
Procalcitonin (PCT) %	0.21	0.04	0.2	0.4
Neutrophils (thou/μL)	2.7	0.55	2	7
Lymphocytes (thou/μL)	2.04	0.56	1	3.5
Monocytes (thou/μL)	0.45	0.09	0.2	1
Eosinophils (thou/μL)	0.25	0.19	0.1	0.5
Basophils (thou/μL)	0.03	0.03	0	0.1
Neutrophils %	49.69	7.91	40	70
Lymphocytes %	38.26	7.43	20	45
Eosinophils %	4.46	2.83	1	6
Basophils %	0.55	0.37	0	2
Erythrocyte sedimentation rate (ESR) (mm/h)	5.06	3.73	2	12
Urea (mg/dL)	33.94	6.43	10	50
Estimated glomerular filtration rate (eGFR) (mL/min/1.73m2)	73.03	13.4	-	-
Uric acid (mg/dL)	5.6	1.45	3.4	7
Glucose (mg/dL)	85.25	17.52	70	99
Total cholesterol (mg/dL)	179.1	32.58	115	190
Cholesterol high-density lipoproteins (HDL) (mg/dL)	58.21	12.17	≥45	-
Cholesterol non-HDL (mg/dL)	119.84	37.31	-	-
Cholesterol low-density lipoproteins (LDL) (mg/dL)	105.46	31.23	0	<115
Triglycerides (mg/dL)	81.36	34.51	0	150
Aspartate transaminase (AST) (U/L)	28.81	22.87	0	40
Alanine aminotransferase (ALT) (U/L)	22.22	7.59	0	41
Alkaline phosphatase (U/L)	59.22	10.44	40	129
Gamma-glutamyl transferase (GGTP) (U/L)	19.89	10.59	8	61
Serum amylase (U/L)	63.58	21.38	28	100
Sodium (mmol/L)	141.46	2.27	136	145
Potassium (mmol/L)	4.53	0.37	3.5	5.1
Total calcium (mmol/L)	2.42	0.11	2.15	2.5
Magnesium (mmol/L)	0.86	0.06	0.66	1.07
Iron (μg/dL)	11.05	50.3	33	193
C-reactive protein (CRP) (mg/dL)	0.71	0.97	0	5
Thyroid-stimulating hormone (μIU/mL)	1.71	0.71	0.27	4.2
Testosterone (ng/dL)	591.94	210.72	239	836
Cortisol (μg/dL) 7–10 AM	14.24	4.32	6.2	19.4

3.2. Correlations for Independent Variables

The VO2 max had significant correlations with five variables. Most of these correlations were moderately strong or strong, and positive. The results are shown in Table 4. Only statistically significant results are presented in the paper.

Table 4. The *p*-values and correlations for the VO2 max of the athletes.

Variable	*p*-Value	Correlation
Monocytes (thou/μL)	0.001	−0.750
Eosinophils (thou/μL)	0.026	0.613
Monocytes %	<0.001	−0.797
Eosinophils %	0.027	0.610
Erythrocyte sedimentation rate (ESR) (mm/h)	0.010	−0.620
Estimated glomerular filtration rate (eGFR) (mL/min/1.73 m^2)	0.041	0.531
Sodium (mmol/L)	0.004	−0.680
Total calcium (mmol/L)	0.035	−0.530

3.3. Regression Model

For the variable under consideration, a model with the highest R^2 coefficient value was selected, for which dependent variables could have influenced the variable. The distribution of the value of the R^2 model adjustment measure depending on the selection of independent variables is presented in Figure 1.

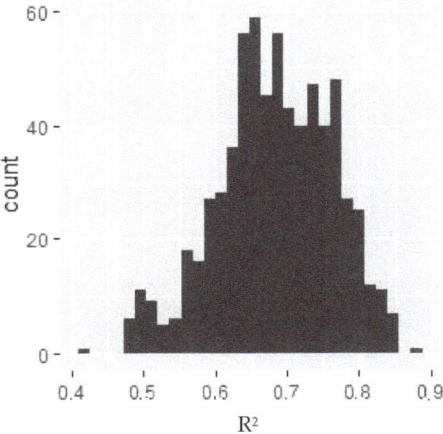

Figure 1. R^2 value histogram for models for VO2 max. Y-axis: the number of models where R^2 of the given value was obtained. The selected model includes the following variables: monocytes %, sodium, and total calcium. All of these parameters negatively affected the relative VO2 max (i.e., as their value increases, the relative VO2 max decreases).

4. Discussion

Studies have shown that athletes have their own inherent hematological and biochemical adaptations. It was also recorded that they are at a higher level compared to non-athletes in terms of physiological parameters [4]. This study investigated the differences in some hematological and biochemical parameters between amateurs, athletes, and non-athletes at rest. Consensus on the variability in hematological variables over time among athletes and non-athletes [5,6] or seasonal differences within the same squad [7] is lacking. This paper is, to our knowledge, the first providing information about amateur cross-country skiers.

A study by Baffour-Awuah et al. [8] showed differences between athletes and non-professional athletes. Comparing the results obtained in these studies, it can be noted that trained amateurs showed higher BMI parameters both compared to the training and non-training groups. According to Gallagher et al. [9], the body fat contents of the subjects were normal for age and gender, but comparing these results to athletes' standards [10] shows higher levels of body fat (15.51 ± 2.59 vs. 10.5 ± 1.8) [11]. This could indicate the possibility of developing diseases associated with the cardiovascular system and, for example, overweight. However, the parameters of the patients' lipid profile were correct. The body fat content should be related to a specific group that consists of amateur athletes. Exercise and regular training have a significant impact on lipid and lipoprotein levels in athletes. In fact, it has previously been documented that participation in sport has a positive effect on athletes compared to non-athletes with regard to lipid status markers [7].

The basic indicators defined in literature as significantly affecting the performance, such as the number of red blood cells, hemoglobin, and hematocrit were within the recommended standards, but were higher than in the study by Baffour-Awuah et al. This may be due to the selection of a group that only included men in this study. Studies in amateur cyclists [12] showed similar results of the red blood system at rest as in this study. Another study [13] suggested that some hematological values, such as the reticulocytes percentage (Ret%) and hemoglobin (Hb), were relatively stable over four consecutive seasons in elite triathletes, implying that in adults variability should be limited.

The results indicate that the immune system rates were lower than those recorded in the literature [7], but were normal. Their growth may indicate the body's response to intense effort, pro-inflammatory factors, as well as immunosuppression resulting from prolonged fatigue. Studies have shown that hematological variables in athletes and non-athletes are subject to different influences after session or training [14].

Higher sodium and potassium values have been shown than in the study by Baffour-Awuah et al. [8], which may be due to lower training activities or other factors such as diet or environmental conditions. The correct concentrations of sodium and potassium determine the proper nerve conductivity and muscle tension.

Monitoring these indicators during the transition period (the period after the starts and before the preparation period in the annual training cycle for skiers takes place in April) can give guidelines in the field of diet, training and health care.

4.1. Predictors for VO2 max

The selected model includes the following variables: monocytes %, sodium, and total calcium (see Table 5). All of these parameters negatively affected the relative VO2 value (max) (i.e., as their value increases, the relative VO2 level (max) decreases).

Table 5. Multivariate linear regression model parameters for r VO2 max, $R^2 = 0.879$.

Variable	Regression Coefficient	Statistical Error	t-Value	p-Value
Intercept	237.147	37.655	6.30	0.000
Monocytes %	−0.902	0.354	−2.55	0.031
Sodium (mmol/L)	−0.980	0.261	−3.76	0.004
Total Calcium (mmol/L)	−18.074	4.387	−4.12	0.03

4.1.1. Monocytes

Monocytes are one of the largest types of blood cells. They make up about 3–7% of leukocytes. They are capable of reducing infectious conditions, as well as red blood cells and other large particles. However, they cannot replace the function of neutrophils in removing and destroying bacteria. Monocytes usually enter areas of the inflammatory tissue later than granulocytes. They are often found at places of chronic infection. They are precursors of the mononuclear macrophage system. After 1–2 days, they pass into the tissues, where they differentiate into macrophages. In addition to the role of scavengers, macrophages play a key role in immunity, taking antigens and processing them so that they can be recognized by foreign lymphocytes as foreign substances. They also release compounds that regulate the inflammatory process and produce interleukins, interferons, and leukotrienes. An increase in the level of monocytes is observed, for example, in bacterial, viral, and parasitic infections, autoimmune diseases at an early stage, cancer, and after intense physical exertion [15]. The importance of changes in monocyte properties in the systemic anti-inflammatory effect of exercise remains undetermined. Monocytes represent a relatively small part of all leukocytes.

This applies, in particular, to resting values in amateur athletes. In people who exercise regularly with moderate intensity, monocytes are less reactive to exogenous stimuli. The expression of TLR4 receptors and the percentage of monocytes with "inflammatory" CD14+/CD16+ after exercise are reduced, and the number of CD14+/CD16 monocytes at rest are also reduced [12]. The increased values of these cells can be affected by the stress that accompanies amateur athletes in everyday life and the result of a lack of adaptation to exercise and low capacity. The release of cortisol (especially after exercise) and catecholamines (during exercise) can stimulate the production of immune cells (in the first line of neutrophils and natural killers cells). This effect is differentiated by lymphocytes and monocytes having receptors for specific endocrine proteins and hormones. The nature of activity and gender determine the magnitude of these changes. Interval and strength training, involving, for example, fast-twitch fibers, can strongly stimulate these systems to work. In men, increased testosterone levels simultaneously affect immune functions through the macrophage system, lymphocytes, and muscle cells with adrenergic receptors, which can affect resting values [16].

According to other hypotheses, the high intensity of training with insufficient resting time will activate monocytes to produce pro-inflammatory cytokines, including IL-6 (Interleukin-6) and TNF-α (Tumor necrosis factor alpha) [17]. Subsequently, this can cause fatigue and negative changes in the immune system. That condition is characteristic for the starting period. High-intensity physical efforts that significantly disrupt homeostasis will contribute to this. At the same time, it can be assumed that the lack of adaptation to exercise can contribute to increased secretion of monocytes. This may be the case during a transitional period.

The results of this study may therefore indicate a weaker mobilization of the immune system during the introduction of cross-country skiers to training. Furthermore, the results of the regression indicate that reducing their number to reference values will have a positive impact on increasing exercise capacity. Changes in the body may result from the introduction of regular physical training after the recovery period or from a previous infection that often occurs during the spring solstice period. This may also be due to the lack of proper recovery. Monocytes can persist for quite a long time in patients' blood after an infection. Most monocytes undergo apoptosis after 24 h. However, some of them may remain in the bloodstream. The half-life can then be up to 71 h [18]. This usually occurs when a patient in the course of the disease decreased the number of inert-absorbent granulocytes.

4.1.2. Sodium

Sodium is responsible for regulating the water content in intercellular spaces. When there is potassium deficiency in the body, the amount of sodium (hypernatremia) increases excessively and the body retains water. Then there are swellings of the body. It can cause hypertension and heart disease, muscle spasms, mood swings. In this study, the value was normal, but these results exceeded those reported in the literature [8]. A favorable shift in the sodium/potassium balance of the diet in the general population may have a substantial impact on hypertension related diseases, including stroke and myocardial infarction [19]. Physical effort leads to increased losses of this mineral from the body along with sweat, which can quickly lead to disruption of water and electrolyte balance, muscle spasms, weakness and reduction of efficiency. Despite this, intake of extra sodium dose is not recommended for athletes. Isotonic drinks maintain hydration and normal mineral levels before, during and after exercise. This is especially true for winter disciplines and marathon runners, as confirmed by the latest research [20,21].

Many intend to consciously increase sodium intake in the days preceding and during competition, although these views appear informed mostly by nonscientific and/or non-evidence-based sources [22].

Sodium is often consumed by athletes during ultramarathons with the belief that sodium losses must be replaced to enhance performance and to prevent EAH, muscle cramping, and dehydration. This study shows that only adequate levels of sodium and potassium will guarantee high exercise capacity. Securing the supply of isotonic drinks during effort is enough. Increasing the amount of sodium in the daily supply will negatively affect the body and exercise capacity.

4.1.3. Calcium

Calcium is needed for bone health, nerve conduction, and muscle excitation and contraction. It is a cofactor in glycogenolysis and works with vitamin K in blood coagulation and wound healing.

Although physical activity promotes bone density, athletes who already have low bone density and possibly longstanding suboptimal calcium intakes are likely to be at high risk of stress fractures when undertaking repetitive activities [23].

Previous studies confirmed the positive effect of calcium on muscle excitability, especially rapidly shrinking fibers. In this study, an increase in calcium levels results in lower exercise capabilities. Adverse effects of over-consumption include kidney disease, vascular calcification, increased risk of cardiovascular diseases, and impaired absorption of other minerals, such as magnesium, zinc, and iron [24]. Calcium also increases the incidence of heart spasms and an increase in its contractility, which increases blood pressure. The use of calcium channel blockers results in greater use of free fatty acids for the energy used in heart muscle contractions instead of glucose. This also translates into higher exercise potential [25]. However, the use of calcium channel inhibitors is prohibited in sports and included in the WADA (World Anti-Doping Agency) World List of Prohibited Substances [26]. Due to increased heart function (with an increase in heart rate and blood pressure), as well as the contraction of coronary vessels and coronary congestion, ischemia and myocardial infarctions may occur. The problem is compounded by too much activity and lack of adaptation to it. This underlines the role of regular and fitted training in amateur athletes (e.g., cross-country skiers) and people at risk of early heart attack [27].

Maintaining homeostasis is crucial. However, it is important to cause damage in the training process. The damage enables adaptation to occur. The supercompensation process is based on the capacity of chronic exercise to induce beneficial adaptive changes. However, it must be properly monitored so as not to lead to overtraining. Physical activity can induce beneficial adaptive changes, constitute a therapeutic tool in cardiovascular diseases, and cause antioxidant and anti-senescent effects in human cells [28].

5. Conclusions

The aim of this study was to identify determinants of the cardiovascular capacity of amateur long-distance skiers during the transition period. Three main predictors have been appointed for maximum oxygen uptake in this group. An increase in the percentage of monocytes, as well as changes in the concentration of sodium and calcium, can impair exercise capabilities in subjects and negatively affect their health. Monitoring these indicators can help to protect the health of amateur athletes and provide guidelines in the training process. This problem is described in detail in the case of professional athletes, but has not yet been studied among amateur athletes. Changes in hematological and biochemical parameters at rest need not be solely related to sports, indicating the need for similar research and special protection for men competing in ultramarathons and ski marathons. Biochemical and physiological monitoring of amateur athletes can help to protect their health and prepare them properly to the effort required to compete in their sport. The growing popularity of long-distance competitions among middle-aged amateur athletes and the lack of guidance on how to assess their health indicate the need for such research. Due to the relatively small sample size in this study, further research could focus on monitoring and assessing changes in other parts of the annual training cycle and in a larger group of athletes, including women.

Funding: The study received financial support by the Ministry of Science and Higher Education (grant No. 71/E-716/S2018) the entity subsidy to maintain the research potential (base subsidy) in 2018 for Vistula School of Hospitality, Vistula Group of Universities in Warsaw.

Conflicts of Interest: The author declares no conflict of interest.

References

1. Sandbakk, Ø.; Holmberg, H.C. Physiological Capacity and Training Routines of Elite Cross-Country Skiers: Approaching the Upper Limits of Human Endurance. *Int. J. Sports Physiol. Perform.* **2017**, *12*, 1003–1011. [CrossRef]
2. Carlsson, M.; Assarsson, H.; Carlsson, T. The influence of sex, age, and race experience on pacing profiles during the 90 km Vasaloppet ski race. *J. Sports Med.* **2016**, *7*, 11–19. [CrossRef] [PubMed]
3. Skattebo, Ø.; Losnegard, T.; Stadheim, H.K. Double-Poling Physiology and Kinematics of Elite Cross-Country Skiers: Specialized Long-Distance Versus All-Round Skiers. *Int. J. Sports Physiol. Perform.* **2019**, *14*, 1190–1199. [CrossRef] [PubMed]
4. Grzebisz, N. Cardiovascular Adaptations to Four Months Training in Middle-Aged Amateur Long-Distance Skiers. *Diagnostics* **2020**, *10*, 442. [CrossRef] [PubMed]
5. Joksimovic, A.; Stankovic, D.; Ilic, D.; Joksimovic, I.; Jerkan, M. Hematological Profile of Serbian Youth National Soccer Teams. *J. Hum. Kinet.* **2009**, *22*, 51–60. [CrossRef]
6. Nikolaidis, M.; Protosygellou, M.; Petridou, A.; Tsalis, G.; Tsigilis, N.; Mougios, V. Hematologic and biochemical profile of juvenile and adult athletes of both sexes: Implications for clinical evaluation. *Int. J. Sports Med.* **2003**, *24*, 506–511.
7. Manna, I.; Khanna, G.; Chandra Dhara, P. Effect of training on physiological and biochemical variables of soccer players of different age groups. *Asian J. Sports Med.* **2010**, *1*, 5–22. [CrossRef]
8. Baffour-Awuah, B.; Addai-Mensah, O.; Moses, M.; Mensah, W.; Ibekwe, B.; Essaw, E.; Acheampong, I. Differences in Haematological and Biochemical Parameters of Athletes and Non-Athletes. *JAMMR* **2017**, *24*, 1–5. [CrossRef]
9. Gallagher, D.; Heymsfield, S.; Heo, M.; Jebb, S.; Murgatroyd, P.; Sakamoto, Y. Healthy percentage body fat ranges: An approach for developing guidelines based on body mass index. *Am. J. Clin. Nutr.* **2000**, *72*, 694–701. [CrossRef]
10. Grzebisz, N.; Piejko, L.; Sulich, A. Determinants of cardiorespiratory fitness in amateur male cross-country skiers. *Russ. J. Cardiol.* **2019**, *12*, 109–113. [CrossRef]
11. Undebakke, V.; Berg, J.; Tjønna, A.E.; Sandbakk, Ø. Comparison of Physiological and Perceptual Responses to Upper-, Lower-, and Whole-Body Exercise in Elite Cross-Country Skiers. *J. Strength Cond. Res.* **2019**, *33*, 1086–1094. [CrossRef] [PubMed]
12. Silva, R.A.S.; Sampaio, N.L.F.; Cruz, C.J.G.; Vianna, B.; Pires, F.O. Haematological Responses on Amateur Cycling Stages Race. In Proceedings of the ICCSS 2018: International Conference on Cycle and Sports Science, Sydney, Australia, 29–30 January 2018.
13. Diaz, E.; Ruiz, F.; Hoyos, I.; Zubero, J.; Gravina, L.; Gil, J.; Irazusta, J.; Gil, S.M. Cell damage, antioxidant status, and cortisol levels related to nutrition in ski mountaineering during a two-day race. *J. Sports Sci. Med.* **2010**, *9*, 338–346.
14. Tayebi, S.; Ghanbari-Niaki, A. Effects of a low intensity circuit resistance exercise session on some hematological parameters of male collage students. *Ann. Appl. Sport Sci.* **2013**, *1*, 6–11.
15. Kurowski, M.; Kowalski, M. Wpływ wysiłku fizycznego na odpowiedź immunologiczną–wybrane zagadnienia. *Alerg. Astma Immunol.* **2014**, *19*, 144–149.
16. Gleeson, M.; Bishop, N.; Oliveira, M.; Tauler, P. Influence of training load on upper respiratory tract infection incidence and antigen-stimulated cytokine production. *Scand. J. Med. Sci. Sports* **2013**, *23*, 451–457. [CrossRef] [PubMed]
17. Smith, L.L. Cytokine hypothesis of overtraining: A physiological adaptation to excessive stress? *Med. Sci. Sports Exerc.* **2000**, *32*, 317–331. [CrossRef] [PubMed]
18. Delves, P.; Roitt, I.M. *Encyclopedia of Immunology*, 2nd ed.; Academic Press: Michigan University, Ann Arbor, MI, USA, 1998; pp. 1793–1802.
19. Geleijnse, J.; Kok, F.; Grobbee, D. Blood pressure response to changes in sodium and potassium intake: A metaregression analysis of randomised trials. *J. Hum. Hypertens.* **2003**, *17*, 471–480. [CrossRef] [PubMed]
20. Chlíbková, D.; Nikolaidis, P.; Rosemann, T.; Knechtle, B.; Bednář, J. Fluid Metabolism in Athletes Running Seven Marathons in Seven Consecutive Days. *Front. Physiol.* **2018**, *9*, 91. [CrossRef] [PubMed]
21. Baker, L. Sweating Rate and Sweat Sodium Concentration in Athletes: A Review of Methodology and Intra/Interindividual Variability. *Sports Med.* **2017**, *47*, 111–128. [CrossRef] [PubMed]

22. McCubbin, A.; Cox, G.R.; Costa, R. Sodium Intake Beliefs, Information Sources, and Intended Practices of Endurance Athletes Before and During Exercise. *Int. J. Sport Nutr. Exerc. Metab.* **2019**, *29*, 371–381. [CrossRef] [PubMed]
23. Wentz, L.; Liu, P.; Ilich, J.; Haymes, E. Dietary and training predictors of stress fractures in female runners. *Int. J. Sport Nutr. Exerc. Metab.* **2012**, *22*, 374–382. [CrossRef] [PubMed]
24. Moe, S. Disorders involving calcium, phosphorus, and magnesium. *Prim. Care* **2008**, *35*, 215–237. [CrossRef] [PubMed]
25. Ulimoen, S.; Enger, S.; Pripp, A.; Abdelnoor, M.; Arnesen, H.; Gjesdal, K.; Tveit, A. Calcium channel blockers improve exercise capacity and reduce N-terminal Pro-B-type natriuretic peptide levels compared with beta-blockers in patients with permanent atrial fibrillation. *Eur. Heart J.* **2014**, *35*, 517–524. [CrossRef] [PubMed]
26. Heuberger, J.; Cohen, A. Review of WADA Prohibited Substances: Limited Evidence for Performance-Enhancing Effects. *Sports Med.* **2019**, *49*, 525–539. [CrossRef]
27. Boisseau, N. Fat mass reduction and weight loss: Strategies and potential risk in Olympic athletes. In Proceedings of the Sport Nutrition Conference, INSEP, Paris, France, 7 May 2011.
28. Russomanno, G.; Corbi, G.; Manzo, V.; Ferrara, N.; Rengo, G.; Puca, A.A.; Latte, S.; Carrizzo, A.; Calabrese, M.C.; Andriantsitohaina, R.; et al. The anti-ageing molecule sirt1 mediates beneficial effects of cardiac rehabilitation. *Immun. Ageing* **2017**, *14*, 7. [CrossRef]

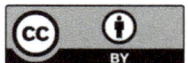

© 2020 by the author. Licensee MDPI, Basel, Switzerland. This article is an open access article distributed under the terms and conditions of the Creative Commons Attribution (CC BY) license (http://creativecommons.org/licenses/by/4.0/).

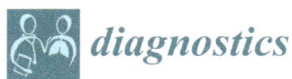 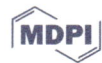

Article

A Pilot Study of the Reliability and Agreement of Heart Rate, Respiratory Rate and Short-Term Heart Rate Variability in Elite Modern Pentathlon Athletes

Bartosz Hoffmann [1], Andrew A. Flatt [2], Luiz Eduardo Virgilio Silva [3], Marcel Młyńczak [4], Rafał Baranowski [5], Ewelina Dziedzic [6], Bożena Werner [7] and Jakub S. Gąsior [7,*]

1. Physiotherapy Division, Faculty of Medical Sciences, Medical University of Warsaw, 02-091 Warsaw, Poland; bartosz.hoffmann@icloud.com
2. Biodynamics and Human Performance Center, Department of Health Sciences and Kinesiology, Georgia Southern University (Armstrong Campus), Savannah, GA 31419, USA; aflatt@georgiasouthern.edu
3. Department of Internal Medicine of Ribeirão Preto Medical School, University of São Paulo, Ribeirão Preto 14049-900, SP, Brazil; luizeduardo@usp.br
4. Faculty of Mechatronics, Institute of Metrology and Biomedical Engineering, Warsaw University of Technology, 02-525 Warsaw, Poland; marcel.mlynczak@pw.edu.pl
5. Department of Heart Rhythm Disorders, National Institute of Cardiology, 04-628 Warsaw, Poland; rb@ikard.pl
6. Medical Faculty, Lazarski University in Warsaw, 02-662 Warsaw, Poland; ewelinadziedzic82@gmail.com
7. Department of Pediatric Cardiology and General Pediatrics, Medical University of Warsaw, 02-091 Warsaw, Poland; bozena.werner@wum.edu.pl
* Correspondence: jgasior@wum.edu.pl or gasiorjakub@gmail.com; Tel.: +48-793-199-222

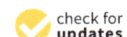

Received: 28 September 2020; Accepted: 14 October 2020; Published: 16 October 2020

Abstract: Research on reliability of heart rate variability (HRV) parameters in athletes has received increasing attention. The aims of this study were to examine the inter-day reliability of short-term (5 min) and ultra-short-term (1 min) heart rate (HR), respiratory rate (RespRate) and HRV parameters, agreement between short-term and ultra-short-term parameters, and association between differences in HR, RespRate and HRV parameters in elite modern pentathletes. Electrocardiographic recordings were performed in stable measurement conditions with a week interval between tests. Relative reliability was evaluated by intra-class correlation coefficients, absolute reliability was evaluated by within-subject coefficient of variation, and agreement was evaluated using Bland–Altman (BA) plot with limits of agreement and defined a priori maximum acceptable difference. Short-term HR, RespRate, log transformed (ln) root mean square of successive normal-to-normal interval differences (lnRMSSD), ln high frequency (lnHF) and SD2/SD1 HRV indices and ultra-short-term HR, RespRate and lnRMSSD presented acceptable, satisfactory inter-day reliability. Although there were no significant differences between short-term and ultra-short-term HR, RespRate and lnRMSSD, no parameter showed acceptable differences with BA plots. Differences in time-domain and non-linear HRV parameters were more correlated with differences in HR than with differences in RespRate. Inverse results were observed for frequency-domain parameters. Short-term HR, RespRate, lnRMSSD, lnHF, and SD2/SD1 and ultra-short-term HR, RespRate and lnRMSSD could be used as reliable parameters in endurance athletes. However, practitioners should interpret changes in HRV parameters with regard to concomitant differences in HR and RespRate and caution should be taken before considering 5 min and 1 min parameters as interchangeable.

Keywords: heart rate; respiratory rate; heart rate variability; reliability; repeatability; modern penthatlon; athletes

1. Introduction

Comprehensive monitoring of fitness and performance as well as accurate diagnosis of fatigue, non-functional overreaching, and overtraining states are crucial for optimizing training and reducing risk of injury in elite professional sport [1–6]. In this regard, sensitive, non-invasive, time-efficient and cost-effective testing methods and biomarkers encompassing a multidimensional approach are being sought by coaches, exercise scientists and sports physicians to improve the evaluation of athletes [4,7–9].

Over the past decade, parameters associated with autonomic nervous system (ANS) regulation such as heart rate (HR) and heart rate variability (HRV), measures assessed during the post-exercise recovery period, have received increasing interest for monitoring training status and cardiovascular fitness [2,4–6,10–25]. Nevertheless, contradictory findings related to methodological inconsistencies and partial misinterpretation of the results limit the widespread implementation of HR and HRV measures in the sports field [4,18,20].

From the perspective of coaches and sports professionals, it is important to evaluate training status in as many athletes as possible relatively quickly and frequently to distinguish intended (e.g., due to training) from unintended (measurement error) changes using reliable measurements and validated tools. This will ensure reproducible results and enable meaningful findings [26,27]. Parameters (or tools) are rated as useful or sensitive based on providing high reliability and low test–retest variation [4].

Previous studies on reliability of HRV measures in athletes focused mainly on looking for an ultra-shortened reliable user-friendly HRV parameter [22,25,28–34]. It was suggested that the root mean square of successive differences between adjacent normal RR intervals (RMSSD), or its log transformed version (lnRMSSD), calculated based on 60 sec recordings is reliable [30] and displays strong agreement with RMSSD criterion derived from 5 min recordings [28,31,32]. Moreover, RMSSD is suggested to be the most appropriate and attractive parameter for use in elite endurance and team sports athletes [2,15,18,22,28,30,31].

Apart from the cardiac measurements, the basic parameter reflecting respiration (another part of the cardiorespiratory fitness) is respiratory rate. The assessment of its reliability and agreement can also be considered relevant, as some moderate causal effects might also influence the measurements of cardiac parameters.

A less-studied group of endurance athletes are elite modern pentathletes. The modern pentathlon is an Olympic sport that consists of five different modalities (fencing, freestyle swimming, equestrian show jumping, and a combination of pistol shooting and cross-country running). Events last up to 8 h in duration, making energy and physiological demands close to maximal [35–38]. To date, there are few studies addressing modern pentathlon athletes [35–41] and we have found no data within the literature on the reliability of HRV in this population. Establishing the typical variation in HRV among this population is necessary to aid coaches in detecting meaningful changes related to pentathletes' training status.

Despite the large number of methodological papers published on HRV [42–51], many studies in this area failed to provide the necessary details concerning data acquisition and measurements, so the experimental design could not be replicated in laboratories, clinical settings and sports field. The lack of details concerning methodological aspects of the study significantly limits confidence in interpretation [52,53]. A recent paper on HRV reliability stated that still little is known about the reliability of baseline 5 min (short-term) measurements of HRV and studies continue to differ with respect to important methodological characteristics [54]. Therefore, the presented study has the following aims: (i) to assess the inter-day reliability of short-term (5 min) HR, respiratory rate and selected time-domain, frequency-domain, and non-linear HRV parameters; (ii) to assess the inter-day reliability of ultra-short-term (1 min) HR, respiratory rate and RMSSD (popular in sports field); (iii) to determine the agreement between short-term (5 min) and ultra-short-term (1 min) parameters, and (iv) to verify the correlations between differences in HR, respiratory rate and HRV parameters in stable conditions in elite modern pentathletes.

2. Materials and Methods

2.1. Participants

A total of 12 elite modern Caucasian pentathletes (8♂) living in Warsaw (Poland), aged 17–26 years, with professional careers ranging from 7 to 15 years, participated in the study. The study group included medalists of the World Championships ($n = 6$) and European Championships ($n = 8$). Inclusion criteria were: being an active athlete [55] currently in possession of the modern pentathlon license from the National Association; being in the pre-season period; acceptance and compliance with the measurement rules (details in Measurement protocol); absence of diseases and/or regular use of medications affecting the cardiopulmonary system and/or interfering with the ANS. The study was approved by the University Ethical Committee (SKE 01-01/2017, 7 March 2017, Warsaw, Poland) and followed the rules and principles of the Helsinki Declaration. All athletes were informed of the aims and risks involved with the protocol and subsequently provided written informed consent prior to data collection.

2.2. Measurement Protocol

Body mass status was measured using Body Mass Index (BMI) defined as body mass (kilograms) divided by the squared height (meters). A questionnaire that supports the collection and control of many confounding variables influencing HRV proposed by Laborde et al. [56] was used. The athletes were informed in detail about the objectives of the study and measurement protocol by telephone conversations 3 months before and 2 weeks before the measurements, and also by e-mail with instructions and study procedures. Briefly, participants were instructed to sleep normally (as usual in the 5 days before examination), refrain from physical activity the day before and on the day of study, eat a light breakfast, and use the toilet (if needed) on the day of study before examinations. The examinations were carried out at least 1 h after home breakfast and before lunch. Each athlete underwent two electrocardiography recordings (ECGs) with 7 day intervals between measurements. Athletes declared participation in one training per day (typical for the pre-season period) within the days between examinations. The first examination was denoted as "Test", and the second one was denoted as "Retest." Both the Test and Retest recordings were performed under the same conditions, i.e., in a quiet, bright university room, with stable temperature and humidity adjusted by the group of researchers (BH, JSG, AK).

2.3. Electrocardiography (ECG) Acquisition

Twelve-lead, 6-min ECGs were performed in a supine position between 8:00 AM to 12:00 PM. All ECGs (sampling frequency = 1000 Hz) were performed using a portable PC with an integrated software system (Custo cardio 100 12-channel PC ECG system; Custo med GmbH, Ottobrunn, Germany). The athletes were cabled by a same-sex researcher [54]. On both study days, in order to stabilize HR and respiratory rate, the participants were asked to lie in the supine position for 10 min [57] before the beginning of the appropriate ECGs (used to calculate HRV parameters). Athletes were encouraged to refrain from speaking and moving during the ECG examination. All ECGs were assessed by an experienced cardiologist (RB). Recordings of ECGs and respiratory rate were started at the same time.

2.4. Respiratory Rate

The athletes were not instructed how to breath during examinations (spontaneous breathing) to increase the applicability of the results in the sports field [11] but were informed that the breathing pattern would be video-recoded. Respiratory rate (RespRate) was monitored using the Sony® HDRAS20 Action Camera with Wi-Fi. A picture from one video capture can be seen in Figure 1. Only the abdomen, thorax and neck were recorded. RespRate was determined from the counted number of respiratory cycles. The beginning of each respiratory cycle was defined as the end of the inspiratory phase when the diaphragm was at the apex. Calculation of the RespRate based on 5 min and 1 min video recordings (first minute of the 5 min recording) was independently performed by two researchers (BH, JSG). The disagreements between them were resolved through discussion.

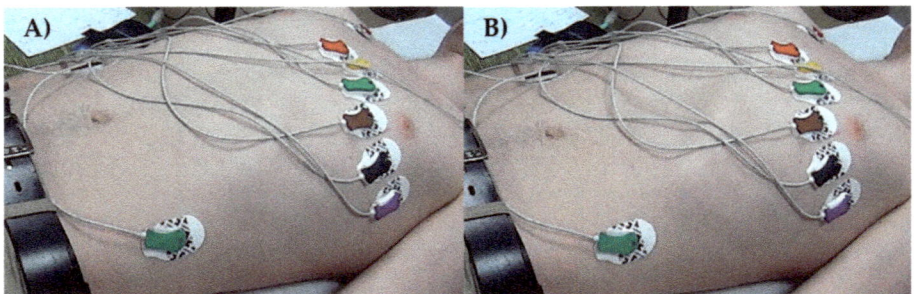

Figure 1. Picture from one of the videos, showing the athlete lying down: (**A**) end of inspiratory phase, (**B**) end of expiratory phase.

2.5. HRV Analysis

The ECGs were visually inspected for potential non-sinus or aberrant beats and such erroneous beats were corrected from the cardiac interval series (RR series) before HRV analysis. The erroneous beats were manually corrected, i.e., one R-R interval before and one after each non-sinus beat were eliminated and replaced by R-R intervals computed by interpolation of degree zero based on the surrounding normal beats [58]. HR and HRV parameters were calculated based on appropriate ECGs (recordings started after stabilization period): (a) 5 min—criterion period (short-term parameters), and (b) 1 min ECGs (first minute of the 5 min recording—ultra-short-term parameters) using Kubios HRV Standard 3.4 software (University of Eastern Finland, Kuopio, Finland) [59,60].

Short-term time-domain, frequency-domain and nonlinear HRV parameters were calculated based on 5 min ECGs. Standard deviation of normal-to-normal RR intervals (SDNN), RMSSD, the log transformed RMSSD (lnRMSSD), log transformation of ratio between RMSSD (in ms) and mean RR interval (mRR, in ms), i.e., lnRMSSD/mRR and pNN50, which denotes the percent of RR intervals differing >50 ms from the preceding one, were determined. The following, popular in sport science, ultra-short-term parameters were calculated and analyzed based on 1 min ECGs: HR, RMSSD, (lnRMSSD) and lnRMSSD/mRR [2,15,18,21,22,28,30,31].

The usefulness of the frequency-domain HRV parameters for monitoring athletes in practice has been questioned. Some authors indicated several limitations of these parameters: (i) sensitivity to alterations in breathing rate and thus lower reliability [17]; (ii) analysis requires technical knowledge for interpretation; (iii) appropriate time needed for calculation may not be a suitable for analyzing athletes in a time-constrained setting [32]. Nevertheless, we decided to include the reliability assessment of the frequency-domain short-term (5 min) in the set of HRV parameters evaluated in this study. The recordings were obtained in stable conditions so that our findings could be considered as reference and prerequisites for future studies performed in the sports field.

Before calculating spectral HRV parameters, smoothness priors based on the detrending approach was applied (smoothing parameter, Lambda value = 500) [61], and then RR interval series were transformed to an evenly sampled time series using a cubic spline interpolation followed by 4-Hz resampling. The detrended and interpolated RR interval series were used to compute HRV spectra by employing a fast-Fourier transform (FFT) with Welch's periodogram method (300 s window width without overlap for 5 min ECGs). This definition ensures that the HRV spectral parameters were estimated from a single window, containing the whole 5 min period of recording. The range for respiratory rate was between 9 and 19 breaths/min in all subjects. Thus, the following bands for spectral components were securely distinguished: low-frequency (LF, 0.04–0.15 Hz) and high-frequency

(HF, 0.15–0.40 Hz). The power at both bands were estimated in absolute (ms^2) and normalized units (nu) [42]. Natural log transformed (ln) absolute powers in the LF (lnLF) and HF (lnHF) bands, the LF/HF ratio, and the powers in normalized units (nLF and nHF) were used for further analysis. From nonlinear HRV parameters, the ratio of Poincaré plot standard deviation along the line of identity to the standard deviation perpendicular to the line of identity (SD2/SD1), approximate entropy (ApEn), sample entropy (SampEn) and short-term fluctuations of detrended fluctuation analysis (DFAα1) were analyzed. Notice that HRV spectral and nonlinear parameters were obtained only for short-term (5 min) recordings.

2.6. Relationships between Differences in HR and RespRate and Differences in HRV Parameters

Most HRV studies have not accounted for the significant correlation between HRV parameters and mean HR [45,62–64]. This is an important consideration for sport practitioners and scientists using HRV to assess training status in athletes who typically present low resting HR [65,66]. Reduction in HRV, indicating, e.g., ANS stress, should be interpreted by taking into account respective changes in resting HR [67,68]. In addition to HR, we also assessed the correlation between differences in RespRate and differences in HRV.

2.7. Statistical Analysis

The Kolmogorov–Smirnov test was used to assess the normality of the data distribution. Natural log transformation (ln) was used if the data were not normally distributed. A paired Student's *t*-test was employed to compare systematic changes between Test and Retest in analyzed parameters. Pearson's correlation coefficient (r) was calculated to illustrate the relationship among differences (values from Retest—values from Test) in HR (HR-diff), RespRate (RespRate-diff) and HRV parameters. Due to the low sample size, the figures with correlations are more useful as illustrative than as analytic. The threshold probability of $p < 0.05$ was taken as the level of significance for all statistical tests. All calculations were performed using the STATISTICA 12 (StatSoft Inc., Tulsa, OK, USA) and MedCalc software version 19.4.1 (MedCalc Software, Ostend, Belgium). The Bland–Altman plots were created using MedCalc software version 19.4.1 (MedCalc Software, Ostend, Belgium). GraphPad Prism 5 (GraphPad Software Inc., San Diego, CA, USA, 2005) was used to create correlation plots.

2.7.1. Reliability Statistics

Inter-day reliability of all parameters was calculated using the intraclass correlation coefficient (ICC), the within-subject coefficient of variation (WSCV) and Cohen's d. The relative reliability of HR, RespRate and HRV parameters was analyzed using the ICC [69]. A priori, an ICC value between 0 to 0.30 was considered small, 0.31 to 0.49 moderate, 0.50 to 0.69 large, 0.70 to 0.89 very large, and 0.90 to 1.00 nearly perfect [70]. The absolute reliability was analyzed using typical error of measurement (WSCV) [71–74]. The WSCV less than 10% was considered highly reliable. Cohen's d was utilized to determine the effect size of the mean differences between Test and Retest [75] with thresholds considered a priori as trivial (<0.2), small (0.2–0.6), moderate (0.6–1.2), large (1.2–2.0) or very large (>2.0) [70]. In general, the combination of a trivial or small Cohen's d, ICC > 0.85 and WSCV < 10% was considered as acceptable, with satisfactory reliability.

2.7.2. Agreement Statistics

Agreement between short-term (5 min) and ultra-short-term (1 min) HR, RespRate and HRV parameters (from Test and Retest separately) was verified using a Bland–Altman plot with limits of agreement (LoA) [76–80] and ICC [81] with interpretation proposed by Hopkins et al. [70]. The smallest worthwhile change (SWC, calculated using formula 0.2 × Test-values standard deviation) [82] was used to define the maximum allowed difference between methods presented in Bland–Altman plots. Two methods are considered in agreement if the LoA do not exceed the maximum allowed difference between methods (SWC).

3. Results

3.1. Participants

Results of four participants (out of 12) were excluded from the analysis due to the detection of cardiac abnormalities in the recorded ECG (prolonged QTc interval > 450 ms, n = 2; left bundle branch block, n = 2). Consequently, results of 8 male athletes were included in the statistical analysis. The mean (± SD) age, weight, height, BMI and duration of professional athletic career were: 21.7 years (±3.1), 75.9 kg (±9.5), 182.6 cm (±6.1), 22.7 kg/m^2 (±2.3) and 10.8 years (±2.9). Athletes declared participating in 19 training sessions (±2) per week during the normal in-season time.

3.2. Reliability of Short-Term (5 min) HR, RespRate and HRV Parameters

Table 1 presents the results of reliability statistics for short-term (5 min) HR, RespRate and HRV parameters. There were no significant differences in all analyzed parameters between Test and Retest (p-values between 0.25 and 0.94). Relative and absolute reliability of HR, RespRate, and all time-domain HRV parameters (with one exception, pNN50) were considered nearly perfect (ICC between 0.96 and 0.99) and high (WSCV% between 1.4 and 7.5), respectively, with trivial effect size (Cohen's d between −0.18 and 0.15). Effect size for frequency-domain parameters were trivial (nLF, lnHF, nHF, LF/HF) or small (lnLF). lnLF presented large, nLF, lnHF, nHF very large, and LF/HF nearly perfect relative reliability (ICC between 0.66 and 0.93). Absolute reliability was considered low for all frequency domain parameters (WSCV% between 10.4 and 55.2) except for lnHF, which presented high absolute reliability (WSCV% = 6.1). The nonlinear parameters presented large (ApEn and SampEn: ICC = 0.63 and 0.67), very large (DFAα1 and SD2/SD1: ICC = 0.77 and 0.87) relative reliability and high (SD2/SD1, ApEn and SampEn: WSCV% = 8.9, 6.1 and 9.1) or low (DFAα1, WSCV% = 17.2) absolute reliability with small (ApEn, DFAα1) and trivial (SD2/SD1 and SampEn) effect size.

3.3. Reliability of Ultra-Short-Term (1 min) HR, RespRate, RMSSD, lnRMSSD and lnRMSSD/mRR

Table 2 presents results of reliability statistics for ultra-short-term (1 min) HR, RespRate and RMSSD indexes. There were no significant differences in all analyzed parameters between Test and Retest (p-value between 0.18 and 0.80). HR and RespRate presented very large or nearly perfect relative reliability and high absolute reliability with trivial effect size. Relative and absolute reliability of lnRMMSD and lnRMSSD/mRR were considered very large and high, respectively, with a small effect size.

3.4. Agreement between Short-Term and Ultra-Short-Term Parameters

Table 3 and Figures 2 and 3 present results of agreement between short-term (5 min) and ultra-short-term (1 min) HR, RespRate and selected HRV parameters from Test and Retest independently. There were no significant differences between short-term (5 min) and ultra-short-term (1 min) parameters in both Test and Retest. HR and RespRate presented nearly perfect agreement (ICC > 0.9) in Test and Retest with a trivial effect size. Small or trivial effect sizes of the mean difference between 5 min and 1 min parameters were observed for all measured time-domain indices in Test and Retest. RMSSD, lnRMSSD and lnRMSSD/mRR presented very large and nearly perfect agreement (ICC > 0.7) in Test and Retest. The Bland–Altman plots are shown in Figure 2 (HR and RespRate) and Figure 3 (RMSSD, lnRMSSD and lnRMSSD/mRR), representing the agreement between the 1 min and 5 min parameters in both Test (column A) and Retest (column B) periods. The LoA are defined as the mean difference ± 1.96 SD of differences. The 95% confidence intervals for upper and lower LoA are presented in Table 3. In all analyzed parameters, in both Test and Retest, LoA exceeded the defined maximum acceptable difference.

3.5. Correlation between Differences in HR or RespRate and Differences in HRV Parameters

The correlations for Retest–Test differences between HRV parameters and HR (column A) or RespRate (column B) are shown in Figure 4 (time-domain short-term parameters), Figure 5 (frequency-domain short-term parameters), Figure 6 (nonlinear short-term parameters) and Figure 7 (ultra-short-term parameters). For short-term (5 min) time-domain and nonlinear HRV parameters, the Retest–Test differences are more correlated to the differences in HR (HR-diff) than to the differences in RespRate (RespRate-diff). Inversely, for short-term (5 min) frequency-domain HRV parameters (except for LF/HF), the Retest–Test differences are more correlated with the RespRate-diff than the HR-diff. Significant correlations were observed for the association between HR-diff and lnRMSSD-diff ($r = -0.86$, $p < 0.01$) and between RespRate-diff and lnHF-diff ($r = 0.80$, $p < 0.05$). For ultra-short-term (1 min) HRV parameters, the Retest–Test differences are more correlated (higher r) with HR-diff than with RespRate-diff.

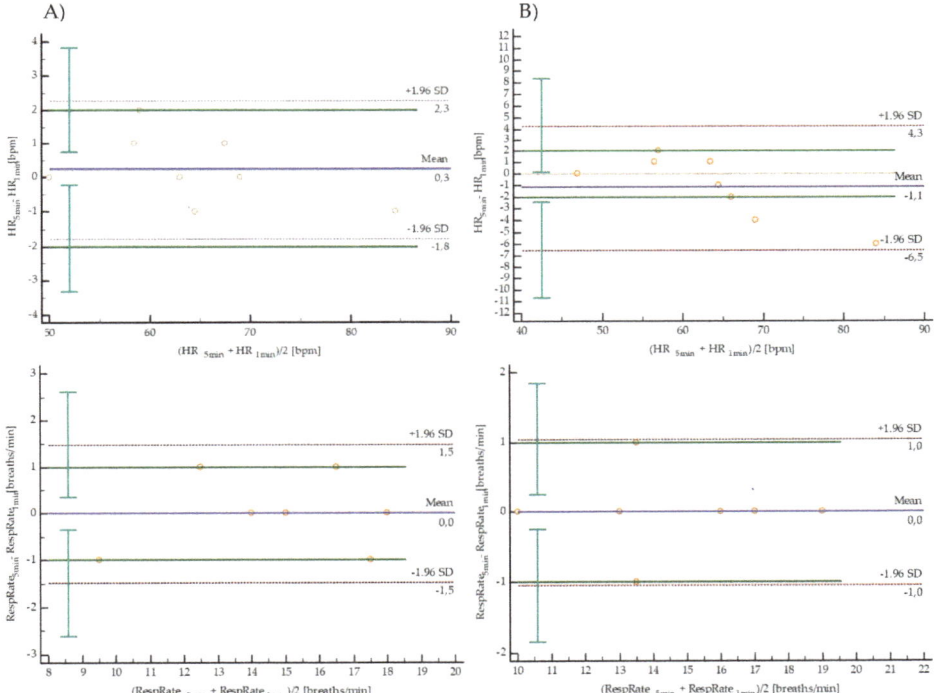

Figure 2. Bland–Altman plots representing the agreement between the 1 min and 5 min in HR and RespRate in both Test (column **A**) and Retest (column **B**) periods. The solid blue line indicates the bias, dotted red lines are the 95% LoA (±1.96 SD), vertical lines are confidence interval LoA limits, solid green lines are a priori defined maximum allowed difference.

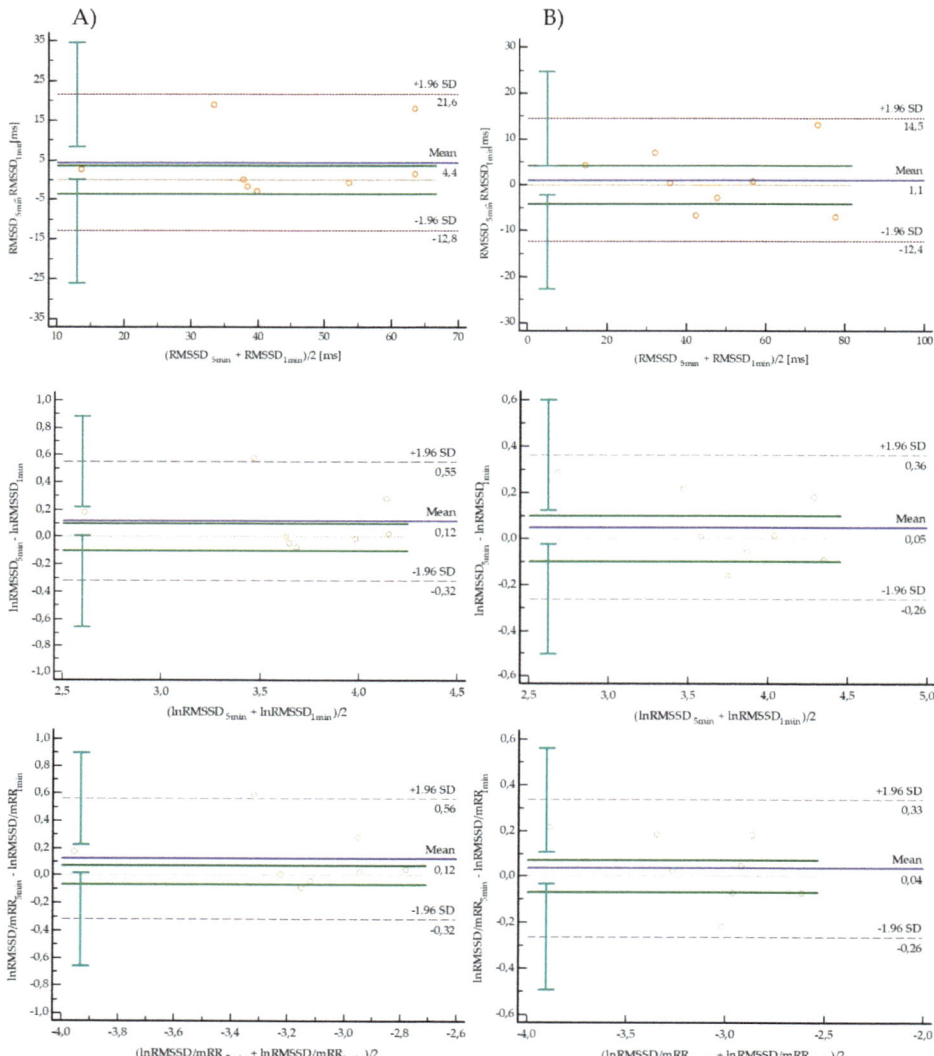

Figure 3. Bland–Altman plots representing the agreement between the 1 min and 5 min in selected HRV parameters in both Test (column **A**) and Retest (column **B**) periods. The solid blue line indicates the bias, dotted red lines are the 95% LoA (±1.96 SD), vertical lines are confidence interval LoA limits, solid green lines are a priori defined maximum allowed difference.

Table 1. Reliability results for HR, RespRate and selected short-term 5 min HRV parameters.

	Test Mean ± SD	Retest Mean ± SD	p	Cohen's d (95% CI)	ICC (95% CI)	WSCV% (95% CI)
HR [bpm]	64.6 ± 9.8	62.9 ± 9.7	0.73	−0.18 (−0.35–−0.04)	0.97 (0.71–0.99)	2.8 (1.2–4.6)
RespRate [breaths/min]	15 ± 3	15 ± 3	0.94	0.04 (−0.18–0.33)	0.96 (0.84–0.99)	3.4 (1.4–5.4)
SDNN [ms]	43.3 ± 16.6	45.9 ± 20.0	0.78	0.14 (−0.11–0.36)	0.96 (0.81–0.99)	7.5 (3.0–12.2)
RMSSD [ms]	45.2 ± 17.9	48.2 ± 21.1	0.76	0.15 (0.01–0.33)	0.97 (0.81–0.99)	6.7 (2.7–10.9)
lnRMSSD	3.72 ± 0.48	3.78 ± 0.49	0.83	0.11 (−0.05–0.25)	0.98 (0.89–0.99)	1.8 (0.7–2.9)
lnRMSSD/mRR	−3.12 ± 0.35	−3.09 ± 0.35	0.88	0.08 (−0.08–0.20)	0.99 (0.94–1.00)	1.4 (0.6–2.2)
pNN50	21.9 ± 16.6	32.1 ± 17.3	0.25	0.60 (−0.03–1.37)	0.61 (−0.02–0.90)	152.4 (46.0–336.2)
lnLF	6.22 ± 1.05	6.51 ± 1.11	0.60	0.27 (−0.50–1.24)	0.66 (0.03–0.92)	10.4 (4.1–17.1)
nLF [nu]	44.8 ± 20.4	48.0 ± 21.7	0.77	0.15 (−0.21–0.95)	0.78 (0.23–0.95)	31.2 (11.8–54.1)
lnHF	6.43 ± 0.94	6.60 ± 1.02	0.74	0.17 (−0.27–0.86)	0.86 (0.47–0.97)	6.1 (2.4–9.8)
nHF [nu]	55.2 ± 20.3	52.0 ± 21.7	0.77	−0.15 (−0.95–−0.21)	0.78 (0.23–0.95)	18.9 (7.4–31.8)
LF/HF	1.17 ± 1.17	1.35 ± 1.28	0.78	0.15 (−0.10–0.89)	0.93 (0.71–0.98)	55.2 (19.7–101.3)
SD2/SD1	1.69 ± 0.37	1.66 ± 0.42	0.89	−0.07 (−0.55–−0.37)	0.87 (0.48–0.97)	8.9 (3.5–14.5)
ApEn	1.09 ± 0.11	1.05 ± 0.09	0.42	−0.42 (−0.91–−0.33)	0.63 (0.02–0.91)	6.1 (2.5–9.9)
SampEn	1.67 ± 0.20	1.69 ± 0.29	0.92	0.05 (−0.63–0.74)	0.67 (−0.05–0.93)	9.1 (3.6–14.9)
DFAα1	0.87 ± 0.23	0.93 ± 0.31	0.67	0.23 (−0.34–0.82)	0.77 (0.26–0.95)	17.2 (6.7–28.7)

HR—Heart rate, RespRate—respiratory rate, HRV—Heart rate variability, SDNN—Standard deviation of the normal-to-normal RR intervals, RMSSD—Root mean square of successive RR interval differences, mRR—Mean RR interval, ln—Natural log transformed, pNN50—Percent of RR intervals differing >50 ms from the preceding one, LF—Low frequency, HF—High frequency, SD—Standard deviation, ApEn—Approximate entropy, SampEn—Sample entropy, DFAα1—Detrended fluctuation analysis (short-term fluctuations), ICC—Intra-class correlation coefficient, WSCV—Within-subject coefficient of variation, CI—confidence interval, bmp—Beats per minute, ms—Milliseconds, nu—Normalized units.

Table 2. Reliability results for ultra-short-term (1 min) HR, RespRate and RMSSD indexes.

	Test Mean ± SD	Retest Mean ± SD	p	Cohen's d	ICC (95% CI)	WSCV% (95% CI)
HR [bpm]	64.4 ± 10.3	64.0 ± 11.9	0.63	−0.03 (−0.24–0.15)	0.98 (0.92–0.99)	2.5 (1.0–3.9)
RespRate [breaths/min]	14.6 ± 2.8	14.8 ± 2.8	0.80	0.05 (−0.36–0.46)	0.89 (0.56–0.98)	6.3 (2.5–10.2)
RMSSD [ms]	40.8 ± 16.7	47.1 ± 21.7	0.18	0.33 (−0.15–0.86)	0.78 (0.29–0.95)	24.8 (9.5–42.2)
lnRMSSD	3.61 ± 0.53	3.73 ± 0.58	0.30	0.22 (−0.21–0.85)	0.84 (0.45–0.97)	6.3 (2.5–10.2)
lnRMSSD/mRR	−3.24 ± 0.40	−3.13 ± 0.44	0.31	0.27 (−0.26–1.01)	0.75 (0.23–0.94)	6.7 (2.7–10.9)

HR—heart rate, RespRate—respiratory rate, RMSSD—Root mean square of successive RR interval differences, mRR—Mean RR interval, ln—Natural log transformed, ICC—Intra-class correlation coefficient, WSCV—Within-subject coefficient of variation, CI—Confidence interval, bmp—Beats per minute, ms—Milliseconds, SD—Standard deviation.

Table 3. Results of agreement between selected short-term (5 min) and ultra-short-term (1 min) parameters in Test and Retest.

	Parameter	Mean ± SD 5 min	Mean ± SD 1 min	p	Mean Difference (95% CI)	SWC	LoA	95% CI for Lower; Upper LoA	ICC (95% CI)
Test	HR [bpm]	64.6 ± 9.8	64.4 ± 10.3	0.52	0.2 (−0.6–1.1)	2.0	−1.8–2.3	−3.3–−0.2; 0.7–3.8	0.99 (0.98–0.99)
	RespRate [breaths/min]	15 ± 3	15 ± 3	0.50	0.0 (−0.6–0.6)	1.0	−1.5–1.5	−2.6–−0.4; 0.4–2.6	0.97 (0.85–0.99)
	RMSSD [ms]	45.2 ± 17.9	40.8 ± 16.7	0.20	4.4 (−2.9–11.7)	3.6	−12.8–21.6	−25.9–−0.3; 8.5–34.7	0.86 (0.48–0.97)
	lnRMSSD	3.72 ± 0.48	3.61 ± 0.53	0.18	0.12 (−0.07–0.30)	0.10	−0.32–0.55	−0.65–−0.01; 0.22–0.88	0.89 (0.58–0.98)
	lnRMSSD/mRR	−3.12 ± 0.35	−3.24 ± 0.40	0.17	0.12 (−0.07–0.31)	0.07	−0.32–0.56	−0.66–−0.02; 0.23–0.90	0.80 (0.32–0.96)
Retest	HR [bpm]	62.9 ± 9.7	64.0 ± 11.9	0.29	−1.1 (−3.4–1.2)	2.0	−6.5–4.3	−10.6–−2.4; 0.2–8.4	0.97 (0.86–0.99)
	RespRate [breaths/min]	15 ± 3	15 ± 3	0.36	0.0 (−0.5–0.5)	1.0	−1.1–1.1	−1.9–−0.3; 0.3–1.9	0.98 (0.92–0.99)
	RMSSD [ms]	48.2 ± 21.1	47.1 ± 21.7	0.68	1.1 (−4.7–6.8)	4.2	−12.4–14.5	−22.6–−2.1; 4.2–24.7	0.95 (0.79–0.99)
	lnRMSSD	3.78 ± 0.49	3.73 ± 0.58	0.42	0.05 (−0.09–0.18)	0.10	−0.26–0.36	−0.50–−0.03; 0.12–0.60	0.96 (0.82–0.99)
	lnRMSSD/mRR	−3.09 ± 0.35	−3.13 ± 0.44	0.53	0.04 (−0.09–0.16)	0.07	−0.26–0.33	−0.49–−0.04; 0.11–0.56	0.93 (0.71–0.99)

HR—Heart rate, RespRate—Respiratory rate, RMSSD—Root mean square of successive RR interval differences, mRR—Mean RR interval, ln—Natural log transformed, ICC—Intra-class correlation coefficient, SWC—Smallest worthwhile change, LoA—Limits of agreement, CI—Confidence interval, bmp—Beats per minute, ms—Milliseconds, SD—Standard deviation.

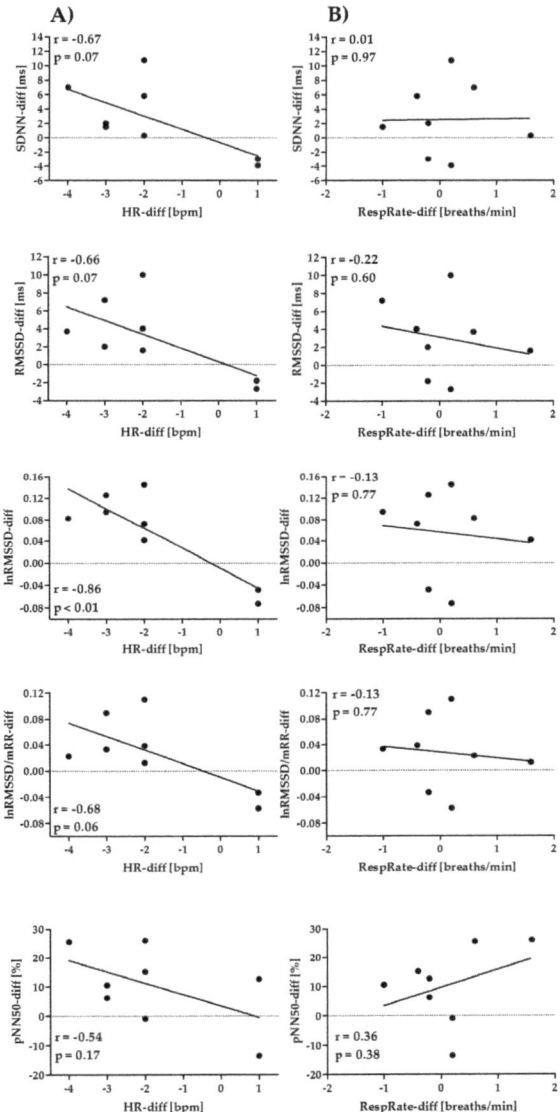

Figure 4. Pearson's correlation coefficient between Retest–Test differences in time-domain short-term (5 min) HRV parameters and differences in HR (HR-diff) (column **A**) or RespRate (RespRate-diff) (column **B**).

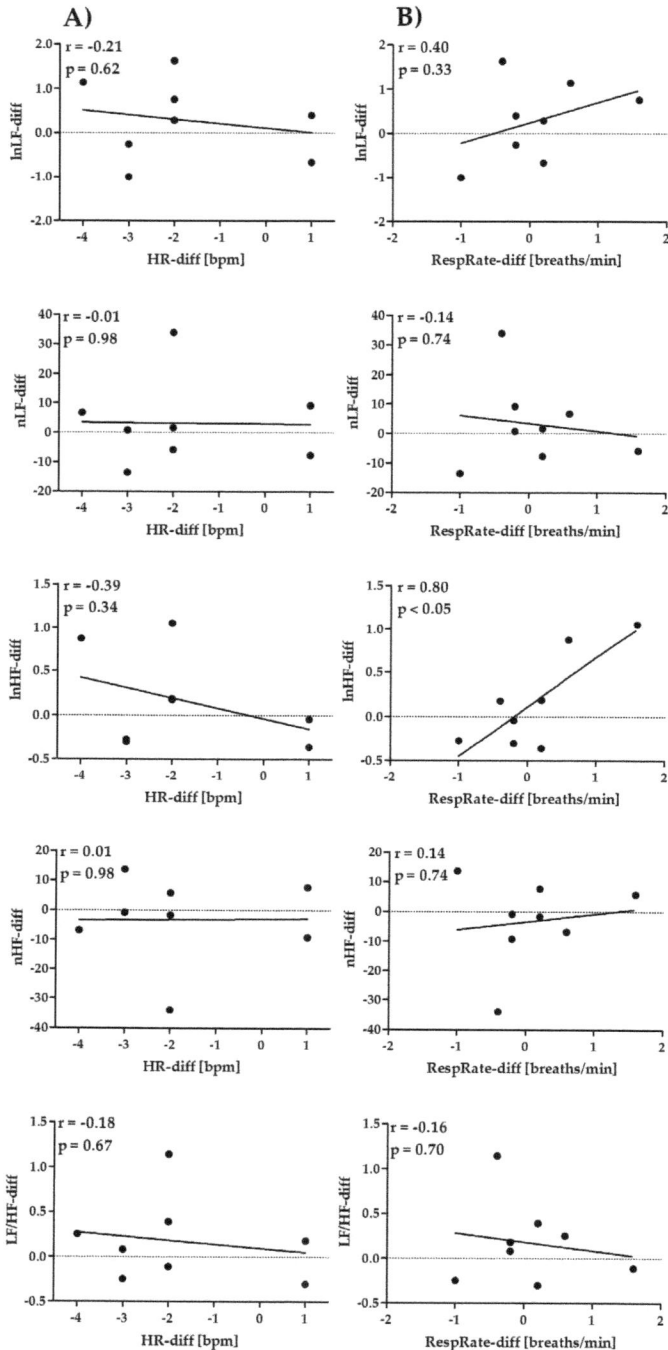

Figure 5. Pearson's correlation coefficient between Retest–Test differences in frequency-domain short-term (5 min) HRV parameters and differences in HR (HR-diff) (column **A**) or RespRate (RespRate-diff) (column **B**).

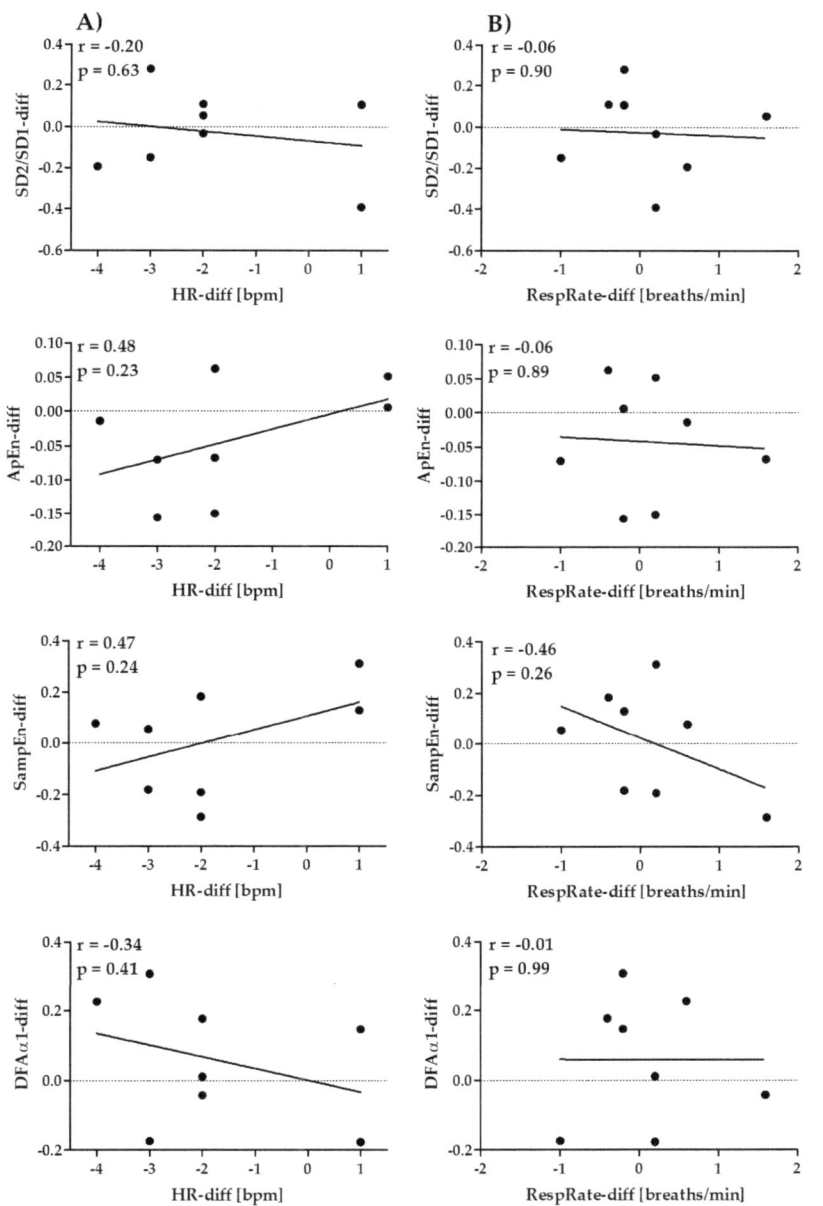

Figure 6. Pearson's correlation coefficient between Retest–Test differences in nonlinear short-term (5 min) HRV indices and differences in HR (HR-diff) (column **A**) or RespRate (RespRate-diff) (column **B**).

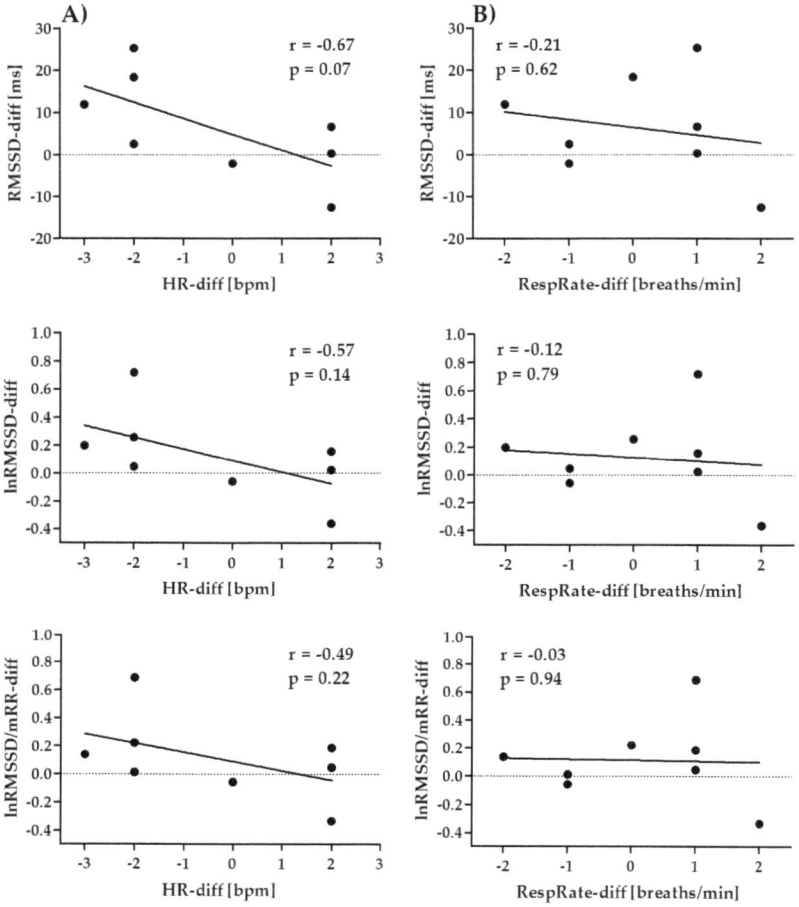

Figure 7. Pearson's correlation coefficient between Retest–Test differences in ultra-short-term (1 min) HRV parameters and differences in ultra-short-term (1 min) HR (HR-diff) (column **A**) or ultra-short-term RespRate (RespRate-diff) (column **B**).

4. Discussion

The purpose of this pilot study was to assess the reliability of short-term (5 min) and ultra-short-term (1 min) HRV parameters derived from ECG recordings performed in stable measurement conditions with one-week time interval between tests in elite modern pentathletes. Agreement between short-term and ultra-short-term parameters and correlation between differences in HR, RespRate and HRV parameters were also assessed.

We showed that short-term (5 min) HR, RespRate, lnRMSSD (time-domain), lnHF (frequency-domain), SD2/SD1 (nonlinear) and ultra-short-term (1 min) HR, RespRate and lnRMSSD presented acceptable, satisfactory reliability. These results indicate that the aforementioned HRV parameters could be used by coaches and researchers as reliable parameters in endurance athletes during baseline periods in laboratory-controlled settings. Methodological differences between published studies, and general lack of studies on test-retest reliability analysis of HR, RespRate, short-term (5 min) and ultra-short-term (1 min) HRV parameters in elite athletes hinder comparisons. The current findings are somewhat in line with previous studies showing that time-domain indices are more reliable than spectral-domain parameters in moderately-trained males [11] and that ultra-short-term (1 min) lnRMSSD demonstrated acceptable interday reliability (ICC = 0.90, CV < 7%) in elite rugby union players [30].

Recently, many authors have adopted ultra-shortened, user-friendly HRV parameters for the evaluation of endurance and team-sport athletes; however, the analysis of the relevance of such parameters focused more on agreement with 5 min criterion parameters than on test-retest reliability [22,25,28,30–34]. Ultra-short-term (1 min) lnRMSSD has been shown to present strong agreement with criterion 5 min recordings [28,31]. No significant differences between short-term (5 min) and ultra-short-term (1 min) HR, RespRate and lnRMSSD were observed in the current study, which is somewhat in line with previous studies with endurance and team-sport athletes [22,28,31,32].

However, in our study, all analyzed ultra-short-term parameters, in both Test and Retest, showed a LoA with short-term parameters that exceeded the defined a priori maximum acceptable difference (SWC). This is contradictory to the high ICC values obtained between 5 min and 1 min HRV parameters. In studies evaluating agreement between short-term and ultra-short-term parameters, authors have not provided the maximum acceptable difference, nor did they report whether it was exceeded by the LoA. Therefore, the criteria for defining strong agreement in these studies are not well defined. Recent reviews have highlighted that important data from the Bland–Altman method are often omitted [79,80]. Abu-Arafeh et al. recently provided a comprehensive list of key items for reporting Bland–Altman analysis [79]. The first key item, not reported in published studies on agreement between ultra-short-term and criterion HRV parameters in athletes, is the definition of the a priori acceptable LoA, to define the minimal agreement needed to consider the new measurement method as interchangeable with another method (often gold standard or criterion method) [79]. lnRMSSD justifiably seems to be the preferred HRV index for monitoring athletic performance and training status due to several advantages described previously [2,15,18,21,22,28,30,31]. We confirm that ultra-short-term (1 min) lnRMSSD, in combination with HR and respiratory rate, can be reliably used in elite modern pentathletes. However, without defining a priori the maximum acceptable difference between 5 min and 1 min parameters, caution should be taken before considering these two methods as interchangeable, at least in this group of participants. From the results of our study, no parameter can be considered interchangeable for 1 min and 5 min, once the LoA between them exceeds the SWC.

On the other hand, although the consideration of LoA < SWC represents an important criterion for agreement analysis, we believe it has an important limitation. Since LoA is calculated from the SD of differences between "Test" and "Retest", LoA will be low whenever the differences from all subjects tend to be homogeneous. This does not happen only when the results from "Test" and "Retest" are the same, but also when they vary by the same amount in all individuals. In other words, the fixed bias is not taken into account in this comparison. We suggest that a more complete analysis would involve the comparison of LoA and SWC together with the one-sample t-test to check if the fixed bias is different from zero. However, since in our study no parameter presented a LoA wider than SWC, the one-sample t-test was needless.

In experimental conditions similar to those of the current study, the reliability of time-domain and frequency-domain HRV parameters was shown to be affected by differences in HR and RespRate in young healthy volunteers. HR was a stronger determinant for HRV reproducibility than RespRate, and even a minimal change of HR considerably altered HRV [83]. In elite athletes, the differences in short-term time-domain and nonlinear HRV parameters, as well as in ultra-short-term HRV parameters, turned out to be more correlated with differences in HR than with differences in RespRate. This supports the notion that changes in HRV indices should be assessed and interpreted with regard to concomitant changes in resting HR [4,15,18]. The normalization of HRV parameters concerning the HR level has already been suggested and we reinforce its importance for comparisons of people with different levels of HR [67,68].

Contrastingly, differences in short-term frequency-domain HRV parameters were more correlated with differences in RespRate than with differences in HR. Indeed, HRV (mostly frequency-domain parameters) is also highly affected by respiratory depth and rate [44,84]. Spectral powers at LF and HF bands are commonly attributed to sympathetic and vagal, and vagal influences alone on HR, respectively. Thus, coaches and sport practitioners should be aware that changes in the respiratory rate may confound spectral indices [53]. It has been suggested that depth of breathing could be even more important than its rate [5]. Młyńczak and Krysztofiak proposed cardiorespiratory temporal causal links with the path for lying supine from tidal volume, through heart activity variation and average heart activity, to respiratory timing [5]. Even if those links appeared rather moderate, the possible differences in the respiratory pattern should be taken into account in the protocol assessing the cardiac parameters. The measurement of tidal volumes using, e.g., mouthpieces may affect HRV data [17,85]. Moreover, there is no optimal solution on how to record and control respiratory depth and rate in HRV studies [44,53]. One possible solution for future studies in athletes could be to implement the Pneumonitor 2 or 3, a portable device that would register respiratory pattern (both depth and rate) together with single-lead ECG (enough to estimate aforementioned parameters), motion, and/or pulse oximetry (saturation, pulse wave) designed for environmental physiology analyses and sports medicine [86,87].

Although HRV parameters are often used as biomarkers of physical conditioning, as well as indicators of the severity of diseases, the physiological meaning of such parameters are not well understood in many situations. While the spectral power at the HF band is widely accepted to represent the vagal modulation (respiratory sinus arrhythmia) to the heart under normal respiratory frequencies (>9 breaths/min), the physiological interpretation of other indices is not so clear. This is the case of most nonlinear HRV parameters. For example, the short-term scaling exponent (DFAα1) represents the fractal correlations present in RR series and was demonstrated to represent one of the best risk factors for patients with heart failure or myocardial infarction [88,89]. However, the changes in fractal structure of RR series in these patients are likely to be the consequence of the global change in cardiovascular function, and not a marker of any specific physiological variable. The living organism can be considered a complex system and, as such, it is difficult to disentangle the influences caused by each mechanism, once their functions are highly interdependent [90]. This is the reason why many nonlinear HRV parameters are considered as "complexity measures", in the sense that, although they are not clearly associated with specific physiological meanings, they are able to represent the general complexity of the system, attested by their important role as risk factors, prognosis and fitness [91,92].

No previous study on inter-day reliability of HRV in athletes with similar methodological characteristics to our study was found. As underlined by many authors, there are still substantial methodological inconsistencies throughout the literature regarding HRV in sports science that limit comparison [4,18,93]. Moreover, the authors of a recent study on test-retest reliability of short-term HRV parameters suggested that the studies differ with respect to important methodological issues and evidence on this topic is far from clear [54]. There are several methodological characteristics that may cause differences in findings among studies on HRV reliability, e.g., reliability statistics adopted, number of tests performed and the time interval between them, and sample heterogeneity [54]. Lack of information about other methodological aspects also limits potential for study replication and confidence in interpretation [52,53], such as the lack of information on ECG acquisition and processing, including device, software, recording duration and conditions, breathing control, and position during recordings. Thus, we emphasize the importance of providing all the necessary information for reproducibility, as well as the standardization of statistics for the analysis of reliability of biomarker parameters in athletes.

Our pilot study was limited by a small homogenous sample size taken at a given moment of the sport season, which limits generalizability of the study's findings. The consequence of low sample size is the illustrative character of the correlation data. HRV data were obtained during supine ECG recordings in controlled laboratory settings. Heart rate monitors or smartphone with HRV application may be more useful to collect RR intervals in athletes than traditional ECG, especially outside of a laboratory setting [94–96]. Nevertheless, as suggested by Lucini et al., caution must be applied when assessing HRV using devices that cannot discriminate RR series between sinus and non-sinus beats, especially in athletes [57]. In our study, four participants were excluded from the analysis due to presence of cardiac abnormalities. Recently, abnormal ECG changes were observed in about 4% of top-level endurance athletes [97]. Therefore, we suggest performing ECG screening among examined athletes before including the data for detailed HRV analysis.

5. Conclusions

Short-term HR, RespRate, short-term lnRMSSD, lnHF, and SD2/SD1 HRV parameters and ultra-short-term HR, RespRate and lnRMSSD could be used by coaches, sport practitioners and researchers as reliable parameters in elite modern pentathlon athletes at baseline examinations in laboratory settings. Without defining the a priori maximum acceptable difference, caution should be taken before considering HR, RespRate and lnRMSSD from 5 min and 1 min recordings as interchangeable. Moreover, differences in short-term and ultra-short-term HRV parameters should be assessed considering the concomitant differences in HR and RespRate.

Author Contributions: B.H. and J.S.G. conceived and designed the experiment. B.H. and J.S.G. acquired the data. R.B. and E.D. analyzed electrocardiography (ECG) recordings. B.H. and J.S.G. analyzed the data (RR intervals) for heart rate variability and statistical analysis. B.H., A.A.F., L.E.V.S., M.M., R.B., E.D., B.W., J.S.G. interpreted the data. B.H., A.A.F., L.E.V.S., M.M., R.B., E.D., B.W., J.S.G. drafted the work and revised it critically for important intellectual content. B.H., A.A.F., L.E.V.S., M.M., R.B., E.D., B.W., J.S.G. approved the final version of the manuscript to be published. All authors have read and agreed to the published version of the manuscript.

Funding: This research received no external funding.

Acknowledgments: This study was completed as a part of a master's thesis by B.H. We thank the athletes for participation in the study and undergraduate student A.K. (Aleksandra Kędziorek) for her help with the electrocardiography data acquisition.

Conflicts of Interest: The authors declare no conflict of interest.

References

1. Meeusen, R.; Duclos, M.; Foster, C.; Fry, A.; Gleeson, M.; Nieman, D.; Raglin, J.; Rietjens, G.; Steinacker, J.; Urhausen, A.; et al. Prevention, diagnosis, and treatment of the overtraining syndrome: Joint consensus statement of the European College of Sport Science and the American College of Sports Medicine. *Med. Sci. Sports Exerc.* **2013**, *45*, 186–205. [CrossRef] [PubMed]
2. Bellenger, C.R.; Fuller, J.T.; Thomson, R.L.; Davison, K.; Robertson, E.Y.; Buckley, J.D. Monitoring Athletic Training Status Through Autonomic Heart Rate Regulation: A Systematic Review and Meta-Analysis. *Sports Med.* **2016**, *46*, 1461–1486. [CrossRef] [PubMed]
3. Kellmann, M.; Bertollo, M.; Bosquet, L.; Brink, M.; Coutts, A.J.; Duffield, R.; Erlacher, D.; Halson, S.L.; Hecksteden, A.; Heidari, J.; et al. Recovery and Performance in Sport: Consensus Statement. *Int. J. Sports Physiol. Perform.* **2018**, *13*, 240–245. [CrossRef] [PubMed]
4. Schneider, C.; Hanakam, F.; Wiewelhove, T.; Döweling, A.; Kellmann, M.; Meyer, T.; Pfeiffer, M.; Ferrauti, A. Heart Rate Monitoring in Team Sports-A Conceptual Framework for Contextualizing Heart Rate Measures for Training and Recovery Prescription. *Front. Physiol.* **2018**, *9*, 639. [CrossRef]
5. Młyńczak, M.; Krysztofiak, H. Cardiorespiratory Temporal Causal Links and the Differences by Sport or Lack Thereof. *Front. Physiol.* **2019**, *10*, 45. [CrossRef]
6. Młyńczak, M.; Krysztofiak, H. Discovery of Causal Paths in Cardiorespiratory Parameters: A Time-Independent Approach in Elite Athletes. *Front. Physiol.* **2018**, *9*, 1455. [CrossRef]
7. Bourdon, P.C.; Cardinale, M.; Murray, A.; Gastin, P.; Kellmann, M.; Varley, M.C.; Gabbett, T.J.; Coutts, A.J.; Burgess, D.J.; Gregson, W.; et al. Monitoring Athlete Training Loads: Consensus Statement. *Int. J. Sports Physiol. Perform.* **2017**, *12*, S2161–S2170. [CrossRef]

8. Gabbett, T.J.; Nassis, G.P.; Oetter, E.; Pretorius, J.; Johnston, N.; Medina, D.; Rodas, G.; Myslinski, T.; Howells, D.; Beard, A.; et al. The athlete monitoring cycle. A practical guide to interpreting and applying training monitoring data. *Br. J. Sports Med.* **2017**, *51*, 1451–1452. [CrossRef]
9. Heidari, J.; Beckmann, J.; Bertollo, M.; Brink, M.; Kallus, W.; Robazza, C.; Kellmann, M. Multidimensional Monitoring of Recovery Status and Implications for Performance. *Int. J. Sports Physiol. Perform.* **2018**, 1–24. [CrossRef]
10. Buchheit, M.; Chivot, A.; Parouty, J.; Mercier, D.; Al Haddad, H.; Laursen, P.B.; Ahmaidi, S. Monitoring endurance running performance using cardiac parasympathetic function. *Eur. J. Appl. Physiol.* **2010**, *108*, 1153–1167. [CrossRef]
11. Al Haddad, H.; Laursen, P.B.; Chollet, D.; Ahmaidi, S.; Buchheit, M. Reliability of resting and postexercise heart rate measures. *Int. J. Sports Med.* **2011**, *32*, 598–605. [CrossRef] [PubMed]
12. Daanen, H.A.; Lamberts, R.P.; Kallen, V.L.; Jin, A.; van Meeteren, N.L. A systematic review on heart-rate recovery to monitor changes in training status in athletes. *Int. J. Sports Physiol. Perform.* **2012**, *7*, 251–260. [CrossRef] [PubMed]
13. Stanley, J.; Peake, J.M.; Buchheit, M. Cardiac parasympathetic reactivation following exercise: Implications for training prescription. *Sports Med.* **2013**, *43*, 1259–1277. [CrossRef]
14. Plews, D.J.; Laursen, P.B.; Kilding, A.E.; Buchheit, M. Heart rate variability in elite triathletes, is variation in variability the key to effective training? A case comparison. *Eur. J. Appl. Physiol.* **2012**, *112*, 3729–3741. [CrossRef] [PubMed]
15. Plews, D.J.; Laursen, P.B.; Stanley, J.; Kilding, A.E.; Buchheit, M. Training adaptation and heart rate variability in elite endurance athletes: Opening the door to effective monitoring. *Sports Med.* **2013**, *43*, 773–781. [CrossRef]
16. Plews, D.J.; Laursen, P.B.; Le Meur, Y.; Hausswirth, C.; Kilding, A.E.; Buchheit, M. Monitoring training with heart rate-variability. How much compliance is needed for valid assessment? *Int. J. Sports Physiol. Perform.* **2014**, *9*, 783–790. [CrossRef]
17. Saboul, D.; Pialoux, V.; Hautier, C. The impact of breathing on HRV measurements: Implications for the longitudinal follow-up of athletes. *Eur. J. Sport Sci.* **2013**, *13*, 534–542. [CrossRef]
18. Buchheit, M. Monitoring training status with HR measures: Do all roads lead to Rome? *Front. Physiol.* **2014**, *5*, 73. [CrossRef]
19. Koenig, J.; Jarczok, M.N.; Wasner, M.; Hillecke, T.K.; Thayer, J.F. Heart rate variability and swimming. *Sports Med.* **2014**, *44*, 1377–1391. [CrossRef]
20. Da Silva, V.P.; de Oliveira, N.A.; Silveira, H.; Mello, R.G.; Deslandes, A.C. Heart rate variability indexes as a marker of chronic adaptation in athletes: A systematic review. *Ann. Noninvasive Electrocardiol.* **2015**, *20*, 108–118. [CrossRef]
21. Schmitt, L.; Regnard, J.; Millet, G.P. Monitoring fatigue status with hrv measures in elite athletes: An avenue beyond rmssd? *Front. Physiol.* **2015**, *6*, 343. [CrossRef] [PubMed]
22. Flatt, A.A.; Esco, M.R. Heart rate variability stabilization in athletes: Towards more convenient data acquisition. *Clin. Physiol. Funct. Imaging* **2016**, *36*, 331–336. [CrossRef] [PubMed]
23. Kiss, O.; Sydó, N.; Vargha, P.; Vágó, H.; Czimbalmos, C.; Édes, E.; Zima, E.; Apponyi, G.; Merkely, G.; Sydó, T.; et al. Detailed heart rate variability analysis in athletes. *Clin. Auton. Res.* **2016**, *26*, 245–252. [CrossRef]
24. Saboul, D.; Balducci, P.; Millet, G.; Pialoux, V.; Hautier, C. A pilot study on quantification of training load: The use of HRV in training practice. *Eur. J. Sport Sci.* **2016**, *16*, 172–181. [CrossRef] [PubMed]
25. Bourdillon, N.; Schmitt, L.; Yazdani, S.; Vesin, J.M.; Millet, G.P. Minimal Window Duration for Accurate HRV Recording in Athletes. *Front. Neurosci.* **2017**, *11*, 456. [CrossRef]
26. Lachin, J.M. The role of measurement reliability in clinical trials. *Clin. Trials* **2004**, *1*, 553–566. [CrossRef]
27. Matheson, G.J. We need to talk about reliability: Making better use of test-retest studies for study design and interpretation. *PeerJ.* **2019**, *7*, e6918. [CrossRef]
28. Esco, M.R.; Flatt, A.A. Ultra-short-term heart rate variability indexes at rest and post-exercise in athletes: Evaluating the agreement with accepted recommendations. *J. Sports Sci. Med.* **2014**, *13*, 535–541.
29. Nakamura, F.Y.; Flatt, A.A.; Pereira, L.A.; Ramirez-Campillo, R.; Loturco, I.; Esco, M.R. Ultra-Short-Term Heart Rate Variability is Sensitive to Training Effects in Team Sports Players. *J. Sports Sci. Med.* **2015**, *14*, 602–605.

30. Nakamura, F.Y.; Pereira, L.A.; Esco, M.R.; Flatt, A.A.; Moraes, J.A.; Cal Abad, C.C.; Loturco, I. Intraday and Interday Reliability of Ultra-Short-Term Heart Rate Variability in Rugby Union Players. *J. Strength Cond. Res.* **2017**, *31*, 548–551. [CrossRef]
31. Pereira, L.A.; Flatt, A.A.; Ramirez-Campillo, R.; Loturco, I.; Nakamura, F.Y. Assessing Shortened Field-Based Heart-Rate-Variability-Data Acquisition in Team-Sport Athletes. *Int. J. Sports Physiol. Perform.* **2016**, *11*, 154–158. [CrossRef]
32. Esco, M.R.; Williford, H.N.; Flatt, A.A.; Freeborn, T.J.; Nakamura, F.Y. Ultra-shortened time-domain HRV parameters at rest and following exercise in athletes: An alternative to frequency computation of sympathovagal balance. *Eur. J. Appl. Physiol.* **2018**, *118*, 175–184. [CrossRef] [PubMed]
33. Vescovi, J.D. Intra-Individual Variation of HRV during Orthostatic Challenge in Elite Male Field Hockey Players. *J. Med. Syst.* **2019**, *43*, 328. [CrossRef] [PubMed]
34. Hung, C.H.; Clemente, F.M.; Bezerra, P.; Chiu, Y.W.; Chien, C.H.; Crowley-McHattan, Z.; Chen, Y.S. Post-Exercise Recovery of Ultra-Short-Term Heart Rate Variability after Yo-Yo Intermittent Recovery Test and Repeated Sprint Ability Test. *Int. J. Environ. Res. Public Health* **2020**, *17*, 4070. [CrossRef] [PubMed]
35. Le Meur, Y.; Hausswirth, C.; Abbiss, C.; Baupi, Y.; Dorel, S. Performance factors in the new combined event of modern pentathlon. *J. Sports Sci.* **2010**, *28*, 1111. [CrossRef] [PubMed]
36. Le Meur, Y.; Dorel, S.; Baup, Y.; Guvomarch, J.P.; Roudaut, C.; Hausswirth, C. Physiological demand and pacing strategy during the new combined event in elite pentathletes. *Eur. J. Appl. Physiol.* **2012**, *112*, 2583–2593. [CrossRef] [PubMed]
37. Coutinho, L.A.; Porto, C.P.; Pierucci, A.P. Critical evaluation of food intake and energy balance in young modern pentathlon athletes: A cross-sectional study. *J. Int. Soc. Sports Nutr.* **2016**, *13*, 15. [CrossRef] [PubMed]
38. Loureiro, L.L.; Fonseca, S., Jr.; Castro, N.G.; Dos Passos, R.B.; Porto, C.P.; Pierucci, A.P. Basal Metabolic Rate of Adolescent Modern Pentathlon Athletes: Agreement between Indirect Calorimetry and Predictive Equations and the Correlation with Body Parameters. *PLoS ONE* **2015**, *10*, e0142859. [CrossRef]
39. Sadowska, D.; Lichota, M.; Sacewicz, T.; Krzepota, J. Influence of Running Phases on the Postural Balance of Modern Pentathlon Athletes in a Laser Run Event. *Int. J. Environ. Res. Public Health* **2019**, *16*, 4440. [CrossRef]
40. Sadowska, D.; Sacewicz, T.; Lichota, M.; Krzepota, J.; Ładyga, M. Static Postural Balance in Modern Pentathletes: A Pilot Study. *Int. J. Environ. Res. Public Health* **2019**, *16*, 1760. [CrossRef]
41. Chirico, A.; Fegatelli, D.; Galli, F.; Mallia, L.; Alivernini, F.; Cordone, S.; Giancamilli, F.; Pecci, S.; Tosi, G.M.; Giordano, A.; et al. A study of quiet eye's phenomenon in the shooting section of "laser run" of modern pentathlon. *J. Cell Physiol.* **2019**, *234*, 9247–9254. [CrossRef] [PubMed]
42. Task Force of the European Society of Cardiology and the North American Society of Pacing and Electrophysiology. Heart rate variability: Standards of measurement, physiological interpretation and clinical use. Task force of the European society of cardiology and the North American society of pacing and electrophysiology. *Circulation* **1996**, *93*, 1043–1065. [CrossRef]
43. Heathers, J.A.J. Everything Hertz: Methodological issues in short-term frequency domain HRV. *Front. Physiol.* **2014**, *5*, 177. [CrossRef] [PubMed]
44. Quintana, D.S.; Heathers, J.A.J. Considerations in the assessment of heart rate variability in biobehavioral research. *Front. Psychol.* **2014**, *5*, 805. [CrossRef]
45. Billman, G.E.; Huikuri, H.V.; Sacha, J.; Trimmel, K. An introduction to heart rate variability: Methodological considerations and clinical applications. *Front. Physiol.* **2015**, *6*, 55. [CrossRef]
46. Shaffer, F.; Ginsberg, J. An Overview of Heart Rate Variability Metrics and Norms. *Front. Public Health* **2017**, *5*, 258. [CrossRef]
47. Ernst, G. Heart-Rate Variability—More than Heart Beats? *Front. Public Health* **2017**, *5*, 240. [CrossRef]
48. Singh, N.; Moneghetti, K.J.; Christle, J.W.; Hadley, D.; Froelicher, V.; Plews, D. Heart Rate Variability: An Old Metric with New Meaning in the Era of Using mHealth technologies for Health and Exercise Training Guidance. Part Two: Prognosis and Training. *Arrhythmia. Electrophysiol. Rev.* **2018**, *7*, 247–255. [CrossRef] [PubMed]
49. Hayano, J.; Yuda, E. Pitfalls of assessment of autonomic function by heart rate variability. *J. Physiol. Anthr.* **2019**, *38*, 3. [CrossRef]
50. Li, K.; Rüdiger, H.; Ziemssen, F. Spectral Analysis of Heart Rate Variability: Time Window Matters. *Front. Neurol.* **2019**, *10*, 545. [CrossRef]

51. Malik, M.; Hnatkova, K.; Huikuri, H.V.; Lombardi, F.; Schmid, R.M.; Zabel, M. CrossTalk proposal: Heart rate variability is a valid measure of cardiac autonomic responsiveness. *J. Physiol.* **2019**, *597*, 2595–2598. [CrossRef] [PubMed]
52. Quintana, D.S.; Alvares, G.A.; Heathers, J.A.J. Guidelines for Reporting Articles on Psychiatry and Heart rate variability (GRAPH): Recommendations to advance research communication. *Transl. Psychiatry* **2016**, *6*, e803. [CrossRef] [PubMed]
53. Gąsior, J.S.; Zamunér, A.R.; Silva, L.E.V.; Williams, C.A.; Baranowski, R.; Sacha, J.; Machura, P.; Kochman, W.; Werner, B. Heart Rate Variability in Children and Adolescents with Cerebral Palsy-A Systematic Literature Review. *J. Clin. Med.* **2020**, *9*, 1141. [CrossRef] [PubMed]
54. Uhlig, S.; Meylan, A.; Rudolph, U. Reliability of short-term measurements of heart rate variability: Findings from a longitudinal study. *Biol. Psychol.* **2020**, *154*, 107905. [CrossRef] [PubMed]
55. Araújo, C.G.; Scharhag, J. Athlete: A working definition for medical and health sciences research. *Scand. J. Med. Sci. Sports* **2016**, *26*, 4–7. [CrossRef] [PubMed]
56. Laborde, S.; Mosley, E.; Thayer, J.F. Heart Rate Variability and Cardiac Vagal Tone in Psychophysiological Research–Recommendations for Experiment Planning, Data Analysis, and Data Reporting. *Front. Psychol.* **2017**, *8*, 89. [CrossRef]
57. Lucini, D.; Marchetti, I.; Spataro, A.; Malacarne, M.; Benzi, M.; Tamorri, S.; Sala, R.; Pagani, M. Heart rate variability to monitor performance in elite athletes: Criticalities and avoidable pitfalls. *Int. J. Cardiol.* **2017**, *240*, 307–312. [CrossRef]
58. Peltola, M.A. Role of Editing of R–R Intervals in the Analysis of Heart Rate Variability. *Front. Physiol.* **2012**, *3*, 148. [CrossRef]
59. Tarvainen, M.P.; Lipponen, J.; Niskanen, J.P.; Ranta-Aho, P.O. Kubios HRV (ver. 3.0.2). User's Guide. 2017. Available online: http://www.kubios.com/downloads/Kubios_HRV_Users_Guide.pdf (accessed on 21 July 2020).
60. Tarvainen, M.P.; Niskanen, J.P.; Lipponen, J.A.; Ranta-Aho, P.O.; Karjalainen, P.A. Kubios HRV-heart rate variability analysis software. *Comput. Methods Programs Biomed.* **2014**, *113*, 210–220. [CrossRef]
61. Tarvainen, M.P.; Ranta-Aho, P.O.; Karjalainen, P.A. An advanced detrending method with application to HRV analysis. *IEEE Trans. Biomed. Eng.* **2002**, *49*, 172–175. [CrossRef]
62. Sacha, J.; Pluta, W. Different methods of heart rate variability analysis reveal different correlations of heart rate variability spectrum with average heart rate. *J. Electrocardiol.* **2005**, *38*, 47–53. [CrossRef] [PubMed]
63. Sacha, J.; Pluta, W. Alterations of an average heart rate change heart rate variability due to mathematical reasons. *Int. J. Cardiol.* **2008**, *128*, 444–447. [CrossRef] [PubMed]
64. Billman, G.E. The effect of heart rate on the heart rate variability response to autonomic interventions. *Front. Physiol.* **2013**, *4*, 222. [CrossRef] [PubMed]
65. Fagard, R. Athlete's heart. *Heart* **2003**, *89*, 1455–1461. [CrossRef]
66. D'Souza, A.; Sharma, S.; Boyett, M.R. CrossTalk opposing view: Bradycardia in the trained athlete is attributable to a downregulation of a pacemaker channel in the sinus node. *J. Physiol.* **2015**, *593*, 1749–1751. [CrossRef]
67. Sacha, J.; Barabach, S.; Statkiewicz-Barabach, G.; Sacha, K.; Müller, A.; Piskorski, J.; Barthel, P.; Schmidt, G. How to strengthen or weaken the HRV dependence on heart rate—Description of the method and its perspectives. *Int. J. Cardiol.* **2013**, *168*, 1660–1663. [CrossRef] [PubMed]
68. Monfredi, O.; Lyashkov, A.E.; Johnsen, A.B.; Inada, S.; Schneider, H.; Wang, R.; Nirmalan, M.; Wisloff, U.; Maltsev, V.A.; Lakatta, E.G.; et al. Biophysical characterization of the underappreciated and important relationship between heart rate variability and heart rate. *Hypertension* **2014**, *64*, 1334–1343. [CrossRef]
69. Shrout, P.E.; Fleiss, J.L. Intraclass correlations: Uses in assessing rater reliability. *Psychol. Bull.* **1979**, *86*, 420–428. [CrossRef]
70. Hopkins, W.G.; Marshall, S.W.; Batterham, A.M.; Hanin, J. Progressive statistics for studies in sports medicine and exercise science. *Med. Sci. Sports Exerc.* **2009**, *41*, 3–13. [CrossRef]
71. Hopkins, W.G. A New View of Statistics. 2000. Available online: http://sportsci.org/resource/stats (accessed on 3 August 2020).
72. Hopkins, W.G. Measures of reliability in sports medicine and science. *Sports Med.* **2000**, *30*, 1–15. [CrossRef]

73. Atkinson, G.; Nevill, A.M. Statistical Methods for Assessing Measurement Error (Reliability) in Variables Relevant to Sports Medicine. *Sports Med.* **1998**, *26*, 217–238. [CrossRef] [PubMed]
74. Bland, J.M.; Altman, D.G. Statistics Notes: Measurement error proportional to the mean. *Br. Med. J.* **1996**, *313*, 106. [CrossRef] [PubMed]
75. Cohen, J. *Statistical Power Analysis for the Behavioral Sciences*, 2nd ed.; Routledge: London, UK, 1988; pp. 179–206.
76. Altman, D.G.; Bland, J.M. Measurement in medicine: The analysis of method comparison studies. *Statistician* **1983**, *32*, 307–317. [CrossRef]
77. Bland, J.M.; Altman, D.G. Statistical methods for assessing agreement between two methods of clinical measurement. *Lancet* **1986**, *1*, 307–310. [CrossRef]
78. Bland, J.M.; Altman, D.G. Measuring agreement in method comparison studies. *Stat. Methods Med. Res.* **1999**, *8*, 135–160. [CrossRef]
79. Abu-Arafeh, A.; Jordan, H.; Drummond, G. Reporting of method comparison studies: A review of advice, an assessment of current practice, and specific suggestions for future reports. *Br. J. Anaesth.* **2016**, *117*, 569–575. [CrossRef]
80. Gerke, O. Reporting Standards for a Bland-Altman Agreement Analysis: A Review of Methodological Reviews. *Diagnostics* **2020**, *10*, 334. [CrossRef]
81. Ranganathan, P.; Pramesh, C.S.; Aggarwal, R. Common pitfalls in statistical analysis: Measures of agreement. *Perspect. Clin. Res.* **2017**, *8*, 187–191. [CrossRef]
82. Buchheit, M. Magnitudes matter more than Beetroot Juice. *Sport Perform. Sci. Rep.* **2018**, *1*, 1–3.
83. Gąsior, J.S.; Sacha, J.; Jeleń, P.J.; Zieliński, J.; Przybylski, J. Heart Rate and Respiratory Rate Influence on Heart Rate Variability Repeatability: Effects of the Correction for the Prevailing Heart Rate. *Front. Physiol.* **2016**, *7*, 356. [CrossRef]
84. Brown, T.E.; Beightol, L.A.; Koh, J.; Eckberg, D.L. Important influence of respiration on human R-R interval power spectra is largely ignored. *J. Appl. Physiol.* **1993**, *75*, 2310–2317. [CrossRef]
85. Bernardi, L.; Wdowczyk-Szulc, J.; Valenti, C.; Castoldi, S.; Passino, C.; Spadacini, G.; Sleight, P. Effects of controlled breathing, mental activity and mental stress with or without verbalization on heart rate variability. *J. Am. Coll. Cardiol.* **2000**, *35*, 1462–1469. [CrossRef]
86. Młyńczak, M.; Niewiadomski, W.; Żyliński, M.; Cybulski, G. Ambulatory devices measuring cardiorespiratory activity with motion. In Proceedings of the 10th International Joint Conference on Biomedical Engineering Systems and Technologies, Porto, Portugal, 21–23 February 2017; pp. 91–97.
87. Młyńczak, M.; Niewiadomski, W.; Żyliński, M.; Cybulski, G.P. Ambulatory Impedance Pneumography Device for Quantitative Monitoring of Volumetric Parameters in Respiratory and Cardiac Applications. In Proceedings of the Computing in Cardiology Conference (CinC), Cambridge, MA, USA, 7–10 September 2014.
88. Huikuri, H.V.; Mäkikallio, T.H.; Peng, C.K.; Goldberger, A.L.; Hintze, U.; Møller, M. Fractal correlation properties of R-R interval dynamics and mortality in patients with depressed left ventricular function after an acute myocardial infarction. *Circulation* **2000**, *101*, 47–53. [CrossRef]
89. Mäkikallio, T.H.; Huikuri, H.V.; Hintze, U.; Videbæk, J.; Mitrani, R.D.; Castellanos, A.; Myerburg, R.J.; Møller, M. Fractal analysis and time-and frequency-domain measures of heart rate variability as predictors of mortality in patients with heart failure. *Am. J. Cardiol.* **2001**, *87*, 178–182. [CrossRef]
90. Goldberger, A. Complex systems. *Proc. Am. Thorac. Soc.* **2006**, *3*, 467–471. [CrossRef]
91. Huikuri, H.V.; Stein, P.K. Heart rate variability in risk stratification of cardiac patients. *Prog. Cardiovasc. Dis.* **2013**, *56*, 153–159. [CrossRef]
92. Fazan, F.S.; Brognara, F.; Fazan Junior, R.; Murta Junior, L.O.; Silva, L.E.V. Changes in the Complexity of Heart Rate Variability with Exercise Training Measured by Multiscale Entropy-Based Measurements. *Entropy* **2018**, *20*, 47. [CrossRef]
93. Michael, S.; Graham, K.S.; Davis Oam, G.M. Cardiac Autonomic Responses during Exercise and Post-exercise Recovery Using Heart Rate Variability and Systolic Time Intervals-A Review. *Front. Physiol.* **2017**, *8*, 301. [CrossRef]

94. Flatt, A.A.; Esco, M.R. Validity of the ithlete™ Smart Phone Application for Determining Ultra-Short-Term Heart Rate Variability. *J. Hum. Kinet.* **2013**, *39*, 85–92. [CrossRef]
95. Perrotta, A.S.; Jeklin, A.T.; Hives, B.A.; Meanwell, L.E.; Warburton, D.E.R. Validity of the Elite HRV Smartphone Application for Examining Heart Rate Variability in a Field-Based Setting. *J. Strength Cond. Res.* **2017**, *31*, 2296–2302. [CrossRef] [PubMed]
96. Hernando, D.; Garatachea, N.; Almeida, R.; Casajús, J.A.; Bailón, R. Validation of Heart Rate Monitor Polar RS800 for Heart Rate Variability Analysis During Exercise. *J. Strength Cond. Res.* **2018**, *32*, 716–725. [CrossRef]
97. Jakubiak, A.A.; Konopka, M.; Bursa, D.; Król, W.; Anioł-Strzyżewska, K.; Burkhard-Jagodzińska, K.; Sitkowski, D.; Kuch, M.; Braksator, W. Benefits and limitations of electrocardiographic and echocardiographic screening in top level endurance athletes. *Biol. Sport* **2020**, *38*, 71–79.

Publisher's Note: MDPI stays neutral with regard to jurisdictional claims in published maps and institutional affiliations.

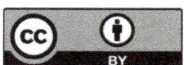 © 2020 by the authors. Licensee MDPI, Basel, Switzerland. This article is an open access article distributed under the terms and conditions of the Creative Commons Attribution (CC BY) license (http://creativecommons.org/licenses/by/4.0/).

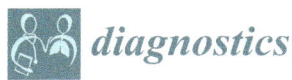

Article

Changes in Short-Term and Ultra-Short Term Heart Rate, Respiratory Rate, and Time-Domain Heart Rate Variability Parameters during Sympathetic Nervous System Activity Stimulation in Elite Modern Pentathlonists—A Pilot Study

Jakub S. Gąsior [1,*], Bartosz Hoffmann [2], Luiz Eduardo Virgilio Silva [3], Łukasz Małek [4], Andrew A. Flatt [5], Rafał Baranowski [6] and Bożena Werner [1]

1. Department of Pediatric Cardiology and General Pediatrics, Medical University of Warsaw, 02-091 Warsaw, Poland; bozena.werner@wum.edu.pl
2. Physiotherapy Division, Faculty of Medical Sciences, Medical University of Warsaw, 02-091 Warsaw, Poland; bartosz.hoffmann@icloud.com
3. Department of Internal Medicine of Ribeirão Preto Medical School, University of São Paulo, Ribeirão Preto 14049-900, SP, Brazil; luizeduardo@usp.br
4. Department of Epidemiology, Cardiovascular Disease Prevention and Health Promotion, National Institute of Cardiology, 04-635 Warsaw, Poland; lmalek@ikard.pl
5. Biodynamics and Human Performance Center, Department of Health Sciences and Kinesiology, Georgia Southern University (Armstrong Campus), Savannah, GA 31419, USA; aflatt@georgiasouthern.edu
6. Department of Heart Rhythm Disorders, National Institute of Cardiology, 04-628 Warsaw, Poland; rb@ikard.pl
* Correspondence: jgasior@wum.edu.pl or gasiorjakub@gmail.com; Tel.: +48-793-199-222

Received: 30 November 2020; Accepted: 16 December 2020; Published: 17 December 2020

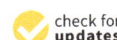

Abstract: Monitoring of markers reflecting cardiac autonomic activity before and during stressful situations may be useful for identifying the physiological state of an athlete and may have medical or performance implications. The study aimed to determine group and individual changes in short-term (5 min) and ultra-short-term (1 min) heart rate (HR), respiratory rate (RespRate), and time-domain heart rate variability (HRV) parameters during sympathetic nervous system activity (SNSa) stimulation among professional endurance athletes. Electrocardiographic recordings were performed in stable measurement conditions (Baseline) and during SNSa stimulation via isometric handgrip in 12 elite modern pentathlonists. Significant increases in short-term HR and decreases in time-domain HRV parameters with no changes in RespRate were observed during SNSa stimulation. Significant differences were observed between Baseline (all minutes) and the last (i.e., 5th) minute of SNSa stimulation for ultra-short-term parameters. Analysis of intra-individual changes revealed some heterogeneity in responses. The study provides baseline responses of HR, RespRate, and time-domain HRV parameters to SNSa stimulation among elite pentathlonists, which may be useful for identifying abnormal responses among fatigued or injured (e.g., concussed) athletes. More attention to individual analysis seems to be necessary when assessing physiological responses to sympathetic stimuli in professional endurance athletes.

Keywords: heart rate variability; heart rate; respiratory rate; modern pentathlon; athletes; physiological state; autonomic nervous system

1. Introduction

Elite athletes' training process demands regular monitoring of fatigue and training response to optimize its effects and avoid over-training [1–3]. Autonomic regulation of the cardiocirculatory system is an important determinant of training adaptation [4,5]. Heart rate (HR) and heart rate variability (HRV) parameters are becoming increasingly popular as non-invasive and inexpensive biomarkers reflecting changes in parasympathetic and sympathetic activity [2,6,7]. Low resting HR and high HRV are beneficial to the performance of the sport [8,9]. It was shown that athletes who practice sports with attention tasks (e.g., pistol shooting, archery) and who presented fewer changes in stress related HRV measures performed better through improved accuracy [10,11]. Therefore, monitoring of parameters reflecting cardiac autonomic activity during the training session, shortly before and/or during professional competition may be useful in identifying the physiological state of an athlete [11,12], which can be further used to improve performance and consequently achieve better sport results.

HRV alterations have been commonly analyzed on the basis of group changes in endurance athletes [13–15], which is ineffective in detecting individual athletes' responses [16]. By analyzing individual HRV changes, one can identify athletes who show large or small responsiveness to the different stressors or challenges [16,17]. Consequently, it was suggested that HRV be assessed in athletes on an individual basis [4].

The isometric handgrip strength test is a non-invasive and validated tool used to stimulate cardiovascular and autonomic function [18–20]. Increased HR during isometric exercise [21] is due to vagal withdrawal [6,18,22,23] concurrent with increased sympathetic activity [6]. Clinicians have analyzed cardiovascular and/or hemodynamic responses to isometric exercise in different groups of patients, mostly using protocols with 2–6 min of sustained handgrip strength exercise [24–29]. There is a lack of studies assessing autonomic response to handgrip isometric exercise in athletes and how the HRV alterations to handgrip exercise can be used to assess the sport performance. Very recently, autonomic responsiveness to isometric handgrip has been investigated as a potential indicator of training fatigue [30]. Further investigation into practical assessment methodologies may influence protocols for monitoring athletic training status and wellbeing.

Coaches and sport practitioners strive for simplification of cardiovascular data acquisition in elite athletes [2,31,32]. Special attention has been given to (i) limiting the time needed to obtain reliable physiological outcomes and (ii) looking for parameters that can be used in the applied sports field. Several authors have demonstrated that vagally-mediated HRV parameters acquired from ultra-short-term 1 min electrocardiography recordings in elite athletes are reliable [31–34]. Recently, it was shown that in addition to commonly used HRV parameters, HR and respiratory rate calculated based on ultra-short-term 1 min recordings could be reliably used in elite endurance athletes [35].

The purpose of this study was to determine group and individual changes during sympathetic nervous system activity stimulation in short-term and ultra-short-term HR, respiratory rate, and HRV parameters commonly used in applied sports settings among elite modern pentathlonists. Determining the sensitivity of these metrics to the isometric stimulus may aid sports practitioners with HRV assessment during similar tasks performed in training and competition.

2. Materials and Methods

Details of the study participants and methods have been presented elsewhere [35]. A total of 12 elite modern pentathlonists (8♂) with professional careers ranging from 7 to 15 years, aged 17–26, participated in the study. Briefly, to be included in the study, participants should be an active athlete [36] currently in possession of the modern pentathlon license from the National Association; be in the pre-season period; declare the absence of diseases and/or regular use of medications affecting the cardiopulmonary system and/or interfering with the autonomic nervous system (ANS); accept and follow the measurement rules and protocol. To collect and control potential confounding variables influencing HRV, a questionnaire proposed by Laborde et al. [37] was used. The athletes were instructed to maintain normal sleep behaviors (as usual in the 5 days before examination), refrain from physical activity the day before and on the day of study, eat a normal, usual light breakfast, and use the toilet (if needed) on the day of study before examinations. The examinations were carried out at least 1 h after home breakfast and before lunch.

The study was approved by the University Ethical Committee and followed the rules and principles of the Helsinki Declaration (SKE 01-01/2017, 7 March 2017, Warsaw, Poland). All athletes gave their informed written consent.

2.1. Electrocardiography Acquisition

Electrocardiography recordings (ECGs) were performed in a quiet, bright university room, with stable temperature and humidity. On the day of the study, each athlete underwent two ECG examinations. The first examination (6 min) was performed under established, controlled measurement conditions and was denoted as "Baseline" (B). The second examination (6 min) was performed during the sympathetic nervous system activity (SNSa) stimulation and was denoted as "SNSa stimulation" (SNSa). When the Baseline examination was finished, the athletes were instructed to grip the dynamometer, and SNSa stimulation examination was started. Twelve-lead ECG recordings (ECGs) (sampling frequency = 1000 Hz) were performed between 8:00 and 12:00 before lunch in a supine position using a portable personal computer with an integrated software system (Custo cardio 100 12-channel PC ECG system; Custo med GmbH, Ottobrunn, Germany). To stabilize HR and respiratory rate before starting appropriate ECG recordings (used to obtain RR intervals), athletes were instructed to lie in a supine position for 10 min [38] before Baseline recordings, and then the appropriate ECGs started. Athletes were encouraged to refrain from speaking and moving during the ECG examination.

2.2. Sympathetic Nervous System Activity Stimulation

To stimulate SNSa, subjects were asked to grip the dynamometer (Saehan hydraulic hand dynamometer, model SH5001, Saehan Corporation, Masan, South Korea, second handle position) at 30% of their maximal voluntary contraction (MVC) using their dominant hand for a 6 min period. The 30% of MVC was controlled by one researcher (B.H.), and the athletes were informed and encouraged to squeeze continuously at 30%, maintaining the adequate value of MVC. To establish the 30% of MVC, a handgrip strength test was performed according to the guideline commonly used in adults [39] seven days before the study.

2.3. Respiratory Rate

Respiratory rate (RespRate) during Baseline and SNSa stimulation was monitored using the Sony® HDRAS20 Action Camera with Wi-Fi. The abdomen, thorax, and neck were recorded. The athletes were not instructed how to breathe but were informed that the breathing pattern would be video-recoded. Calculation of the RespRate based on 5 min and 1 min video recordings was independently performed by two researchers (B.H., J.S.G.).

2.4. HRV Analysis

The detailed ECGs data acquisition and processing have been described in our previous study [35]. Briefly, short-term and ultra-short-term HR and HRV parameters were calculated based on 5 min and 1 min segments, respectively, of appropriate ECGs (recordings started after stabilization period) using Kubios HRV Standard 3.4 software (University of Eastern Finland, Kuopio, Finland) [40,41]. The following parameters were calculated: heart rate (HR), standard deviation of normal-to-normal RR intervals (SDNN), root mean square of successive differences between adjacent normal RR intervals (RMSSD), the log-transformed RMSSD (lnRMSSD), log transformation of the ratio between RMSSD (in ms) and mean RR interval (mRR, in ms), i.e., lnRMSSD/mRR.

Stationarity of the RR intervals and respiratory rate is required for the short-term frequency-domain HRV analysis [42,43]. The low- and high-frequency bands (LF and HF, respectively) of HRV are affected by (i) non-stationarities of the mean RR intervals and (ii) significant alterations or specified frequencies in breathing during recordings [37,44]. For instance, when any participant breathes very slowly, in the range of the LF band (~3 to 9 breaths per minute), the classical interpretation of the HF band as the vagal influence on the HR is flawed. Therefore, in studies where the immediate effect is measured, time-domain analysis is preferred. In the current study, HR increased, and RespRate decreased continuously during SNSa stimulation. Consequently, we assessed only time-domain HRV parameters.

2.5. Relationships between Changes in HR and RespRate and Changes in HRV Parameters

The significant relationship between HRV parameters and mean HR has been usually overlooked in HRV studies [45–47]. HRV alterations should be interpreted by taking into account respective changes in resting HR [48]. In addition to HR, the correlation between differences in RespRate and differences in HRV parameters were also assessed in the present study.

2.6. Statistical Analysis

The Kolmogorov–Smirnov test was used to assess the normality of the data distribution. Natural log transformation (ln) was used if the data were not normally distributed. A paired Student's t-test was employed to compare systematic changes between Baseline and SNSa stimulation in the analyzed parameters calculated based on 5 min recordings. One-way analysis of variance (ANOVA) with repeated measurements (with Tukey's HSD post hoc test) was performed to compare the results of analyzed variables calculated based on 1 min recordings. To illustrate the relationship among differences between SNSa stimulation and Baseline in HRV parameters (Parameter-diff) and (a) participants characteristics (age, body mass index, career time) or (b) differences between SNSa stimulation and Baseline in HR (HR-diff) and RespRate (RespRate-diff) (Figure S1—Supplementary Materials), Pearson's correlation coefficient (r) was calculated. The small sample size resulted in the figures with correlations being more useful as illustrative than as analytic.

To detect individual athletes' responses, tables with directional changes for all athletes individually are presented in Supplementary Materials (Tables S1 and S2). Recently, we showed acceptable reliability between Test and Retest of HR, RespRate, and HRV parameters calculated based on the first minute of the 5 min recordings [35]. In the current study, the parameters calculated based on the first minute of Baseline recordings were considered as a criterion for assessing parameters calculated based on the next minutes of the Baseline or 1st min of SNSa stimulation. The smallest worthwhile change (SWC) was calculated using formula $0.2 \times$ standard deviation [49] of values from the 1st min of Baseline recordings (Criterion) to assess whether parameters: (a) calculated based on the next minutes of Baseline increased (↑) or decreased (↓) more than SWC or did not change (-) in comparison to Criterion; (b) calculated based on the 1st min of SNSa stimulation increased (↑) or decreased (↓) more than SWC or did not change (-) in comparison to the Baseline Criterion. Parameters calculated based on the next minutes of SNSa stimulation (from 2nd to 5th) were compared to the previous min of SNSa stimulation (Supplementary Materials, Tables S1 and S2).

The threshold probability of $p < 0.05$ was taken as the level of significance for all statistical tests. Figure 1 was created and all calculations were performed using STATISTICA 12 (StatSoft Inc., Tulsa, OK, USA). GraphPad Prism 5 (GraphPad Software Inc., San Diego, CA, USA, 2005) was used to create Figures 2 and 3 and Figure S1.

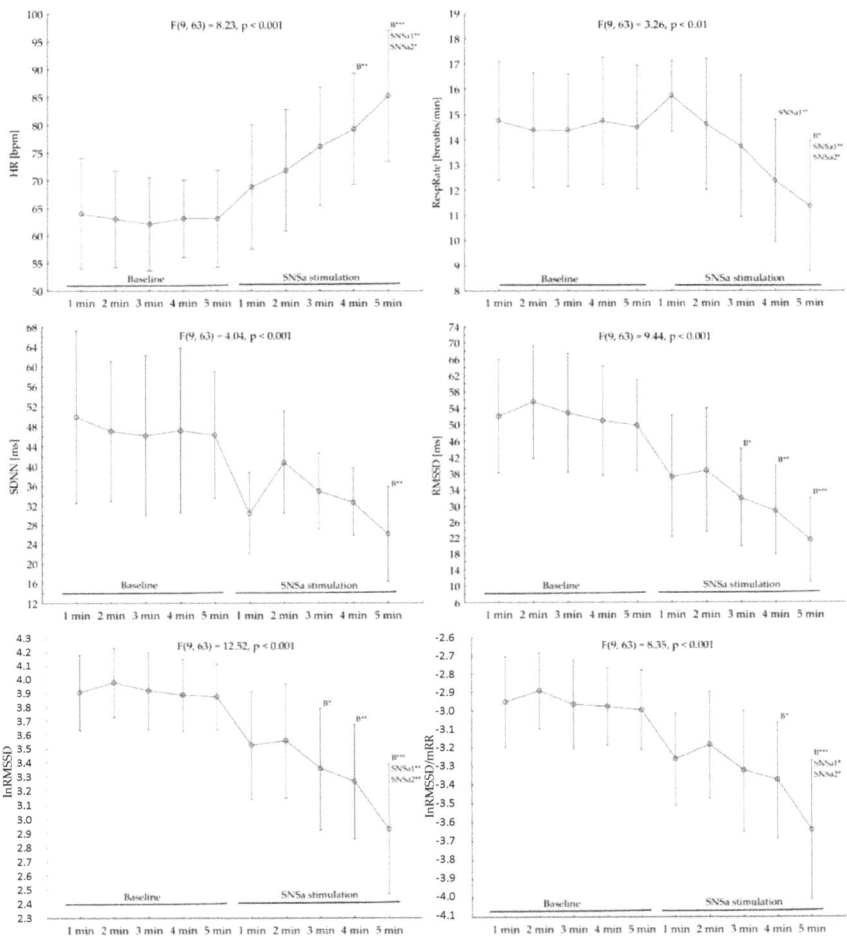

Figure 1. The group changes in heart rate (HR), respiratory rate (RespRate), and time-domain heart rate variability (HRV) parameters minute by minute during the Baseline and sympathetic nervous system activity (SNSa) stimulation recordings. B—significant difference versus Baseline (all minutes), SNSa1—significant difference versus the 1st min from SNSa stimulation, SNSa2—significant difference versus the 2nd min from SNSa stimulation, * $p < 0.05$, ** $p < 0.01$, *** $p < 0.001$.

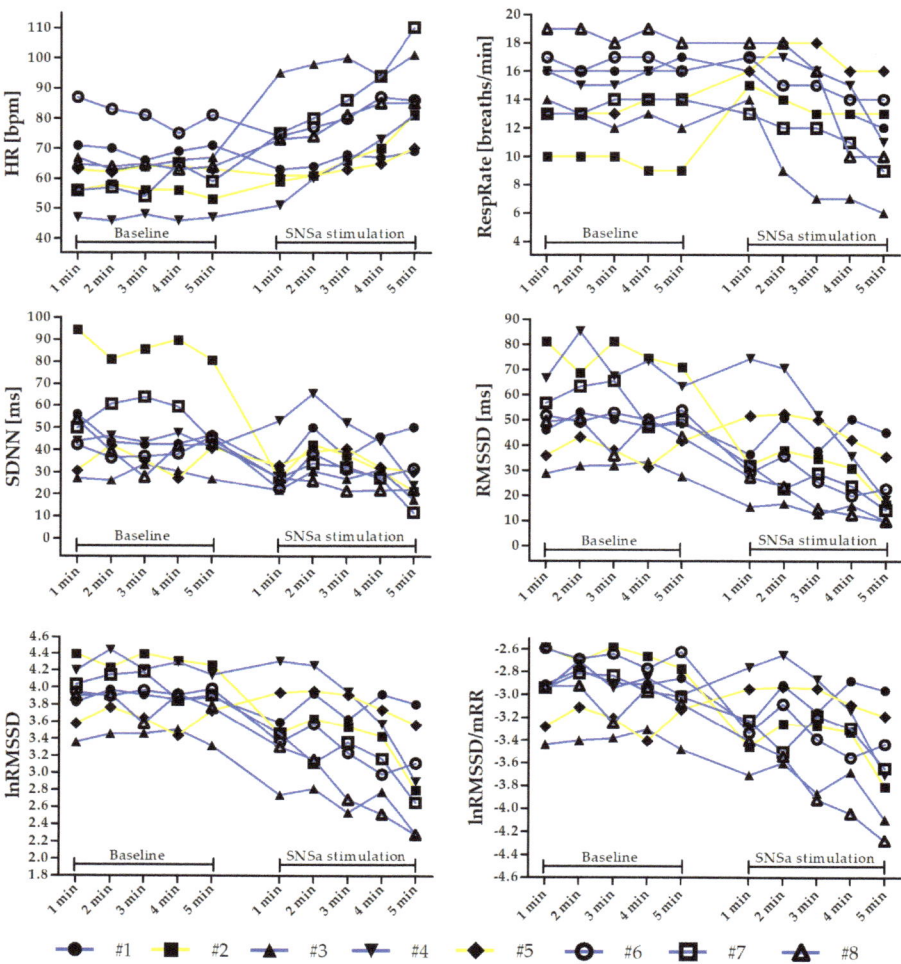

Figure 2. Individual changes in heart rate (HR), respiratory rate (RespRate), and heart rate variability (HRV) parameters minute by minute during the Baseline and sympathetic nervous system activity (SNSa) stimulation recordings. Individuals highlighted in yellow (#2 and #5) are those who increased the RespRate during SNSa stimulation.

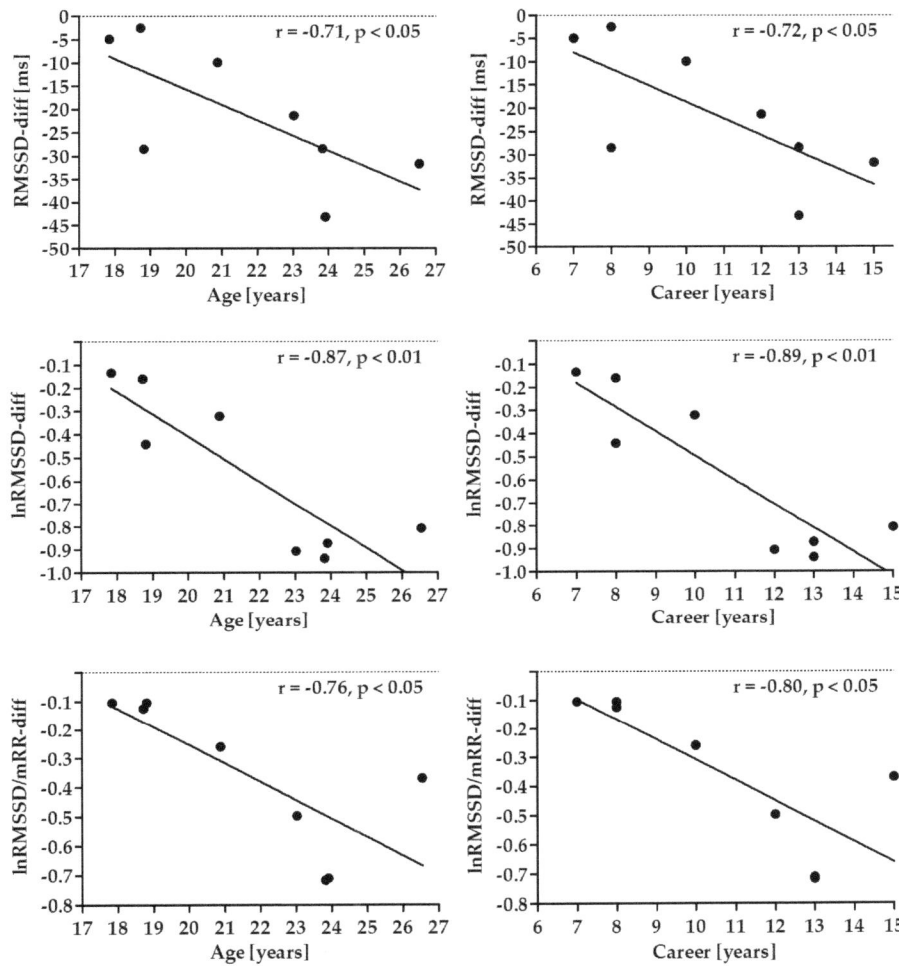

Figure 3. Correlation between differences in root mean square of successive differences (RMSSD) parameters and athlete's age and career time.

3. Results

3.1. Participants Information

Results of 8 male athletes were included in the statistical analysis (results of 4 participants out of 12 were excluded due to the detection of prolonged QTc interval > 450 ms, n = 2; left bundle branch block, n = 2). The mean (±SD) age, weight, height, body mass index (BMI), and duration of professional athletic career were: 21.7 years (±3.1), 75.9 kg (±9.5), 182.6 cm (±6.1), 22.7 kg/m^2 (±2.3), and 10.8 years (±2.9). Athletes declared participating in 19 training sessions (±2) per week during the normal in-season time.

3.2. Changes in Short-Term 5 min Parameters

Table 1 presents the results of short-term 5 min HR, RespRate, and HRV parameters from Baseline and SNSa stimulation. There was a significant increase in HR and a significant decrease in SDNN, RMSSD, lnRMSSD, and lnRMSSD/mRR. No significant changes were observed for RespRate.

Table 1. The effect of sympathetic nervous system activity (SNSa) stimulation on short-term 5 min heart rate (HR), respiratory rate (RespRate), and time-domain heart rate variability (HRV) parameters.

	Baseline	SNSa Stimulation	p
HR [bpm]	62.9 ± 9.7	77.8 ± 12.1	<0.05
RespRate [breaths per min]	15 ± 3	13 ± 3	0.41
SDNN [ms]	45.9 ± 20.0	26.8 ± 6.0	<0.05
RMSSD [ms]	48.2 ± 21.2	26.9 ± 12.2	<0.01
lnRMSSD	3.78 ± 0.49	3.21 ± 0.44	<0.01
lnRMSSD/mRR	−3.09 ± 0.35	−3.45 ± 0.34	<0.01

SNSa—sympathetic nervous system activation; HR—heart rate; RespRate—respiratory rate; SDNN—standard deviation of normal-to-normal RR intervals; RMSSD—root mean square of successive differences between adjacent normal RR intervals; mRR—mean RR interval; ln—log-transformed.

3.3. Changes in Ultra-Short Term 1-min Parameters

A one-way repeated-measures ANOVA revealed that there was a significant main effect of SNSa stimulation in all analyzed parameters (F between 3.26 and 12.52). Post hoc tests showed that there were no significant differences between 1 min parameters from 5 min ECG Baseline recordings in all analyzed indices (Figure 1). However, analysis of intra-individual changes revealed that some athletes presented worthwhile alterations between parameters calculated based on the 1st min (named Criterion) and the next minutes during Baseline recordings (Figure 2 and Tables S1 and S2).

HR gradually increased during SNSa stimulation. $HR_{(SNSa4)}$ (mean: 79.4 ± 12 bpm) and $HR_{(SNSa5)}$ (85.4 ± 14.1 bpm) were significantly higher than $HR_{(B)}$ (all minutes—between 62.1 and 64.0 bpm), and $HR_{(SNSa5)}$ was significantly higher than $HR_{(SNSa1)}$ (68.9 ± 13.5 bpm) and $HR_{(SNSa2)}$ (71.9 ± 13.2 bpm). Interestingly, two athletes (#1 and #6) presented a worthwhile decrease in HR values during the 1st min of SNSa stimulation in comparison to the Criterion from Baseline. A similar pattern of changes during the next minute of SNSa stimulation, i.e., increasing HR values, was observed for most athletes.

RespRate initially increased during SNSa stimulation and then gradually decreased with time. RespRate from the last minute of SNSa stimulation ($RespRate_{(SNSa5)}$ 11 ± 3 breaths/min) was significantly lower than RespRate from Baseline ($RespRate_{(B)}$ all minutes—between 14 and 15 breaths/min), 1st min ($RespRate_{(SNSa1)}$ 16 ± 2 breaths/min) and 2nd min ($RespRate_{(SNSa2)}$ 15 ± 3 breaths/min) of SNSa stimulation. Not all athletes presented the same pattern of breathing rate alterations during SNSa stimulation. Two athletes increased and then slightly decreased the RespRate (#2 and #5—yellow lines), whereas others monotonically decreased the RespRate (blue lines, Figure 2).

Generally, a similar pattern of changes during SNSa stimulation was observed for all time-domain HRV parameters. The first minute of SNSa stimulation was accompanied by a nominal decrease in SDNN, RMSSD, lnRMSSD, and lnRMSSD/mRR compared to Baseline. Then, a nominal increase followed by a gradual decrease in all parameters was observed.

Statistically significant differences were observed between Baseline (all minutes) and last minute (5th) of SNSa stimulation (Figure 1). Detailed results are presented as follows: SDNN: $_{(B)}$ between 46.1 ms and 49.9 ms vs. $_{(SNSa5)}$ 26.1 ± 11.7 ms; RMSSD: $_{(B)}$ between 49.8 ms and 55.6 ms vs. $_{(SNSa5)}$ 21.4 ± 12.5 ms; lnRMSSD: $_{(B)}$ between 3.87 and 3.98 vs. $_{(SNSa5)}$ 2.93 ± 0.55; lnRMSSD/mRR: $_{(B)}$ between −2.89 and −3.00 vs. $_{(SNSa5)}$ −3.64 ± 0.44.

Additionally, $lnRMSSD_{SNSa5}$ and $lnRMSSD/mRR_{SNSa5}$ presented significantly lower values than these parameters calculated based on the 1st min of SNSa stimulation ($lnRMSSD_{SNSa1}$: 3.52 ± 0.46 and $lnRMSSD/mRR_{SNSa1}$: −3.26 ± 0.29) and the 2nd min of SNSa stimulation ($lnRMSSD_{SNSa2}$: 3.55 ± 0.49 and $lnRMSSD/mRR_{SNSa2}$: −3.19 ± 0.35).

A nominal decrease in vagally-mediated time-domain HRV parameters (RMSSD, lnRMSSD) during the 1st min of SNSa stimulation, observed for the group statistic, was not presented by all athletes when assessed individually. Worthwhile increases in these parameters in comparison to Baseline Criterion were noted for two athletes (#4 and #5).

3.4. Relationship among Differences between SNSa Stimulation and Baseline in HRV Parameters and Participants' Characteristics

There were no significant correlations between age, BMI and career time and differences in HR, RespRate, and SDNN. Differences in RMSSD parameters were significantly negatively correlated with age and career time (Figure 3). There were no significant correlations between these parameters and BMI.

3.5. Correlation between Differences in HRV Parameters and Differences in HR or RespRate

The correlations for SNSa–Baseline differences between HRV parameters and HR (column A) or RespRate (column B) are shown as Supplementary Materials in Figure S1. For 5 min short-term RMSSD, lnRMSSD, and lnRMSSD/mRR, SNSa stimulation–Baseline differences are more correlated to the differences in HR (HR-diff) than to the differences in RespRate (RespRate-diff). For short-term SDNN, SNSa stimulation–Baseline difference was more correlated with the RespRate-diff than the HR-diff. Significant, negative correlations were observed for the association between HR-diff and lnRMSSD-diff ($r = -0.72$, $p < 0.05$).

4. Discussion

In the current study, we explored grouped and individual responses of short-term and ultra-short-term HR, RespRate, and time-domain HRV parameters to sympathetic nervous system activity stimulation in elite modern pentathlonists. When analyzing the whole group, we observed a significant increase in short-term (5 min) HR and a significant decrease in short-term SDNN and vagally-mediated HRV parameters. There was no significant group change in RespRate, even though the mean values decreased nominally.

Sustained isometric exercise using a handgrip dynamometer has been commonly used by clinicians to compare cardiovascular and hemodynamic responses between groups of patients and healthy controls [27,29,50–52]. In athletes, isometric handgrip contraction has been used less frequently to evaluate cardiac autonomic modulation during physical exertion [53]. Abaji et al. compared HRV results between groups of concussed and control athletes [53]. Authors observed significantly different responses between groups—post-concussion athletes showed significantly lower vagally-mediated high-frequency power calculated based on the 3 min recordings during isometric handgrip contraction (30% MVC). They concluded that monitoring of HRV in athletes may aid diagnosis and provide insight into the safe return to play [53]. Very recently (2020), a research group in Spain published a protocol with the objective to determine changes in the performance of professional athletes following an HRV-guided training period [3]. By referencing studies published in recent years [54–56], authors stated that HRV-guided training in endurance athletes enables sports practitioners to better adapt training loads to an individual athlete in search of a better recovery and sports outcomes [3].

No significant differences were observed between each 1 min segment and the Criterion 1st min from 5 min ECG Baseline recordings in all analyzed indices, in line with a study by Flatt and Esco from 2016 [31]. Authors also demonstrated that randomly selected 1 min lnRMSSD segments within a standard 5-min ECG recording period were no different from the Criterion among collegiate athletes [32].

In our opinion, the main observation could be focused on parameters calculated based on the last minute from Baseline recordings and the first min of SNSa stimulation recordings. The isometric handgrip exercise is not a sports competition. Nevertheless, the effect and procedure of squeezing the dynamometer's handle may be, to some extent, considered as pre-competition stress and comparable to, e.g., shooting performance. We did not observe statistically significant differences in all measured indices between parameters calculated based on the last min (5th) of the Baseline recordings and the first min of SNSa stimulation recordings. However, the lack of statistical significance does not imply that the intervention/stimulus was not clinically or practically relevant [57]. In the current study, analysis of intra-individual alterations in analyzed parameters during SNSa stimulation revealed different worthwhile athletes' responses to the applied stimulus. In the whole group, HR and RespRate increased, and HRV parameters decreased during 1st min of SNSa stimulation. However, not all of the elite endurance athletes presented the same pattern of alterations. For example, two athletes (#2 and #5) started to breathe faster during SNSa stimulation, and their HRs increased only slightly. However, for athlete #2, a decrease and for athlete #5, an increase in vagally-mediated HRV parameters was observed, respectively. Therefore, our findings support the suggestion that HRV must be assessed in athletes on an individual basis [4,16].

Fewer changes in stress related HRV parameters during attention tasks, such as pistol shooting, improved accuracy [10,11]. Interestingly, changes resulting from SNSa stimulation in short-term (5 min) vagally-mediated HRV parameters were higher in athletes with age and longer careers. A long-term professional career is associated with electrocardiographic alterations in endurance elite athletes [58]. This group has an elevated parasympathetic activity, consequently lower HR and higher baseline HRV compared to, e.g., recreational athletes or non-athletic matched controls [58]. High baseline HRV has a greater margin to decrease. Inversely, low HRV cannot decrease too much lower, especially with concomitant high values of HR. Taylor et al. underlined that a smaller tachycardiac response to isometric exercise in non-athlete older compared to younger men is associated with an inability to decrease cardiac vagal tone below an already reduced baseline level [18]. In our study, there was no significant correlation between baseline HR or HRV and professional career, i.e., athletes with longer professional career did not present lower HR and/or higher HRV than athletes with shorter careers. Therefore, higher changes in short-term vagally-mediated HRV parameters resulted from SNSa stimulation in athletes with longer careers were not related to high baseline values in these groups of athletes.

Not unexpectedly, alterations resulting from SNSa stimulation in lnRMSSD were associated with the changes in HR. A previous study showed that changes in time-domain HRV parameter values obtained from two measurements performed during stable conditions with a one-week interval between tests without external stimulus were shown to be affected by differences in HR in this group of athletes [35]. Even a minimal change in HR considerably altered HRV [59]. Consequently, changes in HRV parameters in sports practitioners should be analyzed, taking into account concomitant changes in HR, such as lnRMSSD/mRR [2,35]. Here, lnRMSSD/mRR also showed differences between Baseline and SNSa stimulation, demonstrating that the vagal modulation is altered during the handgrip test and is not a simple consequence of HR changes.

To check if the autonomic responsiveness, i.e., the HRV differences between SNSa stimulation and Baseline, is related to the athlete's characteristics (age, BMI, and career time), the correlation was analyzed. RMSSD parameters were negatively correlated to the athlete's age and career time. However, since correlation plots are very similar for the two characteristics, it is very likely that the correlation between RMSSD and career time is dependent on the athlete's age. It is known that RMSSD decreases with the natural aging process [60]. Therefore, we believe that the different age is, at least in part, responsible for the individual differences in the autonomic responsiveness to the handgrip test. On the other hand, it does not explain why some individuals increased RespRate during SNSa stimulation while others did not.

Uncontrolled variables within experimental conditions may significantly influence HRV results [61]. Careful consideration of such crucial contextual, environmental, physiological, and methodological factors is required to obtain more accurate and reproducible results. Time of day to record the data (in the case of short-time recordings); subject-characteristic variables (health and physical activity status, control for medication, food and water consumption, voiding of the bladder); the position of the body during short-time recordings; the quality of recorded signals (recording period length, detection or recording method, sampling frequency, breathing pacing—paced or free breathing); as well as the tools used to analyze HRV values (software, removal of artifacts) are examples of such factors [61–64]. In the current study, to collect and control most of the mentioned variables influencing HRV, we used the questionnaire proposed by Laborde et al. [37].

Limitations of the current study were pointed out previously [35]. The small sample of only males and cross-sectional study design limits the generalizability of the study's findings and hinders sex subgroup comparisons. HRV data were obtained during supine ECG recordings performed in controlled laboratory settings. HR monitors may be more practical to collect RR intervals in athletes than traditional ECG, especially during sports competition [65]. However, RR intervals obtained using an HR monitor may add uncertainty to the analysis and interpretation of HRV [66,67]. ECG screening among professional athletes before including the data for detailed HRV analysis was suggested [35].

Electrocardiographic pre-participation screening followed by periodic ECG monitoring in competitive athletes has been established as an easily accessible and effective first-line test in diagnostics of various cardiovascular disorders, which may put athletes at risk of potentially life-threatening events [68]. ECG can be used to detect the signs of a physiological adaptation to exercise called athlete's heart and to differentiate them from potentially pathologic changes, which should require further management [69]. Electrocardiographic monitoring during exercise can be used to assure a linear increase in HR in parallel with increasing exercise intensity until the individual's maximal HR and to analyze HR recovery post-exercise. These data can then be utilized to optimize the training effects or to detect early signs of overtraining characterized, among others, by decreased maximal HR and prolonged HR recovery [70]. Finally, both overtraining and pathological heart conditions may manifest as supraventricular and ventricular arrhythmias during exercise or at rest detected by various ECG monitoring tools, which have been continuously adapted to the sporting environment [71].

In the current study, we did not evaluate cardiac function using echocardiography. Echocardiography is currently not a part of the routine pre-participation assessment of athletes [72]. It is usually performed in cases of suspected abnormalities after personal and family history, physical examination, or ECG. However, it may potentially disclose changes undetected by routine screening, including valvular disease (bicuspid aortic valve, mitral valve prolapse), coronary artery anomalies in younger athletes and dilatation of the aorta, late-onset cardiomyopathies, and wall motion abnormalities due to myocarditis or coronary artery disease in older athletes [73]. For these reasons, there is a growing belief that if it is available and reliable, it may be added to the baseline pre-participation screening panel in athletes.

5. Conclusions

Our findings provide baseline responses of short-term and ultra-short-term HR, RespRate, and time-domain HRV parameters to sympathetic nervous system activity stimulation among elite modern pentathletes that can be used in future studies for comparison with, e.g., concussed pentathletes. These data show "normal" responses, which may, therefore, aid in the identification of abnormal responses (as well as recovery) among concussed athletes. Analysis of inter-individual responses of modifiable parameters (e.g., breathing rate) to a specified stimulus may help in the identification of athletes that will benefit from practical techniques aimed at avoiding pre-performance stress, improve performance in sports and achieve better sport results. The handgrip test can be used as a tool in the analysis of autonomic responsiveness to sympathetic stimulation in pentathletes, with potential application to athletes from other modalities of sports.

Supplementary Materials: The following are available online at http://www.mdpi.com/2075-4418/10/12/1104/s1, Figure S1: Relationship among differences between sympathetic nervous system activity (SNSa) stimulation and Baseline in heart rate variability (HRV) parameters (Parameter-diff) and heart rate (HR) (HR-diff) (A) and respiratory rate (RespRate) (RespRate-diff) (B), Table S1: Individual athletes' responses in heart rate (HR) and respiratory rate (RespRate) during sympathetic nervous system activity (SNSa) stimulation, Table S2: Individual athletes' responses in standard deviation of normal-to-normal RR intervals (SDNN) and root mean square of successive differences (RMSSD) parameters during sympathetic nervous system activity (SNSa) stimulation.

Author Contributions: J.S.G. and B.H. conceived and designed the experiment; B.H. and J.S.G. acquired the data; R.B. analyzed electrocardiography recordings; J.S.G. and B.H. analyzed the data (RR intervals) for heart rate variability and statistical analysis; J.S.G., B.H., L.E.V.S., Ł.M., and A.A.F. interpreted the data; J.S.G., B.H., L.E.V.S., Ł.M., and A.A.F. drafted the work (writing—original draft preparation); J.S.G., B.H., L.E.V.S., Ł.M., A.A.F., R.B., and B.W. revised it critically for important intellectual content (review and editing); Supervision—J.S.G.; Funding acquisition (article processing charge)—B.W.; All authors—J.S.G., B.H., L.E.V.S., Ł.M., A.A.F., R.B., and B.W.—approved the final version of the manuscript to be published. All authors have read and agreed to the published version of the manuscript.

Funding: This research received no external funding.

Acknowledgments: This study was a continuation of a study completed as a part of a Master's thesis by B.H. supervised by J.S.G. We thank the athletes for participation in the study and undergraduate student Aleksandra Kędziorek for her help with the electrocardiography data acquisition.

Conflicts of Interest: The authors declare no conflict of interest.

References

1. Młyńczak, M.; Krysztofiak, H. Discovery of Causal Paths in Cardiorespiratory Parameters: A Time Independent Approach in Elite Athletes. *Front. Physiol.* **2018**, *9*, 1455. [CrossRef]
2. Buchheit, M. Monitoring training status with HR measures: Do all roads lead to Rome? *Front. Physiol.* **2014**, *5*, 73. [CrossRef] [PubMed]
3. Carrasco-Poyatos, M.; González-Quílez, A.; Martínez-González-Moro, I.; Granero-Gallegos, A. HRV-Guided Training for Professional Endurance Athletes: A Protocol for a Cluster-Randomized Controlled Trial. *Int. J. Environ. Res. Public Health* **2020**, *17*, 5465. [CrossRef] [PubMed]
4. Plews, D.J.; Laursen, P.B.; Stanley, J.; Kilding, A.E.; Buchheit, M. Training adaptation and heart rate variability in elite endurance athletes: Opening the door to effective monitoring. *Sports* **2013**, *43*, 773–781. [CrossRef] [PubMed]
5. Vitale, J.A.; Bonato, M.; La Torre, A.; Banfi, G. Heart Rate Variability in Sport Performance: Do Time of Day and Chronotype Play A Role? *J. Clin. Med.* **2019**, *8*, 723. [CrossRef]
6. Iellamo, F.; Pizzinelli, P.; Massaro, M.; Raimondi, G.; Peruzzi, G.; Legramante, J.M. Muscle metaboreflex contribution to sinus node regulation during static exercise: Insights from spectral analysis of heart rate variability. *Circulation* **1999**, *100*, 27–32. [CrossRef]
7. Bourdillon, N.; Schmitt, L.; Yazdani, S.; Vesin, J.M.; Millet, G.P. Minimal Window Duration for Accurate HRV Recording in Athletes. *Front. Neurosci.* **2017**, *11*, 456. [CrossRef]
8. De Meersman, R.E. Heart rate variability and aerobic fitness. *Am. Heart J.* **1993**, *125*, 726–731. [CrossRef]
9. Nummela, A.; Hynynen, E.; Kaikkonen, P.; Rusko, H. High-intensity endurance training increases nocturnal heart rate variability in sedentary participants. *Biol. Sport* **2016**, *33*, 7–13.
10. Thompson, A.G.; Swain, D.P.; Branch, J.D.; Spina, R.J.; Grieco, C.R. Autonomic response to tactical pistol performance measured by heart rate variability. *J. Strength Cond. Res.* **2015**, *29*, 926–933. [CrossRef]
11. Ortega, E.; Wang, C.J.K. Pre-performance Physiological State: Heart Rate Variability as a Predictor of Shooting Performance. *Appl. Psychophysiol. Biofeedback* **2018**, *43*, 75–85. [CrossRef]
12. Schneider, C.; Hanakam, F.; Wiewelhove, T.; Alexander Döweling, A.; Kellmann, M.; Meyer, T.; Pfeiffer, M.; Ferrauti, A. Heart Rate Monitoring in Team Sports—A Conceptual Framework for Contextualizing Heart Rate Measures for Training and Recovery Prescription. *Front. Physiol.* **2018**, *9*, 639. [CrossRef] [PubMed]
13. Schmitt, L.; Willis, S.J.; Fardel, A.; Coulmy, N.; Millet, G.P. Live high-train low guided by daily heart rate variability in elite Nordic-skiers. *Eur. J. Appl. Physiol.* **2018**, *118*, 419–428. [CrossRef] [PubMed]
14. Deus, L.A.; Sousa, C.V.; Rosa, T.S.; Filho, J.M.S.; Santos, P.A.; Barbosa, L.D.; Silva Aguiar, S.; Souza, L.H.R.; Simões, H.G. Heart rate variability in middle-aged sprint and endurance athletes. *Physiol. Behav.* **2019**, *205*, 39–43. [CrossRef] [PubMed]

15. Bentley, R.F.; Vecchiarelli, E.; Banks, L.; Gonçalves, P.E.O.; Thomas, S.G.; Goodman, J.M. Heart rate variability and recovery following maximal exercise in endurance athletes and physically active individuals. *Appl. Physiol. Nutr. Metab.* **2020**, *45*, 1138–1144. [CrossRef] [PubMed]
16. Muñoz-López, A.; Naranjo-Orellana, J. Individual versus team heart rate variability responsiveness analyses in a national soccer team during training camps. *Sci. Rep.* **2020**, *10*, 11726. [CrossRef] [PubMed]
17. Mann, T.N.; Lamberts, R.P.; Lambert, M.I. High responders and low responders: Factors associated with individual variation in response to standardized training. *Sports Med.* **2014**, *44*, 1113–1124. [CrossRef]
18. Taylor, J.A.; Hayano, J.; Seals, D.R. Lesser vagal withdrawal during isometric exercise with age. *J. Appl. Physiol.* **1995**, *79*, 805–811. [CrossRef]
19. Khurana, R.K.; Setty, A. The value of the isometric hand-grip test–studies in various autonomic disorders. *Clin. Auton. Res.* **1996**, *6*, 211–218. [CrossRef]
20. Millar, P.J.; MacDonald, M.J.; McCartney, N. Effects of isometric handgrip protocol on blood pressure and neurocardiac modulation. *Int. J. Sports Med.* **2011**, *32*, 174–180. [CrossRef]
21. Mitchell, J.H.; Wildenthal, K. Static (isometric) exercise and the heart: Physiological and clinical considerations. *Annu. Rev. Med.* **1974**, *25*, 369–381. [CrossRef] [PubMed]
22. Kluess, H.A.; Wood, R.H.; Welsch, M.A. Vagal modulation of the heart and central hemodynamics during handgrip exercise. *Am. J. Physiol. Heart Circ. Physiol.* **2000**, *278*, H1648–H1652. [CrossRef] [PubMed]
23. Tulppo, M.P.; Makikallio, T.H.; Seppanen, T.; Laukkanen, R.T.; Huikuri, H.V. Vagal modulation of heart rate during exercise: Effects of age and physical fitness. *Am. J. Physiol.* **1998**, *274*, H424–H429. [CrossRef] [PubMed]
24. Kurita, A.; Takase, B.; Hikita, H.; Uehata, A.; Nishioka, T.; Nagayoshi, H.; Satomura, K.; Nakao, S. Frequency domain heart rate variability and plasma norepinephrine level in the coronary sinus during handgrip exercise. *Clin. Cardiol.* **1999**, *22*, 207–212. [CrossRef] [PubMed]
25. Stewart, J.M.; Montgomery, L.D.; Glover, J.L.; Medow, M.S. Changes in regional blood volume and blood flow during static handgrip. *Am. J. Physiol. Heart Circ. Physiol.* **2007**, *292*, H215–H223. [CrossRef] [PubMed]
26. Mäki-Petäjä, K.M.; Barrett, S.M.; Evans, S.V.; Cheriyan, J.; McEniery, C.M.; Wilkinson, I.B. The Role of the Autonomic Nervous System in the Regulation of Aortic Stiffness. *Hypertension* **2016**, *68*, 1290–1297. [CrossRef]
27. Almeida, L.B.; Peçanha, T.; Mira, P.A.C.; Souza, L.V.; da Silva, L.P.; Martinez, D.G.; Freitas, I.M.G.; Laterza, M.C. Cardiac Autonomic Dysfunction in Offspring of Hypertensive Parents During Exercise. *Int. J. Sports Med.* **2017**, *38*, 1105–1110. [CrossRef]
28. Cauwenberghs, N.; Cornelissen, V.; Christle, J.W.; Hedman, K.; Myers, J.; Haddad, F.; Kuznetsova, T. Impact of age, sex and heart rate variability on the acute cardiovascular response to isometric handgrip exercise. *J. Hum. Hypertens.* **2020**. [CrossRef]
29. Sherman, S.R.; Schroeder, E.C.; Baynard, T.; Fernhall, B.; Hilgenkamp, T.I.M. Hemodynamic Response to Isometric Handgrip Exercise in Adults with Intellectual Disability. *Med. Sci. Sports Exerc.* **2020**. [CrossRef]
30. Dobson, J.; Harris, B.; Claytor, A.; Stroud, L.; Berg, L.; Chrysosferidis, P. Selected Cardiovascular and Psychological Changes Throughout a Competitive Season in Collegiate Female Swimmers. *J. Strength Cond. Res.* **2020**, *34*, 3062–3069. [CrossRef]
31. Flatt, A.A.; Esco, M.R. Heart rate variability stabilization in athletes: Towards more convenient data acquisition. *Clin. Physiol. Funct. Imaging* **2016**, *36*, 331–336. [CrossRef] [PubMed]
32. Esco, M.R.; Flatt, A.A. Ultra-short-term heart rate variability indexes at rest and post-exercise in athletes: Evaluating the agreement with accepted recommendations. *J. Sports Sci. Med.* **2014**, *13*, 535–541. [PubMed]
33. Nakamura, F.Y.; Flatt, A.A.; Pereira, L.A.; Ramirez-Campillo, R.; Loturco, I.; Esco, M.R. Ultra-Short-Term Heart Rate Variability is Sensitive to Training Effects in Team Sports Players. *J. Sports Sci. Med.* **2015**, *14*, 602–605. [PubMed]
34. Pereira, L.A.; Flatt, A.A.; Ramirez-Campillo, R.; Loturco, I.; Nakamura, F.Y. Assessing Shortened Field-Based Heart-Rate-Variability-Data Acquisition in Team-Sport Athletes. *Int. J. Sports Physiol. Perform.* **2016**, *11*, 154–158. [CrossRef] [PubMed]
35. Hoffmann, B.; Flatt, A.A.; Silva, L.E.V.; Młyńczak, M.; Baranowski, R.; Dziedzic, E.; Werner, B.; Gąsior, J.S. A Pilot Study of the Reliability and Agreement of Heart Rate, Respiratory Rate and Short-Term Heart Rate Variability in Elite Modern Pentathlon Athletes. *Diagnostics* **2020**, *10*, 833. [CrossRef] [PubMed]

36. Araújo, C.G.; Scharhag, J. Athlete: A working definition for medical and health sciences research. *Scand. J. Med. Sci. Sports* **2016**, *26*, 4–7. [CrossRef]
37. Laborde, S.; Mosley, E.; Thayer, J.F. Heart Rate Variability and Cardiac Vagal Tone in Psychophysiological Research—Recommendations for Experiment Planning, Data Analysis, and Data Reporting. *Front. Psychol.* **2017**, *8*, 89. [CrossRef]
38. Lucini, D.; Marchetti, I.; Spataro, A.; Malacarne, M.; Benzi, M.; Tamorri, S.; Sala, R.; Pagani, M. Heart rate variability to monitor performance in elite athletes: Criticalities and avoidable pitfalls. *Int. J. Cardiol.* **2017**, *240*, 307–312. [CrossRef]
39. Fess, E.E.; Casanova, J.S. *Clinical Assessment Recommendations*, 2nd ed.; Grip Strength; American Society of Hand Therapists: Chicago, IL, USA, 1992; pp. 41–45.
40. Tarvainen, M.P.; Lipponen, J.; Niskanen, J.P.; Ranta-Aho, P.O. Kubios HRV (ver. 3.0.2). User's Guide. 2017. Available online: http://www.kubios.com/downloads/Kubios_HRV_Users_Guide.pdf (accessed on 21 July 2020).
41. Tarvainen, M.P.; Niskanen, J.P.; Lipponen, J.A.; Ranta-Aho, P.O.; Karjalainen, P.A. Kubios HRV-heart rate variability analysis software. *Comput. Methods Programs Biomed.* **2014**, *113*, 210–220. [CrossRef]
42. Magagnin, V.; Bassani, T.; Bari, V. Non-stationarities significantly distort short-term spectral, symbolic and entropy heart rate variability indices. *Physiol. Meas.* **2011**, *32*, 1775–1786. [CrossRef]
43. Quintana, D.S.; Alvares, G.A.; Heathers, J.A.J. Guidelines for Reporting Articles on Psychiatry and Heart rate variability (GRAPH): Recommendations to advance research communication. *Transl. Psychiatry* **2016**, *6*, e803. [CrossRef] [PubMed]
44. Hayano, J.; Yuda, E. Pitfalls of assessment of autonomic function by heart rate variability. *J. Physiol. Anthr.* **2019**, *38*, 3. [CrossRef] [PubMed]
45. Sacha, J.; Pluta, W. Alterations of an average heart rate change heart rate variability due to mathematical reasons. *Int. J. Cardiol.* **2008**, *128*, 444–447. [CrossRef] [PubMed]
46. Billman, G.E. The effect of heart rate on the heart rate variability response to autonomic interventions. *Front. Physiol.* **2013**, *4*, 222. [CrossRef]
47. de Geus, E.J.C.; Gianaros, P.J.; Brindle, R.C.; Jennings, J.R.; Berntson, G.G. Should heart rate variability be "corrected" for heart rate? Biological, quantitative, and interpretive considerations. *Psychophysiology* **2019**, *56*, e13287. [CrossRef]
48. Sacha, J.; Barabach, S.; Statkiewicz-Barabach, G.; Sacha, K.; Müller, A.; Piskorski, J.; Barthel, P.; Schmidt, G. How to strengthen or weaken the HRV dependence on heart rate—Description of the method and its perspectives. *Int. J. Cardiol.* **2013**, *168*, 1660–1663. [CrossRef]
49. Buchheit, M. Magnitudes matter more than Beetroot Juice. *Sport Perform. Sci. Rep.* **2018**, *1*, 1–3.
50. Bunsawat, K.; Baynard, T. Cardiac autonomic modulation and blood pressure responses to isometric handgrip and submaximal cycling exercise in individuals with down syndrome. *Clin. Auton. Res.* **2016**, *26*, 253–260. [CrossRef]
51. Idiaquez, J.; Idiaquez, J.F.; Iturriaga, R. Cardiovascular responses to isometric handgrip exercise in young patients with recurrent vasovagal syncope. *Auton. Neurosci.* **2018**, *212*, 23–27. [CrossRef]
52. Stępniewska, A.; Budnik, M.; Krzemiński, K.; Niewiadomski, W.; Gąsiorowska, A.; Opolski, G.; Kochanowski, J.; Mieczkowska, K.; Żukowska, K.; Szepietowska, K.; et al. Impaired hemodynamic response to tilt, handgrip and Valsalva manoeuvre in patients with takotsubo syndrome. *Auton. Neurosci.* **2019**, *220*, 102555. [CrossRef]
53. Abaji, J.P.; Curnier, D.; Moore, R.D.; Ellemberg, D. Persisting Effects of Concussion on Heart Rate Variability during Physical Exertion. *J. Neurotrauma* **2016**, *33*, 811–817. [CrossRef] [PubMed]
54. Nuuttila, O.P.; Nikander, A.; Polomoshnov, D.; Laukkanen, J.A.; Häkkinen, K. Effects of HRV-Guided vs. Predetermined Block Training on Performance, HRV and Serum Hormones. *Int. J. Sports Med.* **2017**, *38*, 909–920. [CrossRef] [PubMed]
55. Javaloyes, A.; Sarabia, J.M.; Lamberts, R.P.; Moya-Ramon, M. Training Prescription Guided by Heart Rate Variability in Cycling. *Int. J. Sports Physiol. Perform.* **2018**, *29*, 1–28. [CrossRef] [PubMed]
56. da Silva, D.F.; Ferraro, Z.M.; Adamo, K.B.; Machado, F.A. Endurance Running Training Individually Guided by HRV in Untrained Women. *J. Strength Cond. Res.* **2019**, *33*, 736–746. [CrossRef] [PubMed]
57. Page, P. Beyond statistical significance: Clinical interpretation of rehabilitation research literature. *Int. J. Sports Phys. Ther.* **2014**, *9*, 726–736. [PubMed]

58. Fagard, R. Athlete's heart. *Heart* **2003**, *89*, 1455–1461. [CrossRef]
59. Gąsior, J.S.; Sacha, J.; Jeleń, P.J.; Zieliński, J.; Przybylski, J. Heart Rate and Respiratory Rate Influence on Heart Rate Variability Repeatability: Effects of the Correction for the Prevailing Heart Rate. *Front. Physiol.* **2016**, *7*, 356. [CrossRef]
60. Natarajan, A.; Pantelopoulos, A.; Emir-Farinas, H.; Natarajan, P. Heart rate variability with photoplethysmography in 8 million individuals: A cross-sectional study. *Lancet Digit. Health* **2020**, *2*, e650–e657. [CrossRef]
61. Quintana, D.S.; Heathers, J. Considerations in the assessment of heart rate variability in biobehavioral research. *Front. Psychol.* **2014**, *5*, 805. [CrossRef]
62. Heathers, J. Everything Hertz: Methodological issues in short-term frequency-domain HRV. *Front. Physiol.* **2014**, *5*, 177. [CrossRef]
63. Fatisson, J.; Oswald, V.; LaLonde, F. Influence Diagram of Physiological and Environmental Factors Affecting Heart Rate Variability: An Extended Literature Overview. *Hear. Int.* **2016**, *11*, e32–e40. [CrossRef] [PubMed]
64. Vila, X.A.; Lado, M.J.; Cuesta-Morales, P. Evidence Based Recommendations for Designing Heart Rate Variability Studies. *J. Med. Syst.* **2019**, *43*, 311. [CrossRef] [PubMed]
65. Hernando, D.; Garatachea, N.; Almeida, R.; Casajús, J.A.; Bailón, R. Validation of Heart Rate Monitor Polar RS800 for Heart Rate Variability Analysis During Exercise. *J. Strength Cond. Res.* **2018**, *32*, 716–725. [CrossRef] [PubMed]
66. Wallen, M.B.; Hasson, D.; Theorell, T.; Canlon, B.; Osika, W. Possibilities and limitations of the polar RS800 in measuring heart rate variability at rest. *Eur. J. Appl. Physiol.* **2012**, *112*, 1153–1165. [CrossRef]
67. Bishop, S.A.; Dech, R.T.; Guzik, P.; Neary, J.P. Heart rate variability and implication for sport concussion. *Clin. Physiol. Funct. Imaging* **2018**, *38*, 733–742. [CrossRef]
68. Pelliccia, A.; Sharma, S.; Gati, S.; Bäck, M.; Börjesson, M.; Caselli, S.; Collet, J.P.; Corrado, D.; Drezner, J.A.; Halle, M.; et al. 2020 ESC Guidelines on sports cardiology and exercise in patients with cardiovascular disease. *Eur. Heart J.* **2020**, ehaa605. [CrossRef]
69. Sharma, S.; Drezner, J.A.; Baggish, A.; Papadakis, M.; Wilson, M.G.; Prutkin, J.M.; La Gerche, A.; Ackerman, M.J.; Borjesson, M.; Salerno, J.C.; et al. International recommendations for electrocardiographic interpretation in athletes. *Eur. Heart J.* **2018**, *39*, 1466–1480. [CrossRef]
70. Urhausen, A.; Kindermann, W. Diagnosis of overtraining: What tools do we have? *Sports Med.* **2002**, *32*, 95–102. [CrossRef]
71. Gajda, R. Is Continuous ECG Recording on Heart Rate Monitors the Most Expected Function by Endurance Athletes, Coaches, and Doctors? *Diagnostics* **2020**, *10*, 867. [CrossRef]
72. Corrado, D.; Basso, C.; Schiavon, M.; Pellicia, A.; Thiene, G. Pre-participation screening of young competitive athletes for prevention of sudden cardiac death. *J. Am. Coll. Cardiol.* **2008**, *52*, 1981–1989. [CrossRef]
73. Niederseer, D.; Rossi, V.A.; Kissel, C.; Scherr, J.; Caselli, S.; Tanner, F.C.; Bohm, P.; Schmied, C. Role of echocardiography in screening and evaluation of athletes. *Heart* **2020**. [CrossRef] [PubMed]

Publisher's Note: MDPI stays neutral with regard to jurisdictional claims in published maps and institutional affiliations.

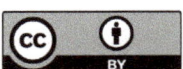

© 2020 by the authors. Licensee MDPI, Basel, Switzerland. This article is an open access article distributed under the terms and conditions of the Creative Commons Attribution (CC BY) license (http://creativecommons.org/licenses/by/4.0/).

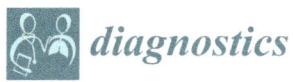

Article

Factors Related to Cardiac Troponin T Increase after Participation in a 100 Km Ultra-Marathon

Łukasz A. Małek [1,*], Anna Czajkowska [2], Anna Mróz [3], Katarzyna Witek [3], Dariusz Nowicki [2] and Marek Postuła [4]

1. Department of Epidemiology, Cardiovascular Disease Prevention and Health Promotion, National Institute of Cardiology, 04-635 Warsaw, Poland
2. Faculty of Tourism and Recreation, University of Physical Education in Warsaw, 00-809 Warsaw, Poland; anna.czajkowska@awf.edu.pl (A.C.); dariusz.nowicki@awf.edu.pl (D.N.)
3. Faculty of Physical Education, University of Physical Education in Warsaw, 00-809 Warsaw, Poland; anna.mroz@awf.edu.pl (A.M.); katarzyna.witek@awf.edu.pl (K.W.)
4. Department of Experimental and Clinical Pharmacology, Medical University of Warsaw, 02-097 Warsaw Poland; mpostula@wum.edu.pl
* Correspondence: lmalek@ikard.pl; Tel.: +48-22-815-65-56 (ext. 214)

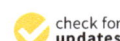

Received: 28 February 2020; Accepted: 16 March 2020; Published: 19 March 2020

Abstract: Background: Intensive and prolonged exercise leads to a rise of troponin concentration in blood. The mechanism responsible for troponin release during exercise remains ill-defined. The study aim was to search for risk factors of troponin increase after a prolonged endurance competition. Methods: The study included a group of 18 amateurs, healthy volunteers (median age 41.5 years, interquartile range – IQR 36–53 years, 83% male) who participated in a 100 km running ultra-marathon. Information on demographic characteristics, pre- and post-race heart rate, blood pressure, body composition and glucose, lactate (L), troponin T (hs-TnT) and C reactive protein (hs-CRP) concentration were obtained. Additionally, data on L and glucose levels every 9.2 km and fluid/food intakes during the race were collected. Results: There was a significant hs-TnT increase after the race exceeding upper reference values in 66% of runners (from 5 IQR 3–7 ng/L to 14 IQR 12–26 ng/L, $p < 0.0001$). None of the baseline parameters predicted a post-race hs-TnT increase. The only factors, correlating with changes of hs-TnT were mean L concentration during the race (rho = 0.52, $p = 0.03$) and change of hs-CRP concentration (rho = 0.59, $p = 0.01$). Conclusions: Participation in a 100 km ultra-marathon leads to a modest, but significant hs-TnT increase in the majority of runners. Among analysed parameters only mean lactate concentration during the race and change in hs-CRP correlated with troponin change.

Keywords: running; exercise; marathon; troponin; risk factor

1. Introduction

Regular physical activity leads to many health benefits including cardio-protective activity [1,2]. Recent guidelines of the European Society of Cardiology have increased the recommended weekly volume of moderate to vigorous exercise from 150 min to 210–420 min as optimal cardiovascular prevention [3]. However, there is a group of athletes who far exceed these recommendations by engaging in long-lasting training and ultra-endurance competitions. The effects of these extreme forms of exercise on health are much less studied [2].

Bouts of intensive or long-lasting exercise (such as marathons or ultra-marathons) have been shown to increase blood levels of cardiac troponin, a known selective marker for myocardial injury and a major component of a current diagnosis of myocardial infarction [4–7]. Troponin rise after exercise is usually discrete with levels returning to reference values within hours [8] and may be accompanied by an increase of natriuretic peptide levels and transient decrease of left or right ventricular systolic function without long-term consequences [9–12]. In line with that, recent studies with new imaging techniques demonstrated that intensive endurance training does not seem to promote myocardial fibrosis [6,13–15].

It is believed that cardiac troponin released after endurance exercise comes from the cytosolic pool and does not signify injury to contractile parts of the cardiomyocytes [4,7]. However, the exact mechanism explaining troponin rise related to physical activity remains ill-defined [4,7]. It has been previously related to athletes age and experience, exercise duration and intensity potentially influencing dehydration, inflammation or pH imbalance during the exercise [4,7]. More detailed knowledge of the risk factors of this form of troponin increase could help in understanding the mechanism behind this phenomenon. They may also improve differential diagnosis in case of post-exercise suspicion of the coronary events in athletes [5,7].

Therefore, the study aimed to search for risk factors of troponin increase after participation in a 100 km ultra-marathon in middle-age, amateur healthy runners.

2. Materials and Methods

2.1. Subjects and Design

The study was conducted during a 100 km running ultra-marathon on flat terrain (asphalt, bitumen track and short parts of cobblestone), which took place on 10th November 2018 at the University of Physical Education in Warsaw (www.supermaraton100lecia.pl). The race consisted of 65.10 laps of 1535.89 m distance and was accredited by the Polish Athletics Association as National Championships on 100 km.

Out of 204 runners taking part in the race, we included 18 amateurs, healthy runners (3 females) who volunteered to participate in the study and to follow the whole protocol of the study.

Each study participant underwent initial screening in the form of a medical questionnaire to exclude any known medical conditions. It was followed by the assessment of (1) body composition including body mass, total body water (TBW), body fat (FAT) and free fatty mass (FFM), (2) resting heart rate (HR) and blood pressure (BP) measurement and (3) blood draw from an antecubital vein for baseline analysis of high-sensitivity troponin T (hs-TnT) and high sensitivity C-reactive protein (hs-CRP) levels. At the same time analysis of baseline capillary lactate (L) and glucose (Glu) concentration was performed.

During the race, we collected data on fluid and food intake. Additionally, every 6 laps (approximately every 9.2 km) runners had fingertip capillary L and Glu assessment. Immediately after the end of running each participant underwent a final assessment of capillary L and Glu concentration followed by venous blood draw for hs-TnT and hs-CRP assessment and BP, HR and body composition analysis. In collaboration with a certified company (datasport.pl) we have collected data on the time of the race, mean pace and total distance covered by each runner participating in the study.

2.2. Methodology

Body composition was analysed with means of a bio-impedance device (Tanita BC 41 MA, Tanita Inc, Tokyo, Japan). To assess hs-TnT and hs-CRP levels an electrochemiluminescence immunoassay method (ECLIA) on Roche Cobas e411 analyser (Roche Diagnostics, Mannheim, Germany) was used. Reference values for this fourth-generation hs-TnT assay were < 14 ng/L and < 5 mg/dL for hs-CRP assay. Fingertip capillary L and Glu assessment were performed with Biosen C-Line Glucose and Lactate analyser (EKF Diagnostics, Cardiff, United Kingdom).

2.3. Study End-Point

The study end-point was a change of hs-TnT concentration, assessed immediately after participation in a running ultra-marathon in comparison to baseline hs-TnT value.

2.4. Statistical Analyses

All results for categorical variables were presented as number and percentage. Continuous variables were expressed as median and interquartile range (IQR). Wilcoxon test for paired samples or Mann-Whitney test for unpaired samples were applied to compare continuous data. To assess the correlation between continuous variables, the Spearman test was applied. All tests were two-sided with the significance level of $p < 0.05$. Statistical analyses were performed with MedCalc statistical software 10.0.2.0 (MedCalc, Mariakerke, Belgium).

2.5. Ethical Considerations

The study had an approval of the Ethics Committee of the Regional Medical Chamber in Warsaw (no 52/17), with written informed consent obtained from all participants.

3. Results

3.1. Baseline Characteristics

Baseline and running characteristics of the runners participating in the study are presented in Table 1. Nine runners (50%) have not participated in any ultra-marathon before. Of those 6 have completed at least one marathon and remaining 3 have run only distances up to 30 km. Eight runners (44%) completed the full distance of 100 km within the time limit of 12 h. Other 10 participants run between 52 and 91 km (median 74 km, IQR 71–89). The median time of running in the studied group was 10.3 h (IQR 8.3–11.5) and the median pace was 8.7 min/km (IQR 8.0–9.4).

Table 1. Baseline and running characteristics of the studied group.

Parameter	Ultra-Marathon Runners $n = 18$
Male sex (%)	15 (83)
Age, yrs (IQR)	41.5 (36–53)
BMI, kg/m2 (IQR)	24.6 (22.7–25.7)
Years of running (IQR)	4.3 (3.5–6.0)
Years of ultra running (IQR)	2 (0–3)
Weekly running distance, km (IQR)	67.5 (40–85)
Number of ultra races completed (IQR)	2 (0–10)
Longest completed race, km (IQR)	58 (42–80)

Data are presented as number and percentage or median and interquartile range (IQR).

3.2. Pre- Vs. Post-Race Values

At baseline, the troponin level was below the upper reference limit (99th percentile) in all runners. In all participants the troponin concentration increased after the race (from 5 IQR 3–7 ng/L ng/L to 14 IQR 12–26 ng/L, $p < 0.0001$). It exceeded upper reference values in 66% of runners. Maximal post-race hs-TnT concentration was 38 ng/L (Figure 1).

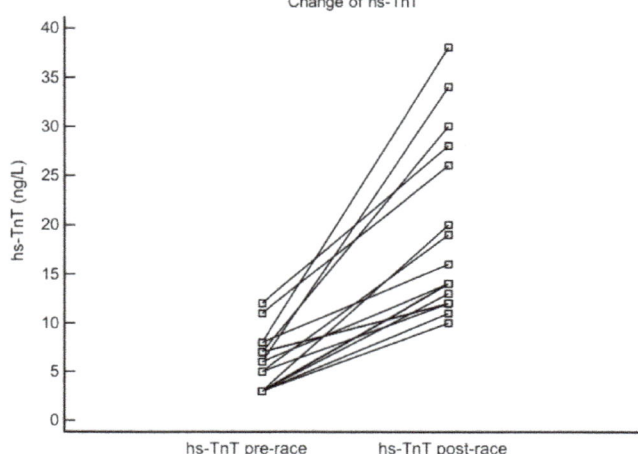

Figure 1. High-sensitivity troponin T (hs-TnT) concentration before and immediately after the end of running.

Table 2 presents the comparison of pre- and post-race values of other parameters. All participants had higher systolic and diastolic BP and lower HR before the race in comparison to post-race values. Running led to a decrease in body mass caused by TBW and FFM loss without significant FAT decrease. During the race, participants drank 1950 mL (IQR 1200–2600 mL) of fluids and ingested 1500 kcal (IQR 919–2340 kcal). There was an increase of CRP after the race, with normal values in all runners before the race and values exceeding the reference values in 6 runners (33%) after the race.

Table 2. Pre- and post-race values of the analysed parameters.

	Pre-Race $n = 18$	Post-Race $n = 18$	p
Body mass, kg	75.0 (69.6–83.3)	74.2 (69.7–82.7)	<0.0001
TBW, kg	44.2 (39.8–49.9)	41.6 (39.2–46.7)	0.008
TBW, %	58.1 (54.4–60.1)	56.6 (54.2–60.1)	0.32
FAT, kg	10.9 (7.9–12.5)	10.5 (7.6–12.2)	0.46
FAT, %	13.7 (11.4–17.5)	14.2 (10.7–18.6)	0.73
FFM, kg	65.7 (61.2–72.0)	64.1 (60.6–70.7)	0.0001
FFM, %	86.3 (82.5–88.7)	85.8 (81.4–89.3)	0.77
HR, bpm	54.5 (50–60)	81.5 (76–93)	<0.0001
SBP, mmHg	137 (130–146)	123 (109–133)	0.0004
DBP, mmHg	84 (92–91)	73 (70–78)	<0.0001
CRP, mg/dL	0.7 (0.43–1.1)	3.2 (1.9–8.1)	<0.0001
hs-TnT, ng/L	5 (3–7)	14 (12–26)	<0.0001
L, mmol/L	2.0 (1.7–2.4)	2.2 (1.4–3.5)	0.22
Glu, mg/dL	89 (86–95)	93 (80–100)	0.83

DBP—diastolic blood pressure, FAT—body fat, FFM—free fatty mass, Glu—glucose, HR—heart rate, hs-CRP—high-sensitivity C reactive protein, L—lactate, SBP—systolic blood pressure, TBW—total body water, hs-TnT—high-sensitivity troponin T.

3.3. Factors Correlating with Troponin Increase

Subsequently, we have analysed, which of the parameters correlated with the change of hs-TnT concentration (Table 3). Interestingly, this was not the case for any of the analysed baseline demographic, clinical and biochemical parameters. We also did not find any correlation between the delta of hs-TnT and the time of running, running pace, fluid and food intake during the race, changes in body composition or pre-post race changes in L and Glu concentration. The only factor correlating with the change of hs-TnT was the change of hs-CRP.

Table 3. Correlation between change in hs-TnT and analysed parameters.

	hs-TnT Change	
	rho	p
Baseline Parameters		
Age, yrs	0.04	0.86
Weekly distance covered, km	0.23	0.34
Body mass pre, kg	0.34	0.16
TBW pre, kg	0.17	0.49
FFM pre, kg	0.31	0.20
HR pre, bpm	0.01	0.96
SBP pre, mmHg	0.04	0.86
DBP pre, mmHg	0.01	0.99
L, mmol/L	0.11	0.66
Glu, mg/dL	−0.26	0.28
Hs-CRP, mg/dL	0.17	0.49
Hs-TnT, mmol/L	0.23	0.32
Race Parameters and Post-Race Changes		
Race time, hours	0.45	0.18
Pace, min/km	0.12	0.62
Water intake during the race, mL	−0.04	0.87
Food intake during the race, kcal	0.07	0.76
Delta body mass, kg	0.08	0.74
Delta TBW, kg	0.31	0.20
Delta FFM, kg	0.29	0.23
Delta L, mmol/L	0.30	0.21
Delta Glu, mg/dL	0.04	0.85
Delta hs-CRP, mg/dL	0.59	0.01

DBP—diastolic blood pressure, FFM—ree fatty mass, Glu—glucose, HR- heart rate, L—lactate concentration, SBP—systolic blood pressure, TBW—total body water, hs-TnT—high-sensitivity troponin T.

3.4. Periodically Assessed Parameters and Troponin Increase

There was no significant change between L values before in comparison to after the race. However, L concentration fluctuated during the race in all runners, with an example demonstrated in Figure 2 affecting mean L concentration during the race rather than post-race L values.

Runners with significant hs-TnT increase after the race had more L peaks > 2 mmol/L during the race (median 7 IQR 4–8 vs. 3.5 IQR 2–5, $p = 0.04$). In consequence, those with mean L concentration during the race above the median of 2.1 mmol/L had a significantly higher increase of hs-TnT (15 IQR 11–19 vs. 8 IQR 7–12 vs. ng/L, $p = 0.02$) as demonstrated on Figure 3. Mean L concentration during the race correlated with change in hs-TnT (rho = 0.52, $p = 0.03$).

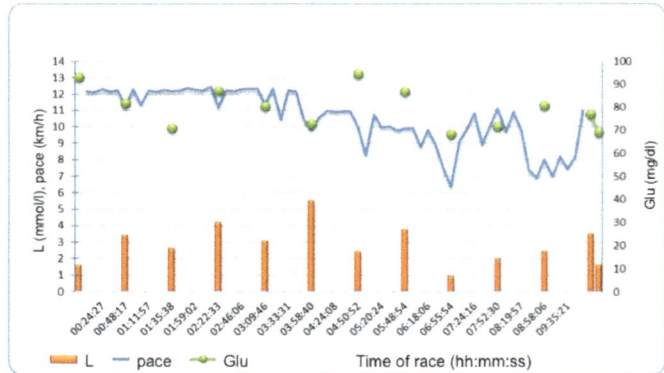

Figure 2. Example of lactate and glucose fluctuations during the race and running pace in one of the runners. L—lactate, Glu- glucose.

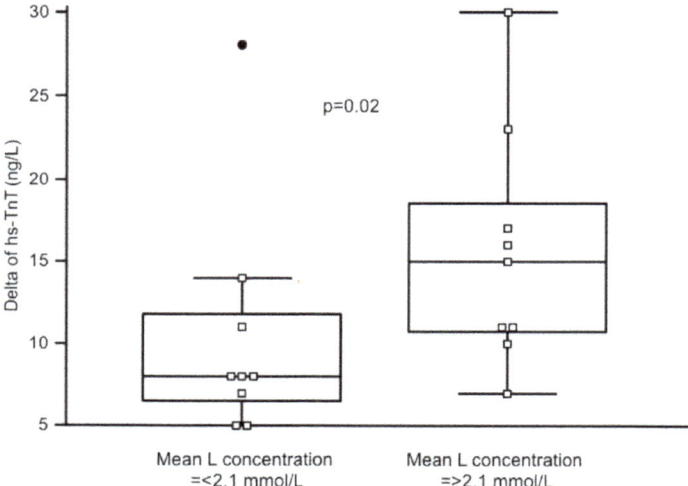

Figure 3. Changes of high-sensitivity TnT (hs-TnT) in runners with mean lactate (L) concentration during the race below and above the median. A black dot on the left is an outstanding result in one of the runners.

At the same time, this was not the case for another periodically assessed parameter—glucose. Glucose fluctuations during the race and mean Glu concentration during the race were unrelated to troponin changes.

4. Discussion

We have demonstrated that participation in a 100 km marathon leads to a significant increase of hs-TnT beyond upper reference limits in 66% of runners. High-sensitivity troponin T measured with a fourth-generation assay, as in our study, is a cardio-selective marker and its increase is believed to have purely cardiac and not skeletal muscle origin [4]. However, it should be noted, that maximal values of post-race hs-TnT in studied runners remained within low probability range of acute coronary syndrome suspicion [5].

Analysis of risk factors of cardiac troponin T increase showed that mean L concentration during the ultra-marathon and hs-CRP increase were the only parameters correlating with troponin T rise after the race. Previous studies have also demonstrated increased hs-CRP levels after prolonged exercise, while L concentrations post-exercise remained unchanged or rose, depending on the physical activity intensity [16–18]. However, lack of pre- and post-exercise difference in L concentration does not exclude fluctuations of L levels during the competition, as in our study, which may affect mean L concentration. Periodic L sampling during long-lasting endurance competitions is rarely performed in clinical studies due to logistic challenges. Therefore our findings regarding fluctuations in lactate concentration and their relation to increased troponin concentration should be considered as a novel finding, not previously reported in the literature.

The exact mechanism connecting lactate fluctuations and hs-CRP to hs-TnT increase is not known. Long-lasting endurance event is usually performed around (or even below) first ventilator threshold. However, periods of anaerobic metabolism during the race may lead to an increase in lactate concentration [18,19]. We postulate that periodic changes in lactate concentration may reflect systemic changes in acid-base and electrolytic balance as described in other studies [18–21]. As shown by our and other research studies, ultra-endurance exercise promotes inflammatory reaction measured in our study by the change of hs-CRP concentration [4,7]. Rise of hs-CRP may be a part of an acute-phase reaction to muscle damage mediated by cytokine system, mainly Il-6, or by lactate increase [16–18]. Acid-base or electrolyte alterations and inflammatory reaction may affect cardiomyocyte cell membrane by increasing its permeability [4,7]. Finally, increased permeability of the cardiomyocyte cell membrane may be responsible for the leakage of hs-TnT from the cytosol to the blood and mild hs-TnT increase observed immediately after the race [4,7]. In line with that, previous research showed a relation between inflammatory markers (including hs-CRP) and troponin increase post-exercise [22,23]. We are aware of the fact that this line of reasoning should be considered as a proposal for future more detailed research, as we were unable to confirm all steps of this hypothesis. In particular, increased cardiomyocyte cell membrane permeability may be also caused by mechanical stress or by oxygen radicals [4,7].

We did not find any correlation between troponin increase and some other previously described risk factors such as younger age, running experience (assessed by weekly covered distance in our study), running intensity (measured with pace and running time) or dehydration [4,7]. It could be caused by the homogeneity of the studied group, which included mainly mid-age, amateur runners with similar experience and comparable race characteristics. Also, unlike in some other studies, none of the analysed baseline biochemical parameters predicted the outcome [24].

Our study has some limitations. First of all, it was conducted on a relatively small number of runners, which precluded any multivariable analysis. However, specifics of the study protocol with a collection of data on fluid and food intake and capillary blood sampling for lactic acid and glucose every 9.2 km with all its logistic challenges made the inclusion of a larger group of participants impossible. We did not want to significantly influence the time of running of the participants, by not causing longer than necessary delays for data collection and blood sampling. For the same reason, we could not include semi-professional or professional runners participating in National Championships of 100 km. Therefore, we focused on amateur athletes only, which could have potentially influence the results. Furthermore, we were unable, as in other similar studies, to correct the post-race biochemical results for the potential changes in plasma volume after long-distance running, which could have affected the results. Finally, we did not analyse the role of potentially interesting cardio-vascular biomarkers such as microRNAs, ST2 protein and others, which could have shed new light on the increase of troponin concentration post-exercise [25]. Nevertheless, we believe that this does not diminish the value of the main findings.

Our results also show that the degree of cardiac troponin T concentration increase after an extreme ultra-marathon remains in the range typical for low cardiovascular risk of an acute event. This can help in the differential diagnosis in this group of patients if deemed necessary [5,7]. Finally, presented observations may help to explain the paradox between cardiac troponin increase after the endurance physical activity and lack of permanent myocardial injury in life-long elite runners observed in other studies [4,6,7,13–15]. As the increase in troponin concentration even after an extremely long race is very mild is it unlikely that it can lead to significant myocardial fibrosis.

5. Conclusions

Participation in a 100 km ultra-marathon leads to a modest, but significant high-sensitivity troponin T increase in the majority of runners. Among analysed parameters only mean lactic acid concentration and change of high-sensitivity C reactive protein correlated with the change of troponin level.

Author Contributions: Conceptualization, Ł.A.M., A.C. and A.M.; Data curation, A.C., A.M. and K.W.; Formal analysis, Ł.A.M., A.C., A.M. and K.W.; Funding acquisition, Ł.A.M.; Investigation, Ł.A.M., A.C., A.M. and K.W. and D.N.; Methodology, Ł.A.M., A.C., A.M. and K.W.; Project administration, Ł.A.M.; Resources, Ł.A.M., A.C., A.M., K.W. and D.N.; Supervision, M.P.; Validation, M.P.; Visualization, K.W.; Writing–original draft, Ł.A.M.; Writing–review & editing, A.C., A.M., K.W., D.N. and M.P. All authors have read and agreed to the published version of the manuscript.

Funding: The study was financed by a statutory grant of the Józef Piłsudski University of Physical Education in Warsaw (DS-296).

Conflicts of Interest: The authors declare no conflict of interest.

References

1. Jee, H.; Jin, Y. Effects of prolonged endurance exercise on vascular endothelial and inflammation markers. *J. Sports Sci. Med.* **2012**, *11*, 719–726. [PubMed]
2. Merghani, A.; Malhotra, A.; Sharma, S. The U-shaped relationship between exercise and cardiac morbidity. *Trends Cardiovasc. Med.* **2016**, *26*, 232–240. [CrossRef] [PubMed]
3. Mach, F.; Baigent, C.; Catapano, A.L.; Koskinas, K.C.; Casula, M.; Badimon, L.; Chapman, M.J.; De Backer, G.G.; Delgado, V.; Ference, B.A.; et al. 2019 ESC/EAS Guidelines for the management of dyslipidaemias: Lipid modification to reduce cardiovascular risk. *Eur. Heart J.* **2019**, *41*, 111–188. [CrossRef] [PubMed]
4. Shave, R.; Baggish, A.; George, K.; Wood, M.; Scharhag, J.; Whyte, G. Exercise-induced cardiac troponin elevation: Evidence, mechanisms, and implications. *J. Am. Coll Cardiol.* **2010**, *56*, 169–176. [CrossRef] [PubMed]
5. Roffi, M.; Patrono, C.; Collet, J.P.; Mueller, C.; Valgimigli, M.; Andreotti, F.; Bax, J.J.; Borger, M.A.; Brotons, C.; Chew, D.P.; et al. 2015 ESC Guidelines for the management of acute coronary syndromes in patients presenting without persistent ST-segment elevation: Task Force for the Management of Acute Coronary Syndromes in Patients Presenting without Persistent ST-Segment Elevation of the European Society of Cardiology (ESC). *Eur. Heart J.* **2016**, *37*, 267–315.
6. Eijsvogels, T.M.; Fernandez, A.B.; Thompson, P.D. Are there deleterious cardiac effects of acute and chronic endurance exercise? *Physiol. Rev.* **2016**, *96*, 99–125. [CrossRef] [PubMed]
7. Stavroulakis, G.A.; George, K.P. Exercise-induced release of troponin. *Clin. Cardiol.* **2020**. [CrossRef]
8. Middleton, N.; George, K.; Whyte, G.; Gaze, D.; Collinson, P.; Shave, R. Cardiac troponin T release is stimulated by endurance exercise in healthy humans. *J. Am. Coll. Cardiol.* **2008**, *52*, 1813–1814. [CrossRef]
9. Gaudreault, V.; Tizon-Marcos, H.; Poirier, P.; Pibarot, P.; Gilbert, P.; Amyot, M.; Rodés-Cabau, J.; Després, J.P.; Bertrand, O.; Larose, E. Transient myocardial tissue and function changes during a marathon in less fit marathon runners. *Can. J. Cardiol.* **2013**, *29*, 1269–1276. [CrossRef]
10. Lord, R.N.; Utomi, V.; Oxborough, D.L.; Curry, B.A.; Brown, M.; George, K.P. Left ventricular function and mechanics following prolonged endurance exercise: An update and meta-analysis with insights from novel techniques. *Eur. J. Appl. Physiol.* **2018**, *118*, 1291–1299. [CrossRef]
11. Vessalle, C.; Masotti, S.; Lubrano, V.; Basta, G.; Prontera, C.; Di Cecco, P.; Del Turco, S.; Sabatino, L.; Pingitore, A. Traditional and new candidate cardiac biomarkers assessed before, early, and late after half marathon in trained subjects. *Eur. J. Appl. Physiol.* **2018**, *118*, 411–417. [CrossRef] [PubMed]
12. Martinez, V.; la Garza, M.S.; Grazioli, G.; Bijnens, B.H.; Trape, J.; Garcia, G.; Corzan, P.; Clemente, A.; González, B.; Sitges, M. Cardiac performance after an endurance open water swimming race. *Eur. J. Appl. Physiol.* **2019**, *119*, 961–970. [CrossRef] [PubMed]

13. Pujadas, S.; Doñate, M.; Li, C.H.; Merchan, S.; Cabanillas, A.; Alomar, X.; Pons-Llado, G.; Serra-Grima, R.; Carreras, F. Myocardial remodelling and tissue characterisation by cardiovascular magnetic resonance (CMR) in endurance athletes. *Bmj. Open Sport Exerc. Med.* **2018**, *4*, e000422. [CrossRef] [PubMed]
14. Małek, Ł.A.; Barczuk-Falęcka, M.; Werys, K.; Czajkowska, A.; Mróz, A.; Witek, K.; Burrage, M.; Bakalarski, W.; Nowicki, D.; Roik, D.; et al. Cardiovascular magnetic resonance with parametric mapping in long-term ultra-marathon runners. *Eur. J. Radiol.* **2019**, *117*, 89–94.
15. Małek, Ł.A.; Buciarelli-Ducci, C. Myocardial Fibrosis in Athletes—Current Perspective. *Clinical. Cardiol.* **2020**, in press.
16. Kyröläinen, H.; Pullinen, T.; Candau, R.; Avela, J.; Huttunen, P.; Komi, P.V. Effects of marathon running on running economy and kinematics. *Eur. J. Appl. Physiol.* **2000**, *82*, 297–304. [CrossRef]
17. Kasapis, C.; Thompson, P.D. The effects of physical activity on serum C-reactive protein and inflammatory markers: A systematic review. *J. Am. Coll Cardiol.* **2005**, *45*, 1563–1569. [CrossRef]
18. Ferguson, B.S.; Rogatzki, M.J.; Goodwin, M.L.; Kane, D.A.; Rightmire, Z.; Gladden, L.B. Lactate metabolism: Historical context, prior misinterpretations, and current understanding. *Eur. J. Appl. Physiol.* **2018**, *118*, 691–728. [CrossRef]
19. Lühker, O.; Berger, M.M.; Pohlmann, A.; Hotz, L.; Gruhlke, T.; Hochreiter, M. Changes in acid-base and ion balance during exercise in normoxia and normobaric hypoxia. *Eur. J. Appl. Physiol.* **2017**, *117*, 2251–2261. [CrossRef]
20. Cooper, D.; Walley, K.; Dodek, P.; Rosenberg, F.; Russel, J.A. Plasma ionized calcium and blood lactate concentrations are inversely associated with human lactic acidosis. *Intensive. Care Med.* **1992**, *18*, 286–289. [CrossRef]
21. Robergs, R.; Ghiasvand, F.; Parker, D. Biochemistry of exercise-induced metabolic acidosis. *Am. J. Physiol. Regul. Intgr. Comp. Physiol.* **2004**, *287*, R502–R516. [CrossRef] [PubMed]
22. Saravia, S.G.; Knebel, F.; Schroeckh, S.; Ziebig, R.; Lun, A.; Weimann, A.; Haberland, A.; Borges, A.C.; Schimke, I. Cardiac troponin T release and inflammation demonstrated in marathon runners. *Clin. Lab.* **2010**, *56*, 51–58, Erratum in: *Clin Lab.* **2011**, *57*, 273. [PubMed]
23. Kłapcińska, B.; Waśkiewicz, Z.; Chrapusta, S.J.; Sadowska-Krępa, E.; Czuba, M.; Langfort, J. Metabolic responses toa 48-h ultra-marathon run in middle-aged male amateur runners. *Eur. J. Appl. Physiol.* **2013**, *113*, 2781–2793. [CrossRef] [PubMed]
24. Katsanos, S.; Mavrogenis, A.F.; Kafkas, N.; Sardu, C.; Kamperidis, V.; Katsanou, P.; Farmakis, D.; Parissis, J. Cardiac biomarkers predict 1-year mortality in elderly patients undergoing hip fracture surgery. *Orthopedics* **2017**, *40*, e417–e424. [CrossRef]
25. Sardu, C.; Paolisso, G.; Marfella, R. Molecular mechanisms and therapeutic targets of inflammatory-related Cardiovascular diseases: From molecular mechanisms to therapeutic targets. *Curr. Pharm. Des.* 2020. [CrossRef]

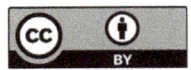

© 2020 by the authors. Licensee MDPI, Basel, Switzerland. This article is an open access article distributed under the terms and conditions of the Creative Commons Attribution (CC BY) license (http://creativecommons.org/licenses/by/4.0/).

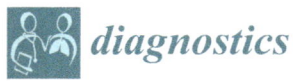

Review

The Cardiac Effects of Performance-Enhancing Medications: Caffeine vs. Anabolic Androgenic Steroids

Sanjay Sivalokanathan [1], Łukasz A. Małek [2] and Aneil Malhotra [1,3,*]

1. Cardiovascular Clinical Academic Group, St. George's University of London and St. George's University Hospitals NHS Foundation Trust, London SW17 0RE, UK; ssivalok@sgul.ac.uk
2. Department of Epidemiology, Cardiovascular Disease Prevention and Health Promotion, National Institute of Cardiology, 04-635 Warsaw, Poland; lmalek@ikard.pl
3. Division of Cardiovascular Sciences, University of Manchester and Manchester University NHS Foundation Trust, Manchester Institute of Health and Performance, Manchester M11 3BS, UK
* Correspondence: aneil.malhotra@manchester.ac.uk

Abstract: Several performance-enhancing or ergogenic drugs have been linked to both significant adverse cardiovascular effects and increased cardiovascular risk. Even with increased scrutiny on the governance of performance-enhancing drugs (PEDs) in professional sport and heightened awareness of the associated cardiovascular risk, there are some who are prepared to risk their use to gain competitive advantage. Caffeine is the most commonly consumed drug in the world and its ergogenic properties have been reported for decades. Thus, the removal of caffeine from the World Anti-Doping Agency (WADA) list of banned substances, in 2004, has naturally led to an exponential rise in its use amongst athletes. The response to caffeine is complex and influenced by both genetic and environmental factors. Whilst the evidence may be equivocal, the ability of an athlete to train longer or at a greater power output cannot be overlooked. Furthermore, its impact on the myocardium remains unanswered. In contrast, anabolic androgenic steroids are recognised PEDs that improve athletic performance, increase muscle growth and suppress fatigue. Their use, however, comes at a cost, afflicting the individual with several side effects, including those that are detrimental to the cardiovascular system. This review addresses the effects of the two commonest PEDs, one legal, the other prohibited, and their respective effects on the heart, as well as the challenge in defining its long-term implications.

Keywords: sports cardiology; athlete; caffeine; anabolic androgenic steroids; heart disease; cardiac magnetic resonance imaging

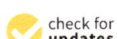

Citation: Sivalokanathan, S.; Małek, Ł.A.; Malhotra, A. The Cardiac Effects of Performance-Enhancing Medications: Caffeine vs. Anabolic Androgenic Steroids. *Diagnostics* **2021**, *11*, 324. https://doi.org/10.3390/diagnostics11020324

Academic Editor: Andrea D. Annoni

Received: 21 December 2020
Accepted: 15 February 2021
Published: 17 February 2021

Publisher's Note: MDPI stays neutral with regard to jurisdictional claims in published maps and institutional affiliations.

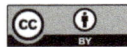

Copyright: © 2021 by the authors. Licensee MDPI, Basel, Switzerland. This article is an open access article distributed under the terms and conditions of the Creative Commons Attribution (CC BY) license (https://creativecommons.org/licenses/by/4.0/).

1. Introduction

Caffeine (1,3,7-Trimethylxanthine) is a popular workplace substance that has been well-researched, with its ergogenic effects being known for centuries [1]. Caffeine has a wide range of acute benefits that includes an increase in alertness and concentration, accompanied by a reduction in fatigue and pain perception [2,3]. As a result, its use has become highly prevalent amongst athletes, especially after 2004, when it was removed from the World Anti-Doping Agency (WADA) list of banned substances; it was, therefore, unsurprising when a study reported that 74% of urine samples from athletes, between 2004 to 2008, demonstrated measurable levels [1]. Common physiological effects of caffeine on the body include an increase in heart rate, catecholamine levels, blood lactate, free fatty acids and glycerol [4]. More significantly, its use has illustrated benefits in both endurance-based and high-intensity exercise, permitting the athlete to train longer and at a greater intensity. A recent meta-analysis yielded a positive relationship of caffeine on muscle strength, muscle endurance and anaerobic power [5]. As a result, it is recommended that ingestion of 3–9 mg/kg approximately 60 min prior to exercise may provide the extra competitive advantage for the athlete [1]. Nonetheless, the response to caffeine is multifaceted, influenced by both genetic and non-genetic predilections, with there being inter-subject variation in response to caffeine consumption, and this heterogeneous response makes it difficult to extrapolate the objective impact of caffeine as a vital ingredient to athletic prowess.

In contrast, anabolic androgenic steroids (AASs), synthetic derivatives of testosterone, have been abused by athletes since the 1950s for their ability to increase muscle mass and improve athletic performance. The terms anabolic and androgenic refer to muscle hypertrophy and increased male sex characteristics, respectively. AASs are artificial substances that act on androgen receptors and are commonly used in the treatment of metabolic or catabolic disorders and other chronic conditions related to low testosterone [6]. More significantly, its misuse stems from the means of achieving a lean and muscular body type, with the potential of shielding the user from muscle fibre damage, through enhanced protein synthesis during recovery. There are multiple manufactured forms, most of which are designed to optimise muscle growth whilst minimising the undesired androgenic effects [6]. Steroid abuse has dramatically increased over the past two decades in the general population who live in an increasingly image-obsessed era. Its users are typically 20–30-year-old males, who participate in recreational exercise largely composed of weight training [6]. Globally, it is estimated that 6.4% of males and 1.6% of females use AASs [7]. The second highest prevalence of users beyond recreational sportspeople (18.4%) are athletes (13.4%) [8]. Whilst anabolic androgenic steroids can play an important role in clinical treatment of endocrine disorders there are several established adverse outcomes, if misused, that includes an increased risk of cardiovascular disease (CVD), risk of tendon ruptures, hepatorenal disorders and psychiatric symptoms. The doses are often 5–15 times higher than recommended levels, with athletes experiencing a higher probability of adverse cardiovascular events that includes stroke and myocardial infarction (MI) [9]. Preceding these events are hypertension and left ventricular (LV) hypertrophy, both independent predictors of cardiovascular mortality and morbidity [10,11]. There are, however, many obstacles to the investigation of the dangers of AASs, due to the dose never being reliably known, to polypharmacy or the ethical restrictions of conducting research studies [6].

Given such a variability in effects of both caffeine and AASs, this review discusses the impact of the two commonest performance-enhancing drugs (PEDs) and its documented cardiac sequalae.

2. Materials and Methods

We performed a comprehensive search on Pubmed, and Scopus focusing on the effects of caffeine and/or AASs to exercise and its subsequent effects on the myocardium (Appendix A Figure A1). Reviews, meta-analyses, prospective, retrospective, interventional and observational studies were included in our search. Exclusion criteria included conference abstracts, or articles where correlation between exercise, the cardiovascular system (CVS) and caffeine or AASs did not exist. The review of AASs was limited to findings after the year of 1986, as widespread testing became available in Europe and the United States at the end of 1986. Key search terms included: "caffeine", "caffeinated", "CAF", "tea", "energy drinks", "anabolic androgenic steroids" in combination with "exercise", "athlete", "myocardium", "cardiac", and "heart".

3. Results

3.1. Caffeine as a Performance Enhancing Agent

In many sports, changes in performance of 1% may be the difference between first or second place [12]. Caffeine is a readily available performance enhancing aid that improves athletic ability across virtually all sporting disciplines. Historically, it was recommended to be banned in 1939, due to its ergogenic properties that may influence sporting accomplishments. Since its legalisation in 2004, it has become a major source for athletes, commonly being in the form of energy drinks, but may vary in the form of a gum, gel, pill or inhaler. Through fat mobilisation and thus sparing of the glycogen reserve, it diminishes the impact of fatigue, pain and effort that is associated with exercise, leading to the more significant motives of athletes for its consumption. A typical 250 mL energy drink (ED) may contain up to 80 mg of caffeine, similar to that in filtered coffee (90 mg), and twice the amount of that in tea (30 mg); additional substances that complement the influence of caffeine include ginseng, taurine and guarana [13–17].

Caffeine use may be classified as low, moderate or high, with ingestion of ~3 mg/kg (~200 mg for a 70 kg individual; 1–2 small cups of coffee) being considered low, 5–6 mg/kg considered moderate and ~10–13 mg/kg viewed as high [17]. It should be noted that the dose-response relationship between caffeine and athletic performance has yet to be established, with low dose caffeine appearing to exhibit the most ergogenic effect on athletes. For instance, caffeine containing drinks, with a dose equivalence to 3 mg/kg, have shown an increased ability of football players in sprinting, jumping and the distance covered [18]. Further meta-analyses investigating the role of caffeine have demonstrated a significant increase in jump height, muscular endurance, aerobic endurance performance and muscle strength [19].

Like most substances, caffeine, when consumed in larger doses, may result in side effects that includes dehydration, seizures, migraines, insomnia, arrhythmias, gastrointestinal problems and psychological permutations [15,16,20].

3.1.1. Caffeine Pharmacology and Cardiac Physiology

Caffeine is rapidly absorbed by the body, with its concentration peaking between 40 to 80 min, and rising to ~15–20 µmol/L with a low caffeine dose, ~40 µmol/L with a moderate and ~60–70 µmol/L with a high dose. It appears in the blood within 5–15 min of ingestion and has a long half-life (3–5 h) [21]. For both female and male athletes, for a given dose of caffeine, it appears that the concentration of caffeine and its metabolites are the same [22,23].

The effects of caffeine are exerted primarily through the blockade of adenosine receptors (subtypes A_1 and A_2), which are found throughout the myocardium and coronary circulation; they are also found in the brain, adipocytes, skeletal and smooth muscle (Figure 1). The result in the competitive blockade of these receptors leads to an increase in peripheral vascular resistance, sympathetic tone and increase in renin, subsequently amplifying the heart rate, cardiac contractility and blood pressure [24]. Secondary metabolic changes of caffeine include stimulating the secretion of epinephrine.

Whilst the concerns of caffeine on overall health has permeated through society, there are many epidemiological studies that have shown its benefit to overall mortality, and in particular cardiac disease [25]. Moreover, although historical studies have demonstrated an increased risk in MI and CVD [26,27], a study of 45,589 men and 85,747 women followed up for 2 and 10 years, respectively, did not show a substantial risk in CVD [28]. Caffeine may, however, conversely attenuate the physiological response to exercise, such that there may be reduced coronary blood flow or response of the endothelial cell in mediating the vascular tone during exercise, which signifies a potential risk to an athlete with silent coronary disease. Other impacts of caffeine include a delayed return of the parasympathetic nervous system, and with a state of sustained sympathetic activity, this may confer an increased risk of life-threatening arrhythmias [21].

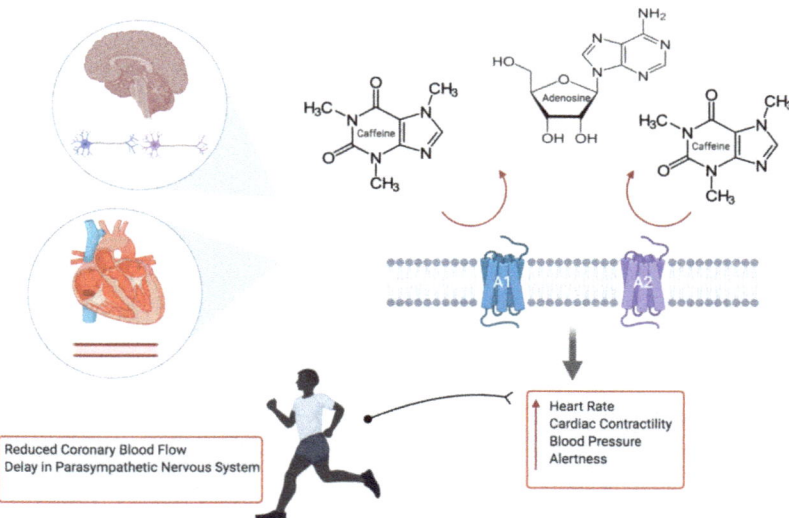

Figure 1. Caffeine inhibits the action of adenosine through the blockade of A_1 and A_2 receptors, resulting in elevated heart rate, blood pressure, cardiac contractility and alertness. Subsequent adverse cardiovascular events during exercise include potentiation of hypoxic damage to cardiac myocytes, through failure in relaxation of the coronary vessels, and arrhythmias (created with BioRender.com).

3.1.2. Caffeine and Risk of Arrhythmia

Whilst many studies have reported the arrhythmogenic effect of caffeine, it has not been replicated on large population studies. With the consumption of caffeine being ubiquitous in Western society, the widely held belief that caffeine may contribute to arrhythmia or the risk and development of coronary heart disease may not be evidence-based [24,25,29–32]. Intoxication of caffeine, however, is still reported, demonstrating its potential in provoking fatal arrhythmias [33]. Physiologically, through the blockade of calcium reuptake into the sarcoplasmic reticulum, and thus a rise in intracellular calcium, the potential of atrial arrhythmia, through enhanced automaticity of atrial pacemaker cells, exists; three cups of coffee (250 mg) have shown to increase both epi- and norepinephrine [34]. More importantly, energy drinks often contain caffeine at a significantly higher concentration than either coffee or tea; the stimulant properties of other compounds in EDs, such as taurine, complicates matters further. Taurine, for instance, is suggested to increase calcium accumulation in the sarcoplasmic reticulum, favouring the excitation-contraction of skeletal muscles, but may also induce unfavourable arrhythmias [35].

It could be argued that the absence of risk may not relate to athletes or those who harbour an underlying abnormal cardiac substrate, especially as the amount of caffeine consumed through energy drinks may be invariably higher. For instance, there has been reports of EDs prolonging QTc and unmasking Brugada syndrome [34]. Another important impact of caffeine includes the augmentation of ryanodine receptors, that may further lead to an increase in calcium release within cardiac cells, affecting the heart's ability to contract and use oxygen, which may predispose to arrhythmias [36].

On the other hand, when attempting to explore the relationship between caffeine and arrhythmias in those with pre-existing cardiac disease, there failed to be a connection, suggesting the complex pharmacodynamics of caffeine [33].

3.1.3. Caffeine Genetics

It is evident that genetic factors demonstrate a huge role on the individual response to the effects of caffeine [37–39]. Whilst its mechanisms may not be well defined, there are certain drivers of these individual differences; notable genes include CYP1A2, ADORA2A and catechol-O-methyltransferase (COMT) [40]. Of the most significance is CYP1A2, which is involved in the breakdown of caffeine and has two alleles (A & C), dichotomising into either fast or slow metabolisers, respectively. The significance of this phenomenon is that those who are slow metabolisers, who consume moderate (3–4 cups) amounts of coffee have a greater risk of hypertension and MI [1]. This is also reflected in athletes, with those who are fast metabolisers showing greater improvement in performance; this may be due a rapid accumulation of caffeine metabolites, and may reflect why timing of caffeine consumption becomes important [1].

In contrast, polymorphisms affecting ADORA2A could lead to an individual to experience greater sleep disturbance, impacting athletes that compete in the evening, or increased anxiety resulting in poor competition performance [12].

3.1.4. Caffeine in Sudden Cardiac Death

Sudden cardiac death (SCD) is defined as an unexpected death or arrest, presumed to be secondary to a cardiac cause, within 1 hour of symptoms or, if unwitnessed, within 24. Energy drinks has been associated with coronary vasospasm and ischaemia, arrhythmias, endothelial dysfunction and increased platelet aggregation [41]. Its use has been a particular concern amongst the younger athletes, where case reports of sudden cardiac death were in part attributed to the consumption of energy drinks [41]. However, whilst no direct link between caffeine and its supposed harmful effects on the heart exist, further studies are required to establish its true safety, particularly in those with underlying electrical or structural cardiac abnormalities. Additional studies would be important in recognising the effects of strength and delivery of caffeine, and the effects of age and genetic expression on the individual's response to caffeine.

3.2. Anabolic Androgenic Steroids as a Performance Enhancing Agent

Anabolic androgenic steroids first gained popularity in the 1954 Olympics and given its potential to improve physical ability, appearance and performance, it has been banned for any sporting use since 1974. Regardless, it is continued to be misused by athletes in sports such as weightlifting, football, cycling and many others to improve both performance and in order to gain a competitive advantage; it is reported that up to 50% of positive doping cases account for AAS use [42]. The lifetime prevalence of AASs ranges from 1–5% in Western countries, and its use has increased four-fold, since 2016, from 0.1% to 0.4% of the population, affecting an extra 19,000 young people (aged 16–24 years old). Although AASs are commonly administered subcutaneously or intramuscularly, it may also be delivered as oral or transdermal preparations or as an implant [43]. Motivators for its use include achieving rapid muscle growth, greater than can be achieved by exercise alone [6]. It can often be problematic to attribute the harmful cardiac effects of AASs, as users often take other compounds such as ephedrine, growth hormone, thyroxine and amphetamines [7,43]. Nonetheless, with mounting evidence in developing several physical and psychological health disorders, its use has become more than a concern restricted to athletes but one of public health.

3.2.1. AASs Pharmacology and Cardiac Physiology

Anabolic androgenic steroids upregulate and increase the number of androgen receptors, increasing the transcription of DNA in skeletal muscle required for muscle growth, thereby contributing to an increase in muscle size and strength. It also includes a direct effect on cardiac muscle metabolism, altering both electrical and structural features of the myocardium [44]. Suraphysiological doses of AASs induces toxicity of the CVS, with the proposed mechanisms including changes in the lipid profile, elevations in blood pressure, myocyte hypertrophy, disarray and apoptosis and a procoagulant state [45]. Thereby, contributing to disorders such coronary artery disease (CAD), hypertension, cardiomyopathy and thromboembolic disorders (Figure 2); the above findings have been correlated with histopathological case reports [46,47]. Physiological changes include alterations in the lipid profile that includes a reduction (up to 20%) in high density lipoprotein (HDL), an increase (up to 20%) in low-density lipoprotein (LDL) and an increase in total cholesterol levels, which is accompanied with an increase in HMG-CoA reductase enzymes [6]. Such changes in lipid characteristics increases the hazard of CAD by 3–6 fold and may occur as quickly as 9 weeks since the onset of AAS use [48]. Hypertension, another commonly reported phenomenon in AAS users, is described to be a consequence of increased sympathetic drive and endothelial dysfunction [6]. The progression of such events is often hard to define, attributed to both dose and drug duration, but some are argued to be non-reversible, resulting in those to require cardiac devices or listed for transplantation.

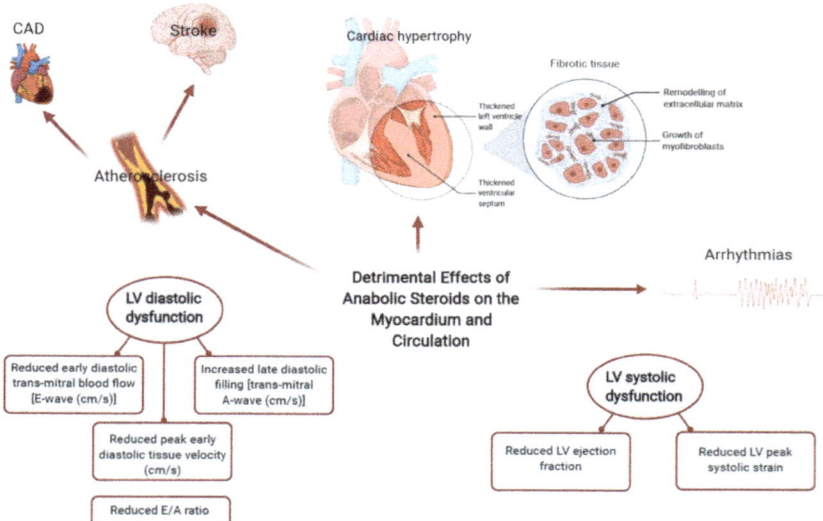

Figure 2. Common adverse cardiovascular effects of anabolic androgenic steroid abuse include vascular calcification, accelerated atherosclerosis, myocardial apoptosis, cardiac hypertrophy and arrhythmias. Impaired LV relaxation is a cardinal feature of the adverse cardiac effects of anabolic androgenic steroids (AASs). With long term abuse, there is evidence of reduced systolic strain and systolic dysfunction with resultant cardiomyopathies. Other sequalae of AAS abuse include increased incidence of thromboembolism and hypertension (created with BioRender.com).

AASs are involved in promoting the growth of cardiac tissue, resulting in significant adverse adaptations such as an increase in wall thickness, and left ventricular cavity size; there has been observable differences in left ventricular posterior wall and septal wall thickness [49]. The induction of myocyte hypertrophy results in counter opposing measures such as the release of apoptogenic factors leading to further deleterious effects on the myocardium (Figure 3). For instance, it has been noted that AAS abusers demonstrate a reduction in peak strain and strain rates of the left posterior and septal walls [50]. Diastolic function also appears to be affected, whereby a reduction in early and late diastolic filling velocity ratios is expected; a reduction in myocardial relaxation through increased collage cross-linking and fibrosis may explain such a phenomenon in anabolic androgenic steroid use [51]. Animal models have been particularly useful in demonstrating such changes. For instance, rats after 8–12 weeks of AAS use demonstrated cardiomegaly [45]. Furthermore, immunohistochemical analyses revealed greater expression of TNF-α and

IL-1β (proinflammatory mediators), signifying ongoing silent myocardial injury in AAS users [52]. Post-mortem studies have also demonstrated adverse phenotypical changes to AASs such as cardiomegaly, myocardial fibrosis and necrosis [49]. Other ramifications include an increase in ventricular rigidity, as its use may reduce myocardial compliance through an apoptogenic effect on the cardiac myocytes [53]. More importantly, the effects of AASs are not limited to the left ventricle and several studies have suggested a global impact. For instance, there is an increase in right ventricular strain, and left atrial dysfunction [54]. As a result, AASs have led to the emergence of acquired cardiac disease in younger and middle-aged athletes.

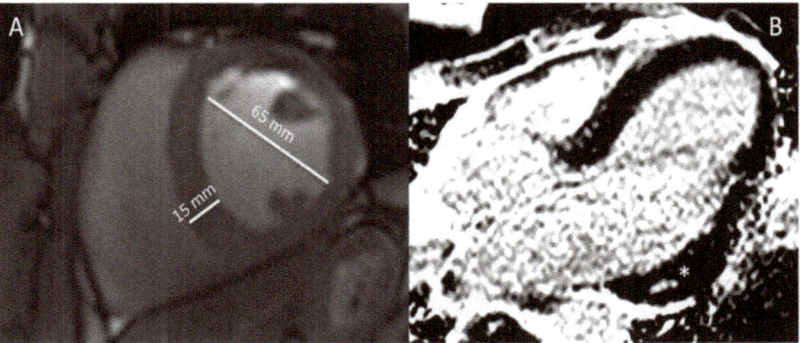

Figure 3. (**A**,**B**). Cardiac magnetic resonance (CMR) images of a 38-year old bodybuilder with anabolic androgenic steroid use—(**A**). Cine steady-state free precession (SSFP) in mid-ventricular short-axis view at end-diastole showing hypertrophied interventricular septum (15 mm) and enlarged left ventricle (62 mm) with decreased systolic function (ejection fracTable 44. not shown), (**B**). Late gadolinium enhancement (LGE) image in 3-chamber view showing midventricular area of fibrosis (non-ischemic) in the basal infero-lateral segment of the left ventricle (asterisk).

Other important manifestations of anabolic androgenic steroid abuse include myocardial infarction and heart failure, secondary to premature atherosclerosis; infarcts may even occur without significant coronary vessel disease [55]. Animal models have illustrated increased androgen-induced vascular calcification, which could be secondary to steroid induced cell damage resulting in loss of tissue elasticity and thus fibrosis [56]. A landmark study among experienced male weightlifters reported that long-term AASs use was associated with myocardial dysfunction and accelerated coronary atherosclerosis [51]. Stroke is a particular risk with AAS use, with current guidelines advocating against the use of testosterone in patients who have experienced MI or stroke within the last 6 months [9]. The proposed mechanisms include hyperaggregation of platelets, increased plasma levels of factor VIII and IX, and heightened fibrinolytic activity through increased tissue plasminogen activator (t-PA) levels. Moreover, AASs can promote polycythaemia, through increased red cell production, leading to potential ischaemic events [9]. These forms of anabolic androgenic steroid-associated adverse cardiovascular phenotypes may represent a previously underrecognized public-health problem.

3.2.2. AASs and Risk of Arrhythmia

Several studies have illustrated how the supraphysiological doses of AASs induces both morphological and electrical ventricular remodelling that results in cardiac autonomic dysfunction [57]. More importantly, hypertrophy, fibrosis and necrosis, repercussions of AAS use, are substrates for arrhythmias that are further compounded by exercise. Testosterone, in particular, has been associated with rhythmic disturbances, possibly through the potentiation of potassium channels involved in ventricular repolarisation, which could explain the presence of QRS-wave delay, sinus tachycardia and supra- and ventricular arrhythmias [44,58,59]. Signal-averaging electrocardiography (SAECG), a method of distinguishing conduction abnormalities has revealed longer QTc interval and QT dispersion in AAS users. Subsequently, increasing the likelihood of abnormal rhythms and SCD after or during exercise [58,59].

3.2.3. AASs Genetics

Interindividual variation in genetics exist and alterations in cytochrome P450 (CYP450) and uridine diphosphate glucuronosyltransferase (UGT) enzymes may explain why certain individuals may require greater amounts of AASs or experience the more harmful effects. To date, no studies have evaluated whether genetic variation in AAS users play a role in the predilection of CVD. There has, however, been studies on the overexpression of molecular mediators, argued to be drivers of CVD. This includes overexpression of calcium/calmodulin dependent protein kinase II delta (CaMKIIδ), beta myosin heavy chain (MHC) and monoamine oxidase (MAO), hallmarks of pathological changes within the myocardium, such as myocyte apoptosis, cardiac hypertrophy, slow shortening velocity of cardiac fibres and arrhythmias [60]. More significantly, imbalance of Ca^{2+} homeostasis and increased CaMKIIδ activity is observed in both human and animal models of heart failure [60]. The overproduction of MAO is also related to ventricular dysfunction, apoptosis and fibrosis [60].

3.2.4. AASs in Sudden Cardiac Death

Anabolic androgenic steroids have the potential of increasing the risk of sudden cardiac death through multiple mechanisms; it is, unfortunately, unclear to the exact nature of these events, especially since those who misuse often use a combination of drugs. Structurally, several modalities of dysfunction that may predispose to sudden cardiac death have been proposed that includes increased coronary artery plaque volume, cardiac hypertrophy, ventricular dilatation, myocardial fibrosis and cardiomyopathy [45,51]. Precisely, four mechanisms have been postulated to describe SCD in AAS users, that includes the thrombosis model, the atherogenic model, the direct myocardial injury model, and model of vasospasm [43]. The thrombosis model suggests that there is an increased risk in thrombus formation as a result of polycythaemia and increased platelet generation and aggregation. More importantly, with ongoing endothelial dysfunction, it precludes AAS users to fatal thrombotic complications, such as ischaemic stroke or pulmonary embolism. Additional physiological changes include the promotion of thromboxane A2 and thrombin, inducing a state of hypercoagulability [45]. In the atherogenic model, the heightened risk in SCD is accounted by the changes in the lipid profile leading to premature atherosclerosis and thus myocardial infarction; the study by Pärssinen accounted as high as 38% to MI [61]. The vasospastic model explains the occurrence of infarction, as a consequence to coronary vasospasm from the release of nitric oxide, in those with no evidence of atherosclerosis or coronary thrombosis [61,62]. The final model describes fatal arrhythmias precipitated by the chronic ischaemic damage brought about by apoptosis, collagen deposition and microcirculatory disturbance [62]. Suggested mechanisms that induces arrhythmias include increased QT interval, Tp-e interval, Tp-e/QT ratio and Tp-e/QTc ratio [45,59]. Furthermore, there have been several case reports of young athletes that have developed rapidly progressive (dilated) cardiomyopathy [45]. Isolated ventricular arrhythmias are another possibility, where it has been suggested that AASs inhibit the re-uptake of catecholamines, and with a combination of exercise, stimulating the nervous system that may increase the likelihood of fatal arrhythmias.

4. Discussion

Our findings suggest that whilst caffeine does not have noticeable structural changes on the myocardium, AASs has several. For instance, imaging and histopathological samples have demonstrated left ventricular hypertrophy, cardiomegaly and interstitial fibrosis, respectively [43]. Such remodelling has ramifications on the CVS, not only immediately but in the long-term as well. Substantial cardiovascular changes include increase in vascular tone and elevation in blood pressure, alterations in lipid profile and direct myocardial toxicity, resulting in reduced left ventricular function, cardiac hypertrophy and arterial and venous thrombosis [43,63]. In contrast, there is a lack of compelling evidence to suggest that caffeine has lasting morphological changes to the myocardium (Figure 4).

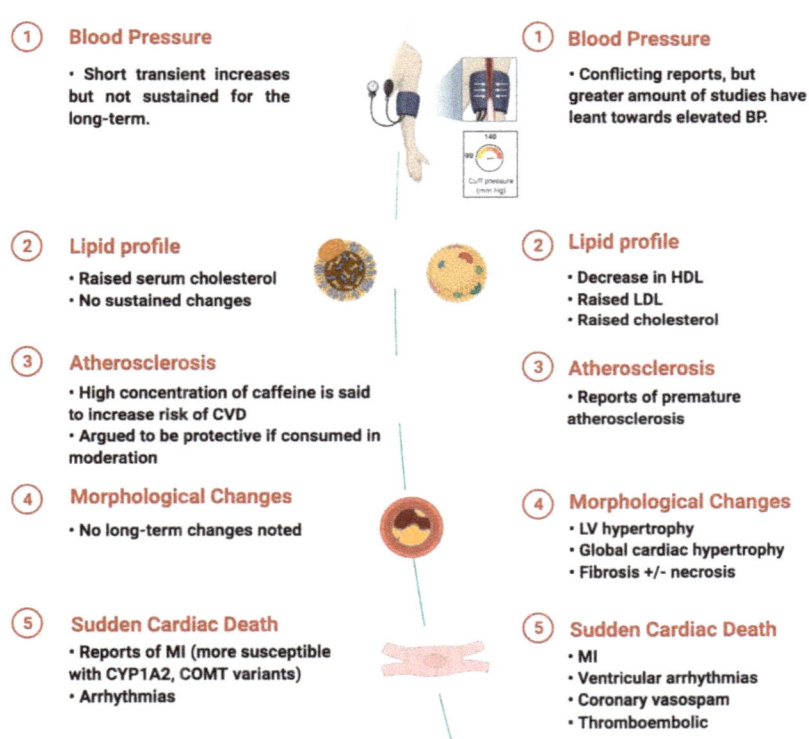

Figure 4. Comparison between caffeine and AASs and its associated cardiovascular effects (created with BioRender.com).

Arrhythmias have also been reported in individuals that consume caffeine or use AASs. Whilst the mechanisms have been discussed, and at length, it is often difficult to reproduce the results in larger studies. In terms of SCD, whilst evidence leans towards AASs, it is less apparent for caffeine. Direct effects of AASs include ventricular remodelling leading to cardiomyopathy. More importantly, left ventricular hypertrophy and fibrosis have both been identified as risk factors to SCD [64,65], and therefore may be argued to be the sequelae of ongoing AASs use that results in the terminal event. More precisely, ventricular arrhythmias, brought about by changes in the myocytes, interstitium and coronary flow reserve could lead to the fatal event [43]. However, it is not uncommon for AASs to stack or combine with other illicit drugs, making it a challenge whether such modifications are solely attributable to AASs. Furthermore, with the presence of physiological remodelling to exercise and thus the presence of the "athlete's heart", that includes left ventricular hypertrophy and increased cavity dimensions, it can be difficult to delineate whether the changes are brought about by AAS use or through exercise. Therefore, detraining could be an option if there is uncertainty to the aetiology.

Ultimately, to negate the suggested adverse cardiovascular effects, both the subject and healthcare professional has to take into consideration the risk of withdrawal if stopped abruptly. Unfavourable symptoms such as headache and irritability would naturally deter the individual in abstaining from caffeine. More importantly, in AAS use, hypogonadism and depression are durable side effects that prevent the user from refraining in its use. Furthermore, it is possible that despite discontinuation, there may be permanent changes from AASs that includes insulin resistance, hypertension and visceral adipose tissue [60].

Clinical Pitfalls and Future Directions

Even though certain physiological mechanisms have been argued to be the benefits or drawbacks of both caffeine and anabolic androgenic steroids, these are still viewed as hypotheses and associations and, thus remain incomplete as explanations without larger randomised controlled trials. To what extent caffeine may be regarded as a drug to the athlete is difficult. There are several preparations, majority of which are in combinations, and there is lack of consistency on both performance and cardiac outcomes. Furthermore, it should be noted that the documented adverse effects of AASs have failed to be replicated in a few studies. For instance, not all AAS users experience left ventricular hypertrophy and/or endothelial dysfunction. Such effects could be explained by the use of allied substances or stimulants, such as cocaine, that are harmful to the CVS. In addition, AAS users often combine different forms of steroids, termed "stacking", as a means of maximising muscle growth, which could account for the adverse cardiac effects experienced in some and not others [6]. More importantly, the varying structure, metabolites and administration patterns of AASs makes it challenging to predict accurate and reproducible physiological consequences on the cardiovascular system. Additionally, the majority of studies are focussed on post-adolescent males, becoming problematic when translating the negative cardiac effects to all users.

Furthermore, the discrepancies observed may depend on the age, sex, coexisting clinical conditions and status of athletic performance. As such this topic requires further studies in different clinical and sport settings. From a methodological point of view, in clinical studies on athletes, it is usually not straightforward to fully confirm or exclude the use of doping agents, which is a serious confounder. Future research may include the use of new promising biomarkers such as microRNAs [66,67]. Those small particles regulate the post-transcription gene expression by RNA-RNA interactions. Circulating microRNAs, due to their high environmental stability and presence in various body fluids, have been already shown to have potential in detection of illicit substances [43]. Several microRNAs have been also linked to heart dysfunction in the form of myocardial ischemia, hypertrophy, fibrosis and arrhythmia [66]. However, many of the same microRNAs also become up-or down- regulated in response to exercise as demonstrated in a recent review [67]. Therefore, their potential future use will depend on the ability to distinguish physiological adaptive changes to exercise from changes related to the use of illicit drugs.

5. Conclusions

There is a large growing body of evidence that describes the impact of both caffeine and anabolic androgenic steroid use on the cardiovascular health of both the athlete and non-athlete. Whilst caffeine may not necessarily give an athlete the essential edge, its use may not disadvantage them either, especially since the majority have consumed such a supplement prior their sporting event. In contrast, AASs have documented improvement in athletic proficiency. However, it does not negate the several adverse cardiovascular effects that is associated with its use. With the continued use of both caffeine and AASs, regular assessment, that includes evaluating the electrical activity and morphology of the myocardium, using non-invasive imaging and functional methods would be important in identifying those who are at an increased risk of cardiovascular disease or an acute cardiac event.

Author Contributions: S.S., Ł.A.M., A.M. contributed to writing, elaboration, editing and approval of the manuscript. S.S. designed the figures and tables. All authors have read and agreed to the published version of the manuscript.

Funding: This research received no external funding.

Conflicts of Interest: The authors declare no conflict of interest.

Appendix A

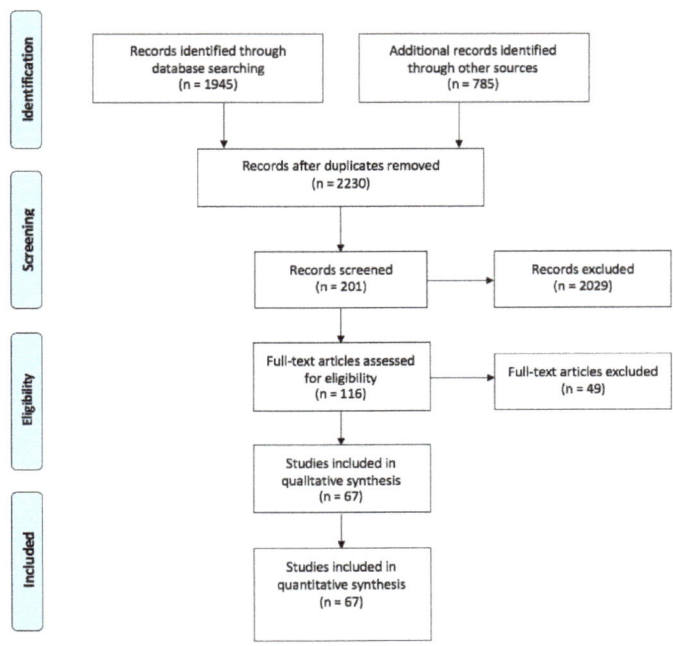

Figure A1. PRISMA flow diagram describing the selection of studies for discussion.

References

1. Pickering, C.; Kiely, J. Are the Current Guidelines on Caffeine Use in Sport Optimal for Everyone? Inter-individual Vari-ation in Caffeine Ergogenicity, and a Move Towards Personalised Sports Nutrition. *Sports Med.* **2018**, *48*, 7–16. [CrossRef]
2. Berglund, B.; Hemmingsson, P. Effects of Caffeine Ingestion on Exercise Performance at Low and High Altitudes in Cross-Country Skiers. *Int. J. Sports Med.* **1982**, *3*, 234–236. [CrossRef] [PubMed]
3. Stadheim, H.K.; Nossum, E.M.; Olsen, R.; Spencer, M.; Jensen, J. Caffeine improves performance in double poling during acute exposure to 2,000-m altitude. *J. Appl. Physiol.* **2015**, *119*, 1501–1509. [CrossRef]
4. Powers, S.K.; Byrd, R.J.; Tulley, R.; Callender, T. Effects of caffeine ingestion on metabolism and performance during graded exercise. *Graefe's Arch. Clin. Exp. Ophthalmol.* **1983**, *50*, 301–307. [CrossRef] [PubMed]
5. Grgic, J.; Grgic, I.; Pickering, C.; Schoenfeld, B.J.; Bishop, D.J.; Virgile, A.; Pedisic, Z. Infographic. Wake up and smell the coffee: Caffeine supplementation and exercise performance. *Br. J. Sports Med.* **2020**, *54*, 304–305. [CrossRef]
6. Mullen, C.; Whalley, B.J.; Schifano, F.; Baker, J.S. Anabolic androgenic steroid abuse in the United Kingdom: An update. *Br. J. Pharmacol.* **2020**, *177*, 2180–2198. [CrossRef] [PubMed]
7. Sagoe, D.; Molde, H.; Andreassen, C.S.; Torsheim, T.; Pallesen, S. The global epidemiology of anabolic-androgenic steroid use: A meta-analysis and meta-regression analysis. *Ann. Epidemiol.* **2014**, *24*, 383–398. [CrossRef]

8. Reyes-Vallejo, L. Current use and abuse of anabolic steroids. *Actas Urológicas Españolas (Engl. Ed.)* **2020**, *44*, 309–313. [CrossRef]
9. Tsatsakis, A.; Docea, A.O.; Calina, D.; Tsarouhas, K.; Zamfira, L.-M.; Mitrut, R.; Sharifi-Rad, J.; Kovatsi, L.; Siokas, V.; Dardiotis, E.; et al. A Mechanistic and Pathophysiological Approach for Stroke Associated with Drugs of Abuse. *J. Clin. Med.* **2019**, *8*, 1295. [CrossRef]
10. McCullough, D.; Webb, R.; Enright, K.J.; Lane, K.E.; McVeigh, J.; Stewart, C.E.; Davies, I.G. How the love of muscle can break a heart: Impact of anabolic androgenic steroids on skeletal muscle hypertrophy, metabolic and cardiovascular health. *Rev. Endocr. Metab. Disord.* **2020**, 1–17. [CrossRef]
11. Payne, J.R.; Kotwinski, P.J.; E Montgomery, H. Cardiac effects of anabolic steroids. *Heart* **2004**, *90*, 473–475. [CrossRef] [PubMed]
12. Southward, K.; Rutherfurd-Markwick, K.J.; Ali, A. The Effect of Acute Caffeine Ingestion on Endurance Performance: A Systematic Review and Meta-Analysis. *Sports Med.* **2018**, *48*, 1913–1928. [CrossRef] [PubMed]
13. Babu, K.M.; Church, R.J.; Lewander, W. Energy Drinks: The New Eye-Opener For Adolescents. *Clin. Pediatr. Emerg. Med.* **2008**, *9*, 35–42. [CrossRef]
14. Espinola, E.; Dias, R.; Mattei, R.; Carlini, E. Pharmacological activity of Guarana (Paullinia cupana Mart.) in laboratory animals. *J. Ethnopharmacol.* **1997**, *55*, 223–229. [CrossRef]
15. Glatter, K.A.; Myers, R.; Chiamvimonvat, N. Recommendations regarding dietary intake and caffeine and alcohol con-sumption in patients with cardiac arrhythmias: What do you tell your patients to do or not to do? *Curr. Treat. Options Cardiovasc. Med.* **2012**, *14*, 529–535. [CrossRef]
16. Seifert, S.M.; Schaechter, J.L.; Hershorin, E.R.; Lipshultz, S.E. Health Effects of Energy Drinks on Children, Adolescents, and Young Adults. *Pediatrics* **2011**, *127*, 511–528. [CrossRef]
17. Spriet, L.L. Exercise and Sport Performance with Low Doses of Caffeine. *Sports Med.* **2014**, *44*, 175–184. [CrossRef]
18. Del Coso, J.; Muñoz-Fernández, V.E.; Muñoz, G.; Fernández-Elías, V.E.; Ortega, J.F.; Hamouti, N.; Barbero, J.C.; Muñoz-Guerraet, J. Effects of a caffeine containing energy drink on simulated soccer performance. *PLoS ONE* **2012**, *7*, e31380. [CrossRef]
19. Pickering, C.; Grgic, J. Caffeine and Exercise: What Next? *Sports Med.* **2019**, *49*, 1007–1030. [CrossRef]
20. Trapp, G.S.; Allen, K.; O'Sullivan, T.A.; Robinson, M.; Jacoby, P.; Oddy, W.H. ENERGY DRINK CONSUMPTION IS ASSOCIATED WITH ANXIETY IN AUSTRALIAN YOUNG ADULT MALES. *Depress. Anxiety* **2013**, *31*, 420–428. [CrossRef]
21. Graham, T.E.; Rush, J.W.E.; Van Soeren, M.H. Caffeine and Exercise: Metabolism and Performance. *Can. J. Appl. Physiol.* **1994**, *19*, 111–138. [CrossRef] [PubMed]
22. Gonzaga, L.A.; Vanderlei, L.C.M.; Gomes, R.L.; Valenti, V.E. Caffeine affects autonomic control of heart rate and blood pressure recovery after aerobic exercise in young adults: A crossover study. *Sci. Rep.* **2017**, *7*, 14091. [CrossRef]
23. Skinner, T.L.; Desbrow, B.; Arapova, J.; Schaumberg, M.A.; Osborne, J.; Grant, G.D.; Anoopkumar-Dukie, S.; Leveritt, M.D. Women Experience the Same Ergogenic Response to Caffeine as Men. *Med. Sci. Sports Exerc.* **2019**, *51*, 1195–1202. [PubMed]
24. Haller, C.A.; Jacob, P.; Benowitz, N.L. Pharmacology of ephedra alkaloids and caffeine after single-dose dietary supplement use*. *Clin. Pharmacol. Ther.* **2002**, *71*, 421–432. [CrossRef]
25. Loftfield, E.; Freedman, N.D.; Graubard, B.I.; Guertin, K.A.; Black, A.; Huang, W.-Y.; Shebl, F.M.; Mayne, S.T.; Sinha, R. Association of Coffee Consumption With Overall and Cause-Specific Mortality in a Large US Prospective Cohort Study. *Am. J. Epidemiol.* **2015**, *182*, 1010–1022. [CrossRef]
26. Rosenberg, L.; Palmer, J.R.; Kelly, J.P.; Kaufman, D.W.; Shapiro, S. Coffee drinking and nonfatal myocardial infarction in men under 55 years of age. *Am. J. Epidemiol.* **1988**, *128*, 570–578. [CrossRef]
27. Lacroix, A.Z.; Mead, L.A.; Liang, K.-Y.; Thomas, C.B.; Pearson, T.A. Coffee Consumption and the Incidence of Coronary Heart Disease. *New Engl. J. Med.* **1986**, *315*, 977–982. [CrossRef]
28. Happonen, P.; Voutilainen, S.; Salonen, J.T. Coffee Drinking Is Dose-Dependently Related to the Risk of Acute Coronary Events in Middle-Aged Men. *J. Nutr.* **2004**, *134*, 2381–2386. [CrossRef]
29. Goldfarb, M.; Tellier, C.; Thanassoulis, G. Review of Published Cases of Adverse Cardiovascular Events After Ingestion of Energy Drinks. *Am. J. Cardiol.* **2014**, *113*, 168–172. [CrossRef] [PubMed]
30. Avcı, S.; Sarıkaya, R.; Büyükcam, F. Death of a young man after overuse of energy drink. *Am. J. Emerg. Med.* **2013**, *31*, 1624.e3–1624.e4. [CrossRef]
31. Frost, L.; Vestergaard, P. Caffeine and risk of atrial fibrillation or flutter: The Danish Diet, Cancer, and Health Study. *Am. J. Clin. Nutr.* **2005**, *81*, 578–582. [CrossRef] [PubMed]
32. Sanchis-Gomar, F.; Pareja-Galeano, H.; Cervellin, G.; Lippi, G.; Earnest, C.P. Energy Drink Overconsumption in Adolescents: Implications for Arrhythmias and Other Cardiovascular Events. *Can. J. Cardiol.* **2015**, *31*, 572–575. [CrossRef]
33. Zuchinali, P.; Zimerman, A.; Giaretta, V.; Salamoni, J.; Fracasso, B.; Pimentel, M.; Souza, G.C.; Chemello, D.; I Zimerman, L.; E Rohde, L. Short-term Effects of High-Dose Caffeine on Cardiac Arrhythmias in Patients With Heart Failure: A Randomized Clinical Trial. *JAMA Intern. Med.* **2016**, *176*, 1752–1759. [CrossRef]
34. Voskoboinik, A.; Kalman, J.M.; Kistler, P.M. Caffeine and Arrhythmias: Time to Grind the Data. *JACC Clin. Electrophysiol.* **2018**, *4*, 425–432. [CrossRef]
35. Souza, D.B.; Del Coso, J.; Casonatto, J.; Polito, M.D. Acute effects of caffeine-containing energy drinks on physical perfor-mance: A systematic review and meta-analysis. *Eur. J. Nutr.* **2017**, *56*, 13–27. [CrossRef]

36. Fletcher, E.A.; Lacey, C.S.; Aaron, M.; Kolasa, M.; Occiano, A.; Shah, S.A. Randomized Controlled Trial of High-Volume Energy Drink Versus Caffeine Consumption on ECG and Hemodynamic Parameters. *J. Am. Hear. Assoc.* **2017**, *6*. [CrossRef]
37. Cornelis, M.C.; Monda, K.L.; Yu, K.; Paynter, N.; Azzato, E.M.; Bennett, S.N.; Berndt, S.I.; Boerwinkle, E.; Chanock, S.; Chatterjee, N.; et al. Genome-Wide Meta-Analysis Identifies Regions on 7p21 (AHR) and 15q24 (CYP1A2) As Determinants of Habitual Caffeine Consumption. *PLoS Genet.* **2011**, *7*, e1002033. [CrossRef]
38. Sulem, P.; Gudbjartsson, D.F.; Geller, F.; Prokopenko, I.; Feenstra, B.; Aben, K.K.H.; Franke, B.; den Heijer, M.; Kovacs, P.; Stumvoll, M.; et al. Sequence variants at CYP1A1- CYP1A2 and AHR associate with coffee consumption. *Hum. Mol. Genet.* **2011**, *20*, 2071–2077. [CrossRef]
39. Denden, S.; Bouden, B.; Khelil, A.H.; Ben Chibani, J.; Hamdaoui, M. Gender and ethnicity modify the association between the CYP1A2 rs762551 polymorphism and habitual coffee intake: Evidence from a meta-analysis. *Genet. Mol. Res.* **2016**, *15*. [CrossRef]
40. Happonen, P.; Voutilainen, S.; Tuomainen, T.-P.; Salonen, J.T. Catechol-O-Methyltransferase Gene Polymorphism Modifies the Effect of Coffee Intake on Incidence of Acute Coronary Events. *PLoS ONE* **2006**, *1*, e117. [CrossRef] [PubMed]
41. Enriquez, A.; Frankel, D.S. Arrhythmogenic effects of energy drinks. *J. Cardiovasc. Electrophysiol.* **2017**, *28*, 711–717. [CrossRef]
42. Bird, S.R.; Goebel, C.; Burke, L.M.; Greaves, R.F. Doping in sport and exercise: Anabolic, ergogenic, health and clinical issues. *Ann. Clin. Biochem.* **2016**, *53*, 196–221. [CrossRef]
43. Torrisi, M.; Pennisi, G.; Russo, I.; Amico, F.; Esposito, M.; Liberto, A.; Cocimano, G.; Salerno, M.; Rosi, G.L.; Di Nunno, N.; et al. Sudden Cardiac Death in Anabolic-Androgenic Steroid Users: A Literature Review. *Medicina* **2020**, *56*, 587. [CrossRef]
44. Marsh, J.D.; Lehmann, M.H.; Ritchie, R.H.; Gwathmey, J.K.; Green, G.E.; Schiebinger, R.J. Androgen receptors mediate hypertrophy in cardiac myocytes. *Circulation* **1998**, *98*, 256–261. [CrossRef]
45. Perry, J.C.; Schuetz, T.M.; Memon, M.D.; Faiz, S.; Cancarevic, I. Anabolic Steroids and Cardiovascular Outcomes: The Controversy. *Cureus* **2020**, *12*, e9333. [CrossRef]
46. Thiblin, I.; Garmo, H.; Garle, M.; Holmberg, L.; Byberg, L.; Michaëlsson, K.; Gedeborg, R. Anabolic steroids and cardiovascular risk: A national population-based cohort study. *Drug Alcohol Depend.* **2015**, *152*, 87–92. [CrossRef]
47. Montisci, M.; El Mazloum, R.; Cecchetto, G.; Terranova, C.; Ferrara, S.D.; Thiene, G.; Basso, C. Anabolic androgenic steroids abuse and cardiac death in athletes: Morphological and toxicological findings in four fatal cases. *Forensic Sci. Int.* **2012**, *217*, e13–e18. [CrossRef] [PubMed]
48. Achar, S.; Rostamian, A.; Narayan, S.M. Cardiac and Metabolic Effects of Anabolic-Androgenic Steroid Abuse on Lipids, Blood Pressure, Left Ventricular Dimensions, and Rhythm. *Am. J. Cardiol.* **2010**, *106*, 893–901. [CrossRef] [PubMed]
49. Sachtleben, T.R.; Berg, K.E.; Elias, B.A.; Cheatham, J.P.; Felix, G.L.; Hofschire, P.J. The effects of anabolic steroids on myocardial structure and cardiovascular fitness. *Med. Sci. Sports Exerc.* **1993**, *25*, 1240–1245. [CrossRef] [PubMed]
50. D'Andrea, A.; Caso, P.; Salerno, G.; Scarafile, R.; De Corato, G.; Mita, C.; Di Salvo, G.; Severino, S.; Cuomo, S.; Liccardo, B.; et al. Left ventricular early myocardial dysfunction after chronic misuse of anabolic androgenic steroids: A Doppler myocardial and strain imaging analysis * COMMENTARY. *Br. J. Sports Med.* **2007**, *41*, 149–155. [CrossRef]
51. Baggish, A.L.; Weiner, R.B.; Kanayama, G.; Hudson, J.I.; Picard, M.H.; Hutter, A.M.; Pope, H.G. Long-Term Anabolic-Androgenic Steroid Use Is Associated With Left Ventricular Dysfunction. *Circ. Hear. Fail.* **2010**, *3*, 472–476. [CrossRef]
52. Riezzo, I.; Di Paolo, M.; Neri, M.; Bello, S.; Cantatore, S.; D'Errico, S.; Dinucci, D.; Parente, R.; Pomara, C.; Rabozzi, R.; et al. Anabolic Steroid - and Exercise - Induced Cardio-Depressant Cytokines and Myocardial β1 Receptor Expression in CD1 Mice. *Curr. Pharm. Biotechnol.* **2011**, *12*, 275–284. [CrossRef]
53. Lieberherr, M.; Grosse, B. Androgens increase intracellular calcium concentration and inositol 1,4,5-trisphosphate and diacylglycerol formation via a pertussis toxin-sensitive G-protein. *J. Biol. Chem.* **1994**, *269*, 7217–7223. [CrossRef]
54. D'Andrea, A.; Radmilovic, J.; Caselli, S.; Carbone, A.; Scarafile, R.; Sperlongano, S.; Tocci, G.; Formisano, T.; Martone, F.; Liccardo, B.; et al. Left atrial myocardial dysfunction after chronic abuse of anabolic andro-genic steroids: A speckle tracking echocardiography analysis. *Int. J. Cardiovasc. Imaging.* **2018**, *34*, 1549–1559. [CrossRef] [PubMed]
55. Hernández-Guerra, A.I.; Tapia, J.; Menéndez-Quintanal, L.M.; Lucena, J.S. Sudden cardiac death in anabolic androgenic ster-oids abuse: Case report and literature review. *Forensic Sci. Res.* **2019**, *4*, 267–273.
56. Zhu, D.; Hadoke, P.W.; Wu, J.; Vesey, A.T.; Lerman, D.A.; Dweck, M.R.; Newby, D.E.; Smith, L.B.; MacRae, V.E. Ablation of the an-drogen receptor from vascular smooth muscle cells demonstrates a role for testosterone in vascular calcification. *Sci. Rep.* **2016**, *20*, 24807. [CrossRef]
57. Liu, J.-D.; Wu, Y.-Q. Anabolic-androgenic steroids and cardiovascular risk. *Chin. Med J.* **2019**, *132*, 2229–2236. [CrossRef] [PubMed]
58. Sculthorpe, N.; Grace, F.; Jones, P.; Davies, B. Evidence of altered cardiac electrophysiology following prolonged an-drogenic anabolic steroid use. *Cardiovasc. Toxicol.* **2010**, *10*, 239–243. [CrossRef] [PubMed]
59. Alizade, E.; Avcı, A.; Fidan, S.; Tabakçı, M.; Bulut, M.; Zehir, R.; Simsek, Z.; Evlice, M.; Arslantaş, U.; Çakır, H.; et al. The effect of chronic anabolic-androgenic steroid use on TpE interval, Tp-E/Qt ratio, and Tp-E/Qtc ratio in male bodybuilders. *Ann. Noninvasive Electrocardiol.* **2015**, *20*, 592–600. [CrossRef]
60. Shirpoor, A.; Heshmatian, B.; Tofighi, A.; Eliasabad, S.N.; Kheradmand, F.; Zerehpoosh, M. Nandrolone administration with or without strenuous exercise increases cardiac fatal genes overexpression, calcium/calmodulin-dependent protein kinaseiiδ, and monoamine oxidase activities and enhances blood pressure in adult wistar rats. *Gene* **2019**, *697*, 131–137. [CrossRef]
61. Pärssinen, M.; Kujala, U.; Vartiainen, E.; Sarna, S.; Seppälä, T. Increased premature mortality of competitive powerlifters suspected to have used anabolic agents. *Int. J. Sports. Med.* **2000**, *21*, 225–227. [CrossRef] [PubMed]

62. Melchert, R.B.; Welder, A.A. Cardiovascular effects of androgenic-anabolic steroids. *Med. Sci. Sports Exerc.* **1995**, *27*, 1252–1262. [CrossRef] [PubMed]
63. Rothman, R.D.; Weiner, R.B.; Pope, H.G.; Kanayama, G.; Hutter, A.M.; A Fifer, M.; Dec, G.W.; Baggish, A.L. Anabolic androgenic steroid induced myocardial toxicity: An evolving problem in an ageing population. *BMJ Case Rep.* **2011**, *2011*. [CrossRef]
64. Finocchiaro, G.; Papadakis, M.; Robertus, J.L.; Dhutia, H.; Steriotis, A.K.; Tome, M.; Mellor, G.; Merghani, A.; Malhotra, A.; Behr, E.; et al. Etiology of Sudden Death in Sports: Insights From a United Kingdom Regional Registry. *J. Am. Coll. Cardiol.* **2016**, *67*, 2108–2115. [CrossRef]
65. Sheppard, M.N. Aetiology of sudden cardiac death in sport: A histopathologist's perspective. *Br. J. Sports Med.* **2012**, *46*, i15–i21. [CrossRef] [PubMed]
66. Sessa, F.; Salerno, M.; Di Mizio, G.; Bertozzi, G.; Messina, G.; Tomaiuolo, B.; Pisanelli, D.; Maglietta, F.; Ricci, P.; Pomara, C. Anabolic Androgenic Steroids: Searching New Molecular Biomarkers. *Front. Pharmacol.* **2018**, *9*, 1321. [CrossRef] [PubMed]
67. Soplinska, A.; Zareba, L.; Wicik, Z.; Eyileten, C.; Jakubik, D.; Siller-Matula, J.M.; De Rosa, S.; Malek, L.A.; Postula, M. MicroRNAs as Biomarkers of Systemic Changes in Response to Endurance Exercise—A Comprehensive Review. *Diagnostics* **2020**, *10*, 813. [CrossRef]

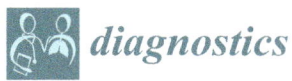

Review

MicroRNAs as Biomarkers of Systemic Changes in Response to Endurance Exercise—A Comprehensive Review

Aleksandra Soplinska [1], Lukasz Zareba [1], Zofia Wicik [1,2], Ceren Eyileten [1], Daniel Jakubik [1], Jolanta M. Siller-Matula [1,3], Salvatore De Rosa [4], Lukasz A. Malek [5] and Marek Postula [1,6,*]

1. Center for Preclinical Research and Technology CEPT, Department of Experimental and Clinical Pharmacology, Medical University of Warsaw, 02-097 Warsaw, Poland; ola@soplinska.pl (A.S.); lukaszzareba01@gmail.com (L.Z.); zofiawicik@gmail.com (Z.W.); ceren.eyileten-postula@wum.edu.pl (C.E.); dr.jakubik@gmail.com (D.J.); jolanta.siller-matula@meduniwien.ac.at (J.M.S.-M.)
2. Centro de Matemática, Computação e Cognição, Universidade Federal do ABC, São Paulo 055080-90, Brazil
3. Department of Cardiology, Medical University of Vienna, 1090 Vienna, Austria
4. Division of Cardiology, Department of Medical and Surgical Sciences, "Magna Graecia" University, 88100 Catanzaro, Italy; saderosa@unicz.it
5. Department of Epidemiology, Cardiovascular Disease Prevention and Health Promotion, National Institute of Cardiology, 04-635 Warsaw, Poland; lmalek@ikard.pl
6. Longevity Center, 00-761 Warsaw, Poland
* Correspondence: mpostula@wum.edu.pl; Tel.: +48-221166160; Fax: +48-221166202

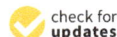

Received: 15 September 2020; Accepted: 9 October 2020; Published: 13 October 2020

Abstract: Endurance sports have an unarguably beneficial influence on cardiovascular health and general fitness. Regular physical activity is considered one of the most powerful tools in the prevention of cardiovascular disease. MicroRNAs are small particles that regulate the post-transcription gene expression. Previous studies have shown that miRNAs might be promising biomarkers of the systemic changes in response to exercise, before they can be detected by standard imaging or laboratory methods. In this review, we focused on four important physiological processes involved in adaptive changes to various endurance exercises (namely, cardiac hypertrophy, cardiac myocyte damage, fibrosis, and inflammation). Moreover, we discussed miRNAs' correlation with cardiopulmonary fitness parameter (VO_{2max}). After a detailed literature search, we found that miR-1, miR-133, miR-21, and miR-155 are crucial in adaptive response to exercise.

Keywords: microRNA; endurance sport; adaptive changes; cardiac hypertrophy; cardiac fibrosis

1. Introduction

The old Latin saying "mens sana in corpore sano" indicates that the beneficial influence of exercise has been known for centuries. Cardiovascular diseases (CVDs) are the leading cause of death worldwide. According to the World Health Organization (WHO) data, they are responsible for approximately 31% of deaths annually. It is estimated that nearly 80% of premature CVDs are preventable by modification of lifestyle including regular physical activity [1]. Regular exercise of moderate intensity has a beneficial influence in cardiovascular health. It is considered to be one of the most valuable nonpharmacological strategies to prevent and reduce the risk of coronary artery disease and myocardial infarction by up to 50% [2]. According to the European Society of Cardiology, adults should engage in at least 150 min per week (min/week) of moderate intensity or 75 min/week of vigorous intensity aerobic exercise to reduce atherosclerotic cardiovascular disease risk. Furthermore, it is recommended to gradually increase aerobic exercise to 300 min/week of moderate intensity or 150 min/week of vigorous intensity for additional benefits [3].

Endurance training can be described as long-time activity characterized by high dynamic and low to high power load such as swimming, rowing, cycling, running, or a combination of those [4]. From a physiological point of view, the main intent of endurance training is to edge the threshold of activation for anaerobic metabolism and lactate production. High-intensity training demands a sustained 5- to 6-fold increase in cardiac output for prolonged time. Repetitive effort is further compensated by electrical, structural, and functional cardiac adaptation called the "athlete's heart" which is characterized by an increase in left ventricular (LV) wall thickness, symmetrical increase in both left and right ventricular and atrial capacity size, and often borderline LV ejection fraction [5].

Despite unarguable beneficial influence, endurance exercise can act as a double-edged sword. Intensive exercise in adolescent and young athletes may be rarely associated with the risk of sudden cardiac death (SCD). The combination of LV hypertrophy, enlargement, and/or low ejection fraction can overlap with inherited cardiomyopathies, which are the most common causes of SCD in young sportsmen [6]. For this reason, the differential diagnosis between athlete's heart and disease using conventional methods remains challenging and new biomarkers are needed to distinguish physiology from pathology.

Over past years, microRNAs (miRNAs) have emerged as potential biomarkers for adaptive changes in response to exercise. MicroRNAs are short noncoding RNAs that regulate post-transcriptional gene expression by inhibiting protein translation or enhancing degradation of messenger RNA (mRNA). MicroRNAs are involved in the development of normal, functional heart tissue. They control cell growth, cell differentiation, apoptosis, and proliferation and are involved in the pathophysiology of cardiovascular pathologies like hypertrophy, fibrosis, and cardiomyocytes' damage [7].

MicroRNAs comprise a leading class of small RNAs in most tissues. MiRNA genes are located in various genomic contexts, however, the majority of human miRNAs are encoded by introns (noncoding transcripts). MiRNA biosynthesis starts by production of primary miRNA by RNA polymerase II. Then, miRNAs are further processed by a complex consisting of the RNA binging protein, DGCR8 microprocessor subunit, and the endoribonuclease, Drosha. Primary miRNAs are exported to the cytoplasm where they are further processed by endoribonuclease Dicer and subsequently loaded onto Argonaute family proteins to form an effector complex [8].

On the strength of their biochemical stability and the ease of access, circulating miRNAs have aroused the interest as potential biomarkers of various pathological states as well as potential therapeutic targets. Multiple studies have been conducted to evaluate their prognostic value in CVDs [9,10].

Circulating miRNAs are altered in response to acute and endurance exercise and can be engaged in the adaptations to exercise. Previous studies assessed miRNA plasma levels in marathon runners and showed increased levels of some miRNAs after marathon runs and their association with standard fitness parameters [11]. Other studies demonstrated correlations between miRNAs expression and cardiac injury markers such as troponin plasma levels, n-terminal b-type natriuretic peptide (NT-pro-BNP), or creatine kinase-MB (CK-MB). Therefore, they are a potential biomarker of cardiac adaptation processes to exercise [12]. Circulating miRNAs may improve exercise evaluation as well as facilitating the differential diagnosis between adaptive changes and pathology [13]. Therefore, in this article, we aim to review the current knowledge of miRNAs' involvement in endurance training.

2. Article Search Process

Electronic databases Pubmed and Scopus were searched up to September 2020. Original studies were reviewed to assess their relevance to our focus, namely the clinical usefulness of miRNAs as biomarkers of adaptive changes in response to endurance exercise based on human studies. We also investigated review articles and meta-analysis and their secondary references were examined for possible inclusion. Papers describing strength exercises were excluded from our review.

The following search syntax was used: "Search ("micrornas" [MeSH Terms] OR "mir" [MeSH Terms] OR "mirna" [MeSH Terms] OR "circulating miRNA" [MeSH Terms] OR "circulating microRNA"

[MeSH Terms]) AND ("endurance training" [MeSH Terms] AND ("adaptation" [MeSH Terms] OR "change" [All Fields]) Filters: Humans. Our search was limited to human studies and did not exclude studies on the basis of ethnicity.

3. Results

3.1. MicroRNAs and Adaptive Cardiac Hypertrophy Versus Hypertrophic Cardiomyopathy

Mild myocardial hypertrophy is considered as one of the structural adaptations to endurance training. Well-trained endurance athletes display an increased wall thickness and relevant dilatation of LV obtained mostly by eccentric hypertrophy. This allows increasing the cardiac output and maximal oxygen uptake (VO_{2max}) and subsequently improves physical fitness [14]. Numerous studies aimed to correlate miRNAs and hypertrophy and allowed a distinction between anti- and prohypertrophic miRNAs (see Figure 1) [15]. It is important also to distinguish adaptive cardiac hypertrophy from hypertrophic cardiomyopathy (HCM) and find the differences in miRNA expression.

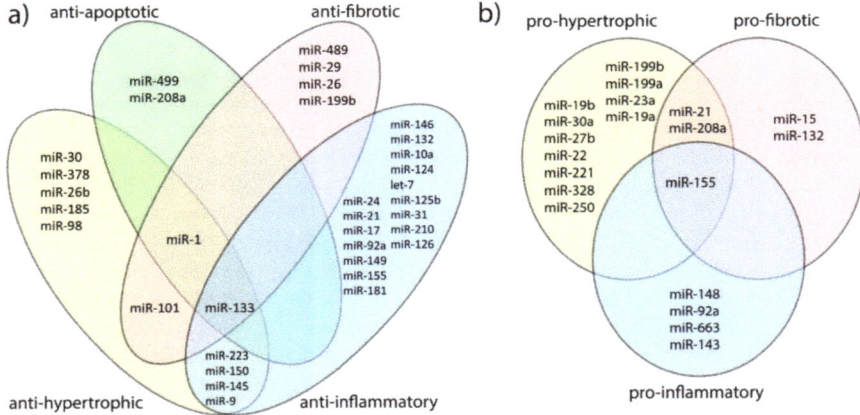

Figure 1. The potential role of microRNAs in cardiac remodeling. (**a**) MicroRNAs associated with ibeneficial response to endurance exercise. (**b**) MicroRNAs associated with pro-inflammatory, pro-fibrotic and pro-hypertrophic processes in cardiac remodeling. miR, microRNA.

Several studies evaluated the involvement of a number of miRNAs in cardiac hypertrophy, however, the results are conflicting [11,16–18]. Moreen et al. investigated a relation of miRNAs with conventional biochemical, cardiovascular, and performance indices in endurance athletes before, immediately after, and 24 h after a marathon run. After the marathon run, significant increases of miR-1, miR-133a, miR-206, miR-208b, and miR-499 were observed. MiR-133a was positively related to the thickness of the intraventricular septum in echocardiography. Interestingly, the expression of miR-1, miR-133a, miR-206 was correlated to themselves ($p < 0.001$), whereas no such correlation was found in the case of miR-208b and miR-499. There is a possibility that the difference occurred due to the stronger skeletal muscle relation of miR-1, miR-133a, and miR-206 than the other measured miRNAs [11]. MiR-1, miR-133, and miR-206 belong to a novel group of miRNAs known as myomiRs. MyomiRNAs are described as striated muscle-specific or muscle-enriched miRNAs that regulate muscle development and homeostasis. They are involved in myoblast proliferation and differentiation as well as muscle regeneration [19]. Interestingly, expression of precursors of the mentioned myomiRs is upregulated in elderly people compared to younger ones. Nevertheless, this difference can no longer be observed while analyzing mature forms of myomiRs [20].

In another study, Ramos et al. hypothesized that miRNAs exhibit dose–response correlation with varying levels of exercise intensity and duration (see details in Table 1). The results showed that miRNAs can be divided into three different expression patterns: (1) responsive, dose-dependent with miR-1 dependent on exercise intensity, and miR-133a, miR-222 dependent on duration of exercise, (2) responsive with no significant dose responsiveness like miR-24, miR-146a, and (3) nonresponsive regardless of intensity or duration of the training (i.e., miR-21, -210). Moreover, using an animal model, it was found that miR-133a correlated positively with increased intraventricular septal thickness and high expression of serum response factor transcripts which play key role in myocyte proliferation and cardiac hypertrophy. Despite the antihypertrophic effect of miR-1 and miR-133a, their plasma level corresponds to the active heart remodeling by a decrease of its intracellular concentration, which may weaken the inhibition effect, activate gene programming, and start the adaptation process [17]. Mooren et al. showed both miR-1 and -133 to be upregulated, which may suggest a similar expression pathway as it was described previously [11,21]. However, in Ramos et al., the gap in expression of those miRNAs was observed. The miR-1 elevation was dependent on the higher intensity of training and was much more increased than miR-133, whereas miR-133 was significantly related to the longer duration of training, which had weaker effect on miR-1 expression [17]. Contradistinctively, Fernandez et al. showed miR-1 correlation with longer exercise (i.e., marathon run) [22]. The difference between studies may occur due to the nature of endurance exertion during marathons, which presents high intensity and long duration features, therefore, simultaneous elevation of miR-1 and miR-133. Additionally, signaling pathways linked to the miR-1 and miR-133 upregulation such as MAPK ERK1/2 or myogenic factors like MyoD or myogenin could be activated by different muscle exertion features, which may result in divergent miRNAs plasma level elevation (see Figure 2) [23,24]. It was shown that ERK1/2 is activated by a hypoxic environment and increases miR-133 expression in cardiomyocytes [23]. Importantly, it was shown that myogenic factors such as myoD and myogenin may regulate the expression of muscle-specific miRNAs, including miR-1, miR-133a/b, and miR-206 in biogenesis and these miRNAs were upregulated during myogenesis [25,26]. On the other hand, Denham et al. [18] demonstrated contrary results; downregulation of miR-1 and miR-133 expressions after acute treadmill exercise was observed. In addition, Baggish et al. [16] detected no miR-133 elevation at the baseline and after the acute exercise at the start and at the end of the 90-day sustained training program. This observation may correspond to the previous finding, as the acute exercise protocol was performed on an upright cycle ergometer and was relatively short. Different results could be obtained due to different features of participants and the training program. However, there is also one relevant difference: the participants have undergone the acute exertion on treadmills not by running. The reason for contrary results can be due to different types of acute exercise. More studies should be conducted to determine the difference in miRNA expression after varied types of endurance exertion.

It is worth mentioning that miR-1 and miR-133 were previously described to be significantly downregulated in heart tissue in patients with HCM [27]. Similar to the endurance athletes, HCM patients showed a significantly increased level of miR-133, but surprisingly, no significant result was observed for miR-1 [28]. This finding may suggest that the poverty of in-tissue miR-1 and miR-133 is important for development of both adaptive hypertrophy and HCM. However, the difference of miR-1 concentration suggests that in the pathological state, miR-1 expression is downregulated in cardiomyocytes, whereas in adaptive hypertrophy, it is probably stable or induced but there is a loss due to sarcolemma damage. This hypothesis should be investigated in the future in athletes and also elderly people, who were proven to develop muscle hypertrophy in response to the training [29].

Importantly, out of 17 articles which aimed to analyze the importance of miRNAs in endurance training, only one study used mRNA–miRNA targeting in silico prediction tool by using bioinformatic analysis via KEGG (Kyoto Encyclopedia of Genes and Genomes) to identify possible molecular pathways. Interestingly, based on functional enrichment analysis, the study identified 31 molecular pathways (enriched with the targets of the miRNA profiles) after a 10 km run, and 61 molecular pathways after the marathon races. These molecular pathways were relatively associated to heart physiology and pathophysiology, including cardiac hypertrophy, cardiac remodeling and function, fibrosis, response to injury, and cell survival and proliferation, which suggests that endurance training may be linked to not only physiological adaptive cardiac hypertrophy, but also pathophysiological cardiac hypertrophy [30].

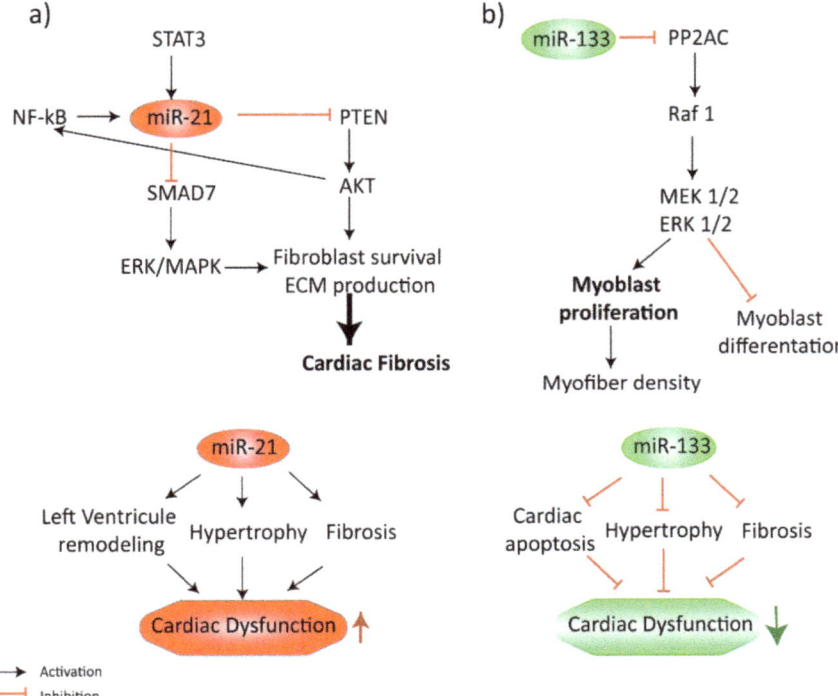

Figure 2. Regulation of cardiac remodeling by microRNAs and the functions of their target mRNAs. MAPK/ERK pathway plays a crucial impact on signal transduction for myosin growth. PI3K/AKT signaling pathway regulates cell proliferation, metabolism, survival, and angiogenesis and controls the development and transformation of left ventricular hypertrophy. The ERK signaling pathway, a member of the MAPK family, comprises a cascade of a series of successively acting kinases. (**a**) The role of miR-21 in cardiac remodeling. Regulation of ERK is mediated by miR-21 via inhibiting PTEN and SMAD7 gene expression. (**b**) The role of miR-133 in cardiac remodeling. MicroRNA-133 plays a role in determining cardiomyocyte hypertrophy by targeting PP2AC. Abbreviations: miR, microRNA; STAT3, signal transducer and activator of transcription 3; NF-κB, nuclear factor-κB; PTEN, phosphatase and tensin homolog; ERK, extracellular signal-regulated kinase; MAPK, mitogen-activated protein kinase; PP2AC, protein phosphatase 2A; Raf-1, Raf-1 proto-oncogene, serine/threonine kinase.

Table 1. Characteristics of microRNA studied in endurance sports.

First Author	miRNAs	Material	Exercise	Training Protocol and Samples Collection	Methodology	Subjects	Results ($p < 0.05$)
Alack 2019 [31]	miR-24, miR-27a, miR-21, miR-15a, miR-23a, miR-221, miR-125b	Leukocytes	-	At rest	qRT-PCR, miRNAeasy Mini kit, TaqTM Universal SYBR Green Supermix	13 trained triathletes and marathon runners ($VO_{2max} > 59$ mL/kg × min) and 12 untrained healthy controls ($VO_{2max} < 45$ mL/kg × min)	Endurance athletes: downregulated: miR-21, miR-23a
Backes 2014 [32]	1205 different miRNAs	Whole blood	Cycling	Before and after exhaustive exercise on cyclic ergometer in each group	Microarray, qRT-PCR miScript SYBR Green	12 elite endurance athletes (6 males, 6 females; 10 triathletes, 2 cyclists) and 12 age- and sex-matched controls; included 8 athletes and 8 controls	Endurance/control after exercise miR-181a, miR-320b were decreased in athletes
Baggish 2011 [16]	miR-20a, miR-210, miR-221, miR-222, miR-328, miR-21, miR-146a, miR-21, miR-133a, miR-21, miR-146a, and miR-210	Blood (plasma)	Cycling	At rest and during acute exhaustive exercise testing on upright cycle ergometer, before and after a 90-day period of aerobic exercise training	qRT-PCR	10 competitive male rowers ($n = 10$, age = 19.1 ± 0.6 years)	Elevated by acute exercise before and after sustained training: miR-146a, miR-222 elevated by acute exercise before but not after sustained training: miR-21, miR-221 elevated after sustained training: miR-20a nonresponsive: miR-133a, miR-210, miR-328
Baggish 2014 [12]	miR-1, miR-133a, miR-499-5p, miR-208a, miR-126, miR-146a	Blood (plasma)	Running	At rest, immediately after marathon and 24 h after	qRT-PCR, TaqMan miRNA	21 healthy male marathon runners	Upregulated after the race: miR-126, miR-1, miR-133a, miR-499-5p, miR-208a, miR-146a
Bye 2013 [33]	miR-210, miR-21, miR-125a, miR-652, miR-151, miR-29a, Let-7d, miR-222	Blood (plasma)	VO_{2max} test	Before the start of the exercise test	qRT-PCR	Screening cohort: 12- high VO_{2max}, 12- low VO_{2max} validation cohort: 38- high VO_{2max}, 38- low VO_{2max}	Low VO_{2max} group: upregulated: miR-210, miR-222, miR-21 (with only males)
Danese 2018 [34]	miR-133a, miR-206	Blood (plasma)	Half-marathon	Before and immediately after the half-marathon—21.1 km	qRT-PCR, TaqMan MicroRNA assay	28 middle-aged, recreation athletes (11 women and 17 men; mean age, 46 years)	Elevated after the half-marathon run: miR-133a and miR-206

164

Table 1. Cont.

First Author	miRNAs	Material	Exercise	Training Protocol and Samples Collection	Methodology	Subjects	Results ($p < 0.05$)
Fernandez-Sanjurjo 2020 [22]	Global miRNA screening (752 miRs)	Blood (plasma)	Running	Before and immediately after: 10 km race, half-marathon, and marathon	qRT-PCR	9 runners	After 10 km run Upregulated: miR-199b-5p, miR-424-3p, miR-33a-5p, miR-551a, miR-1537, miR-223-5p, miR-1260q, let-7b-3p, miR-150-5p, miR-423-5p, miR-223-3p, miR-345-5p, miR-505-3p Downregulated: miR-346 After half-marathon: Upregulated: miR-425-3p, miR-33a-5p, miR-338-3p, miR-339-5p, miR-106b-3p, miR-502-3p, miR-27a-3p, miR-660-5p, miR-505-3p, miR-100-5p, miR-22-3p, miR-30e-5p, miR-497-5p After marathon: Upregulated:miR-1972, miR-940, miR-424-3p, miR-130b-5p, miR-223-5p, miR-145-3p, miR-181c-30, miR-501-3p, miR1260a, miR675-3p, miR345-5p, miR-424-5p, miR-1-3p, miR-34a-5p, miR-629-5p, miR-30a-5p, miR-148a-3p, miR-596, miR-10b-5p, miR-304-5p, miR-320d Downregulated: miR-192-5p, miR-206-5p, miR-103a-3p, miR-106b-5p, miR144-3p, miR-665, miR-486-3p
Gomes 2014 [13]	miR-1, miR-133a, miR-206	Blood (plasma)	Half-marathon	Before warm-up and up to 10 min after the run	qRT-PCRIaq Man miRNA	5 male recreational runners	Upregulated: miR-1, miR-133a, miR-206
Gonzalo-Calvo 2018 [30]	Panel of 74 c-miRNAs	Blood (plasma)	10 km, half-marathon, marathon	Before and after (0 h, 24 h, 72 h): 10-km, half-marathon, and marathon separated by one-month break	qRT-PCR miScript SYBR Green	9 healthy, highly trained middle-aged amateur subjects	10 km run: immediately after – increased miRNAs: miR-132-3p, miR-150-5p, decreased miRNAs: miR-103a-3p and miR-139-5p 24 h after – decreased miRNA: miR-590-5p Marathon run: immediately after – increased miRNAs: miR-21-3p, miR-27a-3p, miR-29a-3p, miR-30a-5p, miR-34a-5p, miR-126-3p, miR-142-5p, miR-143-3p, miR-195-5p, miR-199a-3p 24 h after– decreased miRNAs: miR-25-3p, miR-29b-3p, miR-30b-5p, miR-106b-5p, miR-107, miR-497-5p downregulated immediately after and remained downregulated for 24 h: miR-103a-3p and miR-375-5p

165

Table 1. Cont.

First Author	miRNAs	Material	Exercise	Training Protocol and Samples Collection	Methodology	Subjects	Results ($p < 0.05$)
Denham 2016 [18]	miR-1, miR-133a, miR-181a, miR-486, and miR-494	Whole blood	Running-sprint	Before and after 4 weeks (thrice weekly) of sprint interval training and a single bout of maximal aerobic treadmill exercise	qRT-PCR, TaqMan miRNA	67 endurance athletes and 61 healthy controls; 19 young men—acute exercise trial	Endurance athletes, increased: miR-1, miR-486, and miR-494 after endurance training Healthy, young men decreased: miR-1, miR-133a, and miR-486 immediately after maximal aerobic exercise
Kern 2020 [35]	Global miRNA	Blood (plasma)	Running	Before, after 8 weeks of endurance training, after 8 weeks of wash-out phase, and after another 8 weeks of endurance training	Microarray	23 healthy untrained volunteers	Most important miRNA associated with VO_{2max} Cluster 1: miR-4465, miR-5581-5p, miR-6879-5p, miR-6869-5p Cluster 2: miR-7975 Cluster 6: miR-326-5p, miR-502-5p, miR-502-3p, miR-340-5p
Kraviinen 2019 [36]	miR-21, miR-26, miR-126, miR-146, miR-221, miR-222	Blood (serum and extracellular vesicles, EV) and sweat (EV)	Cycling	Sweat collection during, blood collection before and after each protocol: (1) maximal aerobic capacity test (2) anaerobic threshold, and (3) aerobic threshold (AerT) tests. Sauna—control	qRT-PCR, miRNAeasy Mini kit, miScript II RT Kit	8 healthy trained subjects (all protocols)	Elevated In sweat: All endurance exercise: miR-26 Protocol 3 vs. control: miR-21 In serum EVs: Protocol 2 vs. control: miR-21, miR-222
Mooren 2013 [11]	miR-1, miR-133, miR-206, miR-499, miR-208b, miR-21, and miR-155	Blood (plasma)	Marathon	2 days before in the morning, directly after, and 24 h after a public marathon run	qRT-PCR TaqMan miRNA	14 male endurance athletes	Increased after race: miR-1, miR-133a, miR-206, miR-208b, miR-499 Elevated 24 h after race: miR-1, miR-133a, miR-206
Nielsen 2013 [37]	global miRNA (742 miRNA)	Blood (plasma)	Cycling	Before (at rest) and immediately after 1 h, post 1 h, post 3 h an acute exercise training (60 min cycle ergometer exercise at 65% of Pmax) and following 12 weeks of endurance training (cycle ergometer with frequency of 5 times per week for 12 weeks)	Microarray, RT-PCR, miScript SYBR green and ROX, Exiqons miRNome panel V2, ViiA7 Sequence Detection	13 healthy men—acute exercise training, 7 healthy men—endurance training	Immediately after: all downregulated: miR-106a, miR-221, miR-30b, miR-151-5p, Let7, miR-146a, miR-652, miR-151-3p upregulated 1 h–3 h: miR-330-3p, miR-223, miR-139-5p, miR-143, miR-145, miR-424 after 1 h: miR-1, miR-424, miR-133a, miR-133b after 12-week training: (a) upregulated: miR-103, miR-107 (b) downregulated: miR-342-3p, Let-7d, miR-766, miR-25, miR-148a, miR-185, miR-21, miR-148b, miR-133a, miR-92a, miR-29b

Table 1. Cont.

First Author	miRNAs	Material	Exercise	Training Protocol and Samples Collection	Methodology	Subjects	Results ($p < 0.05$)
Ramos 2017 [17]	miR-21, miR-210, miR-24, miR-146, miR-1, miR-133, miR-222	Blood (plasma)	Running	Two studies: 1) controlled intensity 1-week intervals at 3 intensities (6,7,8 miles/h) and final 5-mile test 2) duration test speed 7 miles/h, 30,60, 90 min duration, final 5-mile treadmill run. Blood samples collected immediately after treadmill running	qRT-PCR, TaqMan miRNA	26 healthy young men—12 in intensity trial and 14 in duration trial	Elevated in both groups and not intensity- or duration-dependent: miR-24, miR-146a Elevated and intensity-responsive: miR-1 Elevated and duration-responsive: miR-133, miR-222
Uhlemann 2014 [38]	miR-126, miR-133	Blood (plasma)		Three studies regarding endurance exercise: Study 1: maximal symptom-limited exercise test, Study 2: bicycling for 4 h, Study 3: running a marathon	qRT-PCR, TaqMan miRNA	Study 1: 13 healthy participants, Study 2: 12 healthy well-trained men, Study 3: 22 male middle-aged marathon runners with no history of coronary artery disease	Study 1: increased miR-126 at maximum power Study 2: increased miR-126 Study 3: increased miR-126 and miR-133
Yin 2020 [39]	miR-1-3p, miR-133a-3p, miR-133b, miR-206	Blood (plasma)	Running	Before, immediately after, and 24 h after 8 km run	qRT-PCR	18 healthy trained young men	Immediately after run elevated: miR-1-3p, miR-133a-3p, and miR-133b 24 h after run: elevated: miR-133a-3p

Abbreviations: microRNA, miR; high-intensity interval training, HIIT; maximal oxygen uptake, VO_{2max}; hour, h; maximal power, P_{max}; minutes, min; second, s; $p < 0.05$; extracellular vesicles (EV).

3.2. MicroRNAs and Cardiomyocytes Damage

It is well known that excessive sustained endurance exercises may lead to increased plasma levels of troponin-I, creatine kinase myocardial band (CK-MB), myoglobin, and B-type natriuretic peptide (BNP), but the cause of this elevation is not clearly understood. Those biomarkers reflect the myocardial cells damage and loss of integrity of their desmosomal connections [40]. In addition, it was shown that elevated cardiac biomarkers such as high-sensitivity cardiac troponin T (hs-cTnT), the N-terminal prohormone of brain natriuretic peptide (NT-proBNP), return to their normal levels within 72 h after excessive exercise such as a marathon without complications [41]. It suggests that excessive endurance exercises can cause temporary, reversible cardiomyocytes sarcolemma damage. Exhaustive endurance exertion can also elevate the plasma levels of muscle-specific miRNA, which are abundantly present in the cardiomyocytes (Figure 1) [42]. In line with that, miR-499, miR-208, miR-133, and miR-1 are reflecting cardiomyocyte damage, and miRNA-1, miR-133, miR-499, and miR-208 possess antiapoptotic function, whereas miR-34 is proapoptotic [43–45].

In the study, running induced overexpression of miR-1-3p, miR-133a-3p, miR-133b-3p in young healthy adults. Moreover, miR-133a-3p was still elevated after 24 h of rest, whereas miR-1-3p and miR-133b-3p returned to their baseline. Levels of miR-1-3p and miR-133a-3p were correlated with myoglobin at 24 h after the run [39]. Baggish et al. showed that the concentration of cardiac-tissue-specific circulating miR-208a was significantly upregulated before, but it was substantially decreased 24 h after completing the marathon. Additionally, the conventional biomarkers of the cardiac injury such as hs-cTnT, hs-cTnI, and NT-pro-BNP were increased immediately after the run and remained elevated at the second time point; however, no correlation was found with miR-208a [12]. Similarly, in another study, there was no correlation between cardiac-specific miR-208, as well as miR-1, miR-133a, and miR-499, and the cardiac biomarkers (i.e., CK-MB, troponin T and I, and pro-BNP) measured after the marathon run [11]. Danese et al. found the elevation of miR-133a, miR-206 and CK, hs-cTnT levels after completing a half-marathon run but again no correlation was found. Interestingly, the highest elevation was detected in the miR-133 and hs-cTnT plasma levels, 7.5-fold and 4.2-fold, respectively. The enhanced plasma value of miR-133a may be interpreted as a potential physiological response to high-intensity and/or prolonged exercise, probably aimed to facilitate immediate regeneration or recovery of cardiac and skeletal muscle tissues [34].

All studies showed a significant elevation of specific miRNAs in response to the endurance exercise. MicroRNA-1, miR-133a/b, miR-208, and miR-499 were significantly upregulated immediately after the excessive endurance exertion, however, there was no correlation with the conventional cardiac damage markers at this time point. This lack of correlation may be explained by the different pattern of release into the circulation after cardiomyocyte injury. In line with that, one study found a correlation of miR-1a-3p and miR-133a-3p with myoglobin at 24 h after exercise, which indicates a faster release of those miRNAs than myoglobin, but a similar maintenance in plasma. miRNAs should be considered not only as the direct muscle damage biomarkers but also as indicators of reparative processes in response to external stimulus such as stress. In this scenario, the reason could be the upregulation of miRNA concentration is not correlated with the classic cardiac damage biomarkers [34]. The value of the above-mentioned miRNAs as cardiomyocytes damage or reparative processes biomarkers should be assessed in future studies. In particular, it is of key importance to understand whether a panel of circulating miRNAs might be able to differentiate hypoxic myocardial damage from myocardial injury induced by overload.

3.3. MicroRNAs and Fibrosis

Endurance exertion requires a significant increase of cardiac output usually for several hours, thereby enforcing prolonged and high-degree stress to all myocardial structures. This might lead to the positive cardiac training adaptations, but there is also a possibility of pathophysiological cardiac remodeling processes. Nowadays, still there is a discussion in the literature whether myocardial fibrosis may occur in elite endurance athletes due to regular excessive training or such an effect does not exist [46,47]. The fibrosis is a well-known risk factor for the major adverse cardiac events (MACE) and is specifically strongly correlated to the increased risk of arrhythmias [48]. Biomarkers have been established which are correlated with the cardiac fibrosis process, including matrix metalloproteinase (MMP)-1,-2,-3,-8,-9, tissue inhibitor of metalloproteinase (TIMP)-1,-4, TGFbeta1, growth differentiation factor 1 (GDF1), connective tissue growth factor (CTGF), osteopontine, periostine, galactine-3, ST2, and miRNAs [49]. Fibrosis-involved miRNAs, such as miR-1, miR-133, miR-26, miR-29, miR-21, miR-34 can be distinguished into those which are expressed mainly in fibroblasts like miR-29 and miR-21, and the rest of them which are expressed in different types of cells. Moreover, some miRNAs may play an important role as an antifibrotic or profibrotic regulator (Figure 1) [15,50,51].

One of the latest studies analyzed the expression of several miRNAs in response to different doses of endurance running. A significant increase of galectin-3 secretion (a prognostic biomarker in patients with heart failure) was observed immediately after a 10 km run, a half-marathon, and a marathon in a dose–response manner. Also, plasma expression of miR-21-5p was increased twofold, miR-29a-3p fourfold, and miR-34a-5p fourfold after a marathon compared to the baseline, however, all measured parameters returned to baseline values after 24 hours [30]. It may suggest that prolonged myocardial stress during a long endurance exertion could induce signaling towards myocardial fibrosis presented by galectine-3 and miR-21 upregulation. However, antifibrotic miRNAs such as miR-29a, miR-34a were also highly expressed, probably possessing a preventive role. Finally, the study may indicate that an endurance exertion-related fibrosis is rare in amateur athletes due to a preserved balance of pro- and antifibrotic agents. On the contrary, a previously described study may indicate that no profibrotic signaling was present in participants after acute endurance exertion, as fibrosis/inflammation-related miR-21 and miR-155 showed no significant response to exercise [11]. This finding could have occurred due to the features of participants. The study did not determine precisely how well trained runners were, which may indicate that most of them might have been amateur athletes. Furthermore, another study demonstrated that in elite runners, only miR-26 plasma expression was decreased, but no significant difference was observed in nonelite runners [52]. It may indicate that well-trained endurance athletes express weaker antifibrotic reaction after the exertion. It was hypothesized that it may predispose to the occurrence of myocardial fibrosis and arrhythmias like atrial fibrillation in some elite endurance athletes [53]. Another study showed upregulation of miR-29c, miR-222, and TGF-β1 mRNA after a high-intensity interval training program (for details, see Table 1) [54]. As miR-29 is considered to prevent fibrosis by targeting the TGFβ/SMAD3 signaling pathway, TGFβ mRNA expression after the training was evaluated and compared to the miRNA expression [55]. The results may implicate that trained endurance athletes express induced profibrotic signaling through the TGFβ pathway after acute exertion compared to the untrained ones.

Hence, we hypothesize that amateur endurance athletes present no or weak pro-/antifibrotic reaction after acute exertion, while well-trained ones express significant pro-/antifibrotic reaction and finally elite athletes show significant pro- and, in some cases, weaker antifibrotic response, however, due to an insufficient number of participants, such a conclusion should be drawn with caution. All studies showed that miRNAs are emerging important biomarkers of myocardial fibrosis in endurance athletes and should be further investigated. Moreover, regular measurements of c-miRNAs levels during a training program in professional endurance athletes may give crucial information for training customizations and myocardial fibrosis prevention.

3.4. MicroRNAs and Inflammatory Response

Inflammation is considered as a key factor of atherosclerosis, the leading CVD disease. It was proven that oxidative stress in vascular endothelial cells leads to accumulation of macrophages and increased production of inflammatory markers like IL-6, IL-1, and TNF-alpha [56]. Depending on the form, exercise seems to have a different influence on the immune system. Endurance training shows a tendency to upregulate the inflammatory biomarkers after an acute bout of exercise and downregulate in long-term programs, however, a previous systematic review on this topic failed to confirm these observations [57].

MicroRNAs are considered as potential biomarkers of inflammation and can be divided into anti-inflammatory and proinflammatory (see Figure 1) and they can correlate with classical markers of inflammatory response (such as leukocyte count, IL-6, IL-10, c-reactive protein-CRP, etc.) [9,58]. Gonzalo-Calvo et al. assessed the classical inflammatory and inflammation-related miRNA response to a 10 km run and a marathon [30]. Total leukocyte and neutrophil counts were elevated after the 10 km run and after the marathon, however, the increase was more pronounced in the marathon group. Furthermore, significant differences were observed in the miRNA expression pattern (after 10 km run, miR-150-5p levels were significantly increased, and after the marathon, let-7d-3p, let-7f-2-3p, miR-29-3p, miR-34a-5p, miR-125b-5p, miR-132-3p, miR-143-3p, miR-148-3, miR-223-5p, miR-424-3p, and miR-424-5p) (for details, see Table 1). Interestingly, miR-150-5p was positively correlated with leukocyte and neutrophil counts after the 10 km run. MiR-150-5p was shown to play an anti-inflammatory role by inhibiting the activation of PI3K and Akt and subsequently the NF-κB pathway detected by in silico analysis, as described by Grabarek et al. [59]. Let-7f-3p was positively correlated with hs-CRP, and miR-29-3p was negatively correlated with IL-10 levels after the marathon. The study suggests that acute endurance exercise induces a dose-dependent circulating inflammatory miRNA response. This might be a reason for the difference in magnitude of the inflammatory response between the race distances. Furthermore, the marathon run seemed to induce higher expression of let-7 family members involved in initiation and development of inflammatory response. Also, Baggish et al. found that inflammation-specific miR-146a, but not hs-CRP, was significantly elevated after the marathon run and returned to baseline value within 24 h (for details, see Table 1). This different temporal pattern of miR-146a rise in comparison to hs-CRP emphasizes a potential role of the miRNAs as novel marker of exercise physiology [12].

In another study using cycle-ergometer expression of two inflammation-related miRNAs in response to acute 60 min long endurance exercise, miR-146 and let-7i were downregulated (for details, see Table 1) [37]. Interestingly, let-7d, miR-21, -29b, -148 expressions were significantly lower after 12-week training. The following observations indicate that both small-dose acute exercise and long-term training may induce an anti-inflammatory response, irrespective of endurance exercise form [30,37]. This is in line with the latest observation where the expression of miR-146 showed the tendency to be increased after different cycling training protocols [36]. Furthermore, a study by Backes et al. showed significantly lower levels of proinflammatory let-7c in endurance athletes compared to controls on baseline [32]. It indicates that regularly training sportsmen have lower immune system reactivity which is in line with de Gonzalo-Calvo's conclusion that long-term endurance sports induce anti-inflammatory response [46]. A recent study showed that lymphocytes adapt to repetitive endurance exercise by increasing their resistance to apoptosis by upregulation of antiapoptotic and downregulation of proapoptotic miRNAs (especially miR-221) [31]. The alterations in apoptotic pathways might be the reason for the above-mentioned studies observing an attenuated immune response as a result of endurance exercise.

As a conclusion, the presented studies show different results of miRNA expression depending on exercise duration but not type. Acute aerobic exercise in small doses induces anti-inflammatory response whereas exhaustive endurance exercise (such as a marathon) increases proinflammatory miRNAs [12,30,37]. It seems that the NF-κB pathway plays a crucial role in exercise-mediated inflammatory response. In de Gonzalo-Calvo's study, miR-150-5p targeted the PI3K/Akt pathway and subsequently suppressed the NF-κB pathway after a 10 km run, whereas after a marathon, miR-146, which is known to enhance production of transcriptional factors of the NF-κB pathway, was upregulated [12,30]. Another important miRNA that takes part in exercise-dependent immune response is the let-7 family upregulating the toll-like receptor (TLR) pathway which initiates and develops inflammatory response. The let-7 family is upregulated in response to exhaustive endurance exercise, however, repetitive doses of aerobic exercises in training programs inhibit inflammation by downregulation of this family [30,32]. It seems that the NF-κB pathway, TLR pathway, and miRNAs related to them (miR-146, miR-150-5p, miR-21, miR-148, miR-223, let-7 family) are most important in exercise-dependent inflammatory response. However, more studies focusing on miRNAs and gene expression are needed to confirm such observations.

3.5. MicroRNAs and VO_{2max}

Maximal oxygen uptake (VO_{2max}) is defined as a maximal rate of oxygen consumption during incremental exercise. It is an indicator for integrated pulmonary, cardiovascular, and muscular capacity to uptake and utilize O_2. Various exercises increase the VO_{2max} capacity, however, aerobic high-intensity training was proven to be the most effective [60]. VO_{2max} was identified as a strong predictor of cardiovascular death and all-cause mortality in healthy adults and in patients with CAD [61].

Elite endurance athletes present high VO_{2max} due to large left cardiac chamber capacity and subsequently high cardiac output. Several miRNAs were identified which were correlated with the parameters of aerobic performance. An exercise-induced increase of miR-1, miR-133a, miR-206, miR-208b, and miR-499 was demonstrated directly after a marathon run. Further analysis revealed that miR-1, miR-133a, and miR-206 were positively correlated with both VO_{2max} and running speed at individual anaerobic lactate threshold (VIAS) [11]. MicroRNA-1, miR-133a, and miR-206 are typical miRNAs enriched from muscles. MicroRNA-1 and miR-206 regulate differentiation of skeletal myoblasts and miR-1 and miR-133a are considered as antihypertrophic factors. Probably, this unique ability to influence both tissues makes the mentioned miRNAs suitable as biomarkers for cardiopulmonary fitness.

Denham et al. confirmed a potential role of miR-1 in aerobic performance capacity, and suggested that together with miR-486, they may constitute an independent predictor of VO_{2max}. MicroRNA-1 and miR-486 were elevated and correlated significantly with the VO_{2max} values, and miR-486 was inversely correlated with heart rate at rest, after completing a four-week training program [18]. Moreover, inflammation-related miRNA such as miR-146a was correlated linearly with the increase of peak oxygen consumption before, as well as after, the training program. A similar expression pattern was observed with miR-20 indicating that both miR-146a and miR-20a could be plasma-based markers of cardiopulmonary fitness (see details in Table 1) [16]. Finally, 12 patients with the highest and 12 with the lowest VO_{2max} were selected out of 4631 patients from HUNT Fitness Study in order to perform the miRNA expression profiling. As a result, miR-210 was significantly higher in a validation cohort and therefore it was negatively correlated with VO_{2max} values. MicroRNA-21 and miR-222 presented weak correlation with VO_{2max}, however, their value was considered predictive of CVD [33].

Kern et al. showed that miRNA expression can be altered due to regular endurance training and highlighted six possible miRNA clusters that can be utilized to predict phenotypic VO_{2max} levels, where clusters 1, 2, and 6 were mostly depleted in the top list of negative feature coefficients (see Table 1). Furthermore, it was suggested that miR-532-5p could be a potential biomarker of VO_{2max} changes after carbohydrate uptake. It is in line with their miRNA enrichment analysis findings as VO_{2max} was significantly associated with the insulin signaling pathway [35].

In conclusion, miR-1, miR-133, miR-206, miR-146a, miR-20 were positively correlated with the VO_{2max} values, which suggests their significance as potential biomarkers for cardiopulmonary fitness. Interestingly, discrepant results were observed regarding miR-486 and its correlation with VO_{2max}. These inconsistencies are likely to be the product of many factors that vary across studies: (1) differences in participants (e.g., healthy endurance athletes who trained more than three times per week for at least one year versus young healthy subjects with no regular exercise regimen); (2) differences in training protocols (e.g., short-term VO_{2max} ergometer test versus long-term steady-state cycling program); (3) differences in blood samples collection schedules; and (4) differences in data analysis. In view of these many differences, it is not surprising that the literature is inconsistent. More studies should be conducted to estimate miR-486 value as a biomarker of cardiopulmonary fitness.

4. Conclusions

In the present article, we summarized the current knowledge of miRNA involvement in endurance training comprehensively, and also discussed the miRNAs that are regulated upon cardiac hypertrophy, cardiac myocyte damage, fibrosis, and inflammatory response during and after the endurance training. After a detailed literature search, we found that miR-1, miR-133, miR-21, and miR-155 are crucial in adaptive response to exercise. Studies available in the literature showed different effects on inflammatory-related miRNA expression depending on exercise duration but not its type [30]. Further studies are needed in order to determine interactions between miRNAs and genes involved in adaptive changes depending on the type and duration of the training.

Author Contributions: A.S., L.Z., and D.J. contributed to the data collection and elaboration, writing, and approval of manuscript; and are guarantors of the article. C.E. and L.A.M. contributed writing, editing, and approval of manuscript. S.D.R., J.M.S.-M., and M.P. contributed to supervising, revising, and approval of the manuscript. C.E., Z.W. contributed valuable graphical designs. The corresponding author attests that all listed authors meet authorship criteria and that no others meeting the criteria have been omitted. All authors have read and agreed to the published version of the manuscript.

Funding: This research received no external funding.

Acknowledgments: Research subject was implemented with CEPT infrastructure financed by the European Union—the European Regional Development Fund within the Operational Program "Innovative Economy" for 2007–2013. The manuscript was published as a result of the collaboration within the I-COMET team.

Conflicts of Interest: The authors declare no conflict of interest.

Abbreviations

ACS	acute coronary syndrome
CAD	coronary artery disease
c-miRNA	circulating microRNA
CRP	c-reactive proteins
CTGF	connective tissue growth factor
CVD	cardiovascular disease
GDF1	growth differentiation factor 1
HCM	hypertrophic cardiomyopathy
hs-cTnT	high-sensitivity cardiac troponin T
ISH	ischemic heart disease
LA	left atrium
LV	left ventricle
MACE	major adverse cardiac events
min/week	minutes per week
miR	microRNA
MMP	matrix metalloproteinase
mRNA	messenger RNA
NT-pro-BNP	n-terminal b-type natriuretic peptide
RNA	ribonucleotide acid
SCD	sudden cardiac death
TIMP	tissue inhibitor of metalloproteinase
TLR	toll-like receptors
WHO	World Health Organization

References

1. World Health Organization (WHO). *World Health Statistics 2019: Monitoring Health for the SDGs, Sustainable Development Goals*; WHO: Geneva, Switzerland, 2019.
2. Booth, F.W.; Gordon, S.E.; Carlson, C.J.; Hamilton, M.T. Waging war on modern chronic diseases: Primary prevention through exercise biology. *J. Appl. Physiol. 1985* **2000**, *88*, 774–787. [CrossRef] [PubMed]

3. Pelliccia, A.; Sharma, S.; Gati, S.; Back, M.; Borjesson, M.; Caselli, S.; Collet, J.P.; Corrado, D.; Drezner, J.A.; Halle, M.; et al. 2020 ESC Guidelines on sports cardiology and exercise in patients with cardiovascular disease. *Eur. Heart J.* **2020**. [CrossRef] [PubMed]
4. Hughes, D.; Ellefsen, S.; Baar, K. Adaptations to Endurance and Strength Training. *Cold Spring Harb. Perspect. Med.* **2018**, *8*, a029769. [CrossRef] [PubMed]
5. Sharma, S.; Merghani, A.; Mont, L. Exercise and the heart: The good, the bad, and the ugly. *Eur. Heart J.* **2015**, *36*, 1445–1453. [CrossRef]
6. Mavrogeni, S.I.; Bacopoulou, F.; Apostolaki, D.; Chrousos, G.P. Sudden cardiac death in athletes and the value of cardiovascular magnetic resonance. *Eur. J. Clin. Investig.* **2018**, *48*, e12955. [CrossRef] [PubMed]
7. Wojciechowska, A.; Osiak, A.; Kozar-Kamińska, K. MicroRNA in cardiovascular biology and disease. *Adv. Clin. Exp. Med.* **2017**, *26*, 868–874. [CrossRef] [PubMed]
8. Ha, M.; Kim, V.N. Regulation of microRNA biogenesis. *Nat. Rev. Mol. Cell Biol.* **2014**, *15*, 509–524. [CrossRef]
9. Feinberg, M.W.; Moore, K.J. MicroRNA Regulation of Atherosclerosis. *Circ. Res.* **2016**, *118*, 703–720. [CrossRef]
10. Romaine, S.P.R.; Tomaszewski, M.; Condorelli, G.; Samani, N.J. MicroRNAs in cardiovascular disease: An introduction for clinicians. *Heart* **2015**, *101*, 921–928. [CrossRef]
11. Mooren, F.C.; Viereck, J.; Krüger, K.; Thum, T. Circulating microRNAs as potential biomarkers of aerobic exercise capacity. *Am. J. Physiol. Circ. Physiol.* **2014**, *306*, H557–H563. [CrossRef]
12. Baggish, A.L.; Park, J.; Min, P.K.; Isaacs, S.; Parker, B.A.; Thompson, P.D.; Troyanos, C.; D'Hemecourt, P.; Dyer, S.; Thiel, M.; et al. Rapid upregulation and clearance of distinct circulating microRNAs after prolonged aerobic exercise. *J. Appl. Physiol. 1985* **2014**, *116*, 522–531. [CrossRef] [PubMed]
13. Gomes, C.P.D.C.; Oliveira, G.P., Jr.; Madrid, B.; Almeida, J.A.; Franco, O.L.; Pereira, R.W. Circulating miR-1, miR-133a, and miR-206 levels are increased after a half-marathon run. *Biomarkers* **2014**, *19*, 585–589. [CrossRef] [PubMed]
14. Hellsten, Y.; Nyberg, M. Cardiovascular Adaptations to Exercise Training. *Compr. Physiol.* **2015**, *6*, 1–32. [CrossRef] [PubMed]
15. Wang, J.; Liew, O.W.; Richards, A.M.; Chen, Y.T. Overview of MicroRNAs in Cardiac Hypertrophy, Fibrosis, and Apoptosis. *Int. J. Mol. Sci.* **2016**, *17*, 749. [CrossRef]
16. Baggish, A.L.; Hale, A.; Weiner, R.B.; Lewis, G.D.; Systrom, D.; Wang, F.; Wang, T.J.; Chan, S.Y. Dynamic regulation of circulating microRNA during acute exhaustive exercise and sustained aerobic exercise training. *J. Physiol.* **2011**, *589*, 3983–3994. [CrossRef]
17. Ramos, A.E.; Lo, C.; Estephan, L.E.; Tai, Y.Y.; Tang, Y.; Zhao, J.; Sugahara, M.; Gorcsan, J., III; Brown, M.G.; Lieberman, D.E.; et al. Specific circulating microRNAs display dose-dependent responses to variable intensity and duration of endurance exercise. *Am. J. Physiol. Circ. Physiol.* **2018**, *315*, H273–H283. [CrossRef]
18. Denham, J.; Prestes, P.R. Muscle-Enriched MicroRNAs Isolated from Whole Blood Are Regulated by Exercise and Are Potential Biomarkers of Cardiorespiratory Fitness. *Front. Genet.* **2016**, *7*, 196. [CrossRef]
19. Zilahi, E.; Adamecz, Z.; Bodoki, L.; Griger, Z.; Póliska, S.; Nagy-Vincze, M.; Dankó, K. Dysregulated expression profile of myomiRs in the skeletal muscle of patients with polymyositis. *EJIFCC* **2019**, *30*, 237–245.
20. Fochi, S.; Giuriato, G.; De Simone, T.; Gomez-Lira, M.; Tamburin, S.; Del Piccolo, L.; Schena, F.; Venturelli, M.; Romanelli, M.G. Regulation of microRNAs in Satellite Cell Renewal, Muscle Function, Sarcopenia and the Role of Exercise. *Inallt. J. Mol. Sci.* **2020**, *21*, 6732. [CrossRef]
21. Chen, J.F.; Mandel, E.M.; Thomson, J.M.; Wu, Q.; Callis, T.E.; Hammond, S.M.; Conlon, F.L.; Wang, D.Z. The role of microRNA-1 and microRNA-133 in skeletal muscle proliferation and differentiation. *Nat. Genet.* **2006**, *38*, 228–233. [CrossRef]
22. Fernández-Sanjurjo, M.; Úbeda, N.; Fernández-García, B.; Del Valle, M.; De Molina, A.R.; Crespo, M.C.; Martin-Hernández, R.; Casas-Agustench, P.; Martínez-Camblor, P.; De Gonzalo-Calvo, D.; et al. Exercise dose affects the circulating microRNA profile in response to acute endurance exercise in male amateur runners. *Scand. J. Med. Sci. Sports* **2020**, *30*, 1896–1907. [CrossRef]
23. Zhang, L.; Wu, Y.; Li, Y.; Xu, C.; Li, X.; Zhu, D.; Zhang, Y.; Xing, S.; Wang, H.; Zhang, Z.; et al. Tanshinone IIA Improves miR-133 Expression Through MAPK ERK1/2 Pathway in Hypoxic Cardiac Myocytes. *Cell. Physiol. Biochem.* **2012**, *30*, 843–852. [CrossRef] [PubMed]
24. Mitchelson, K.R.; Qin, W.Y. Roles of the canonical myomiRs miR-1, -133 and -206 in cell development and disease. *World J. Biol. Chem.* **2015**, *6*, 162–208. [CrossRef] [PubMed]

25. Liu, W.; Wen, Y.; Bi, P.; Lai, X.; Liu, X.S.; Liu, X.; Kuang, S. Hypoxia promotes satellite cell self-renewal and enhances the efficiency of myoblast transplantation. *Development* **2012**, *139*, 2857–2865. [CrossRef] [PubMed]
26. Rao, P.K.; Kumar, R.M.; Farkhondeh, M.; Baskerville, S.; Lodish, H.F. Myogenic factors that regulate expression of muscle-specific microRNAs. *Proc. Natl. Acad. Sci. USA* **2006**, *103*, 8721–8726. [CrossRef] [PubMed]
27. Palacín, M.; Reguero, J.R.; Martín, M.; Molina, B.D.; Moris, C.; Alvarez, V.; Coto, E. Profile of MicroRNAs Differentially Produced in Hearts from Patients with Hypertrophic Cardiomyopathy and Sarcomeric Mutations. *Clin. Chem.* **2011**, *57*, 1614–1616. [CrossRef] [PubMed]
28. Roncarati, R.; Anselmi, C.V.; Losi, M.A.; Papa, L.; Cavarretta, E.; Martins, P.D.C.; Contaldi, C.; Jotti, G.S.; Franzone, A.; Galastri, L.; et al. Circulating miR-29a, Among Other Up-Regulated MicroRNAs, Is the Only Biomarker for Both Hypertrophy and Fibrosis in Patients With Hypertrophic Cardiomyopathy. *J. Am. Coll. Cardiol.* **2014**, *63*, 920–927. [CrossRef]
29. Karlsen, A.; Soendenbroe, C.; Malmgaard-Clausen, N.M.; Wagener, F.; Moeller, C.E.; Senhaji, Z.; Damberg, K.; Andersen, J.L.; Schjerling, P.; Kjaer, M.; et al. Preserved capacity for satellite cell proliferation, regeneration, and hypertrophy in the skeletal muscle of healthy elderly men. *FASEB J.* **2020**, *34*, 6418–6436. [CrossRef]
30. De Gonzalo-Calvo, D.; Dávalos, A.; Fernández-Sanjurjo, M.; Amado-Rodriguez, L.; Diaz-Coto, S.; Tomás-Zapico, C.; Montero, A.; García-González, Á.; Llorente-Cortés, V.; Heras, M.E.; et al. Circulating microRNAs as emerging cardiac biomarkers responsive to acute exercise. *Int. J. Cardiol.* **2018**, *264*, 130–136. [CrossRef]
31. Alack, K.; Krüger, K.; Weiss, A.; Schermuly, R.; Frech, T.; Eggert, M.; Mooren, F.C. Aerobic endurance training status affects lymphocyte apoptosis sensitivity by induction of molecular genetic adaptations. *Brain Behav. Immun.* **2019**, *75*, 251–257. [CrossRef]
32. Backes, C.; Leidinger, P.; Keller, A.; Hart, M.; Meyer, T.; Meese, E.; Hecksteden, A. Blood Born miRNAs Signatures that Can Serve as Disease Specific Biomarkers Are Not Significantly Affected by Overall Fitness and Exercise. *PLoS ONE* **2014**, *9*, e102183. [CrossRef] [PubMed]
33. Bye, A.; Røsjø, H.; Aspenes, S.T.; Condorelli, G.; Omland, T.; Wisloff, U. Circulating MicroRNAs and Aerobic Fitness—The HUNT-Study. *PLoS ONE* **2013**, *8*, e57496. [CrossRef]
34. Danese, E.; Benati, M.; Sanchis-Gomar, F.; Tarperi, C.; Salvagno, G.L.; Paviati, E.; Montagnana, M.; Schena, F.; Lippi, G. Influence of middle-distance running on muscular micro RNAs. *Scand. J. Clin. Lab. Investig.* **2018**, *78*, 165–170. [CrossRef]
35. Kern, F.; Ludwig, N.; Backes, C.; Maldener, E.; Fehlmann, T.; Suleymanov, A.; Meese, E.; Hecksteden, A.; Keller, A.; Meyer, T. Systematic Assessment of Blood-Borne MicroRNAs Highlights Molecular Profiles of Endurance Sport and Carbohydrate Uptake. *Cells* **2019**, *8*, 1045. [CrossRef] [PubMed]
36. Karvinen, S.; Sievänen, T.; Karppinen, J.E.; Hautasaari, P.; Bart, G.; Samoylenko, A.; Vainio, S.J.; Ahtiainen, J.P.; Laakkonen, E.K.; Kujala, U.M. MicroRNAs in Extracellular Vesicles in Sweat Change in Response to Endurance Exercise. *Front. Physiol.* **2020**, *11*, 676. [CrossRef] [PubMed]
37. Nielsen, S.; Akerstrom, T.; Nielsen, A.R.; Yfanti, C.; Scheele, C.; Pedersen, B.K.; Laye, M.J. The miRNA Plasma Signature in Response to Acute Aerobic Exercise and Endurance Training. *PLoS ONE* **2014**, *9*, e87308. [CrossRef] [PubMed]
38. Uhlemann, M.; Möbius-Winkler, S.; Fikenzer, S.; Adam, J.; Redlich, M.; Möhlenkamp, S.; Hilberg, T.; Schuler, G.C.; Adams, V. Circulating microRNA-126 increases after different forms of endurance exercise in healthy adults. *Eur. J. Prev. Cardiol.* **2014**, *21*, 484–491. [CrossRef]
39. Yin, X.; Cui, S.; Li, X.; Li, W.; Lu, Q.J.; Jiang, X.H.; Wang, H.; Chen, X.; Ma, J.Z. Regulation of Circulatory Muscle-specific MicroRNA during 8 km Run. *Int. J. Sports Med.* **2020**, *41*, 582–588. [CrossRef]
40. Patil, H.R.; O'Keefe, J.H.; Lavie, C.J.; Magalski, A.; Vogel, R.A.; McCullough, P.A. Cardiovascular Damage Resulting from Chronic Excessive Endurance Exercise. *Mo. Med.* **2012**, *109*, 312–321.
41. Scherr, J.; Braun, S.; Schuster, T.; Hartmann, C.; Moehlenkamp, S.; Wolfarth, B.; Pressler, A.; Halle, M. 72-h Kinetics of High-Sensitive Troponin T and Inflammatory Markers after Marathon. *Med. Sci. Sports Exerc.* **2011**, *43*, 1819–1827. [CrossRef]
42. Fernandes, T.; Barauna, V.G.; Negrao, C.E.; Phillips, M.I.; De Oliveira, E.M. Aerobic exercise training promotes physiological cardiac remodeling involving a set of microRNAs. *Am. J. Physiol. Circ. Physiol.* **2015**, *309*, H543–H552. [CrossRef]

43. Wang, X.; Yang, C.; Liu, X.; Yang, P. Ghrelin Alleviates Angiotensin II-Induced H9c2 Apoptosis: Impact of the miR-208 Family. *Med. Sci. Monit.* **2018**, *24*, 6707–6716. [CrossRef] [PubMed]
44. Sun, T.; Dong, Y.H.; Du, W.; Shi, C.Y.; Wang, K.; Akram, J.; Wang, J.; Li, P.F. The Role of MicroRNAs in Myocardial Infarction: From Molecular Mechanism to Clinical Application. *Int. J. Mol. Sci.* **2017**, *18*, 745. [CrossRef] [PubMed]
45. Guo, Y.; Luo, F.; Liu, Q.; Xu, D. Regulatory non-coding RNAs in acute myocardial infarction. *J. Cell. Mol. Med.* **2017**, *21*, 1013–1023. [CrossRef] [PubMed]
46. Baggish, A.L. Focal Fibrosis in the Endurance Athlete's Heart. *JACC Cardiovasc. Imaging* **2018**, *11*, 1271–1273. [CrossRef] [PubMed]
47. Malek, A.L.; Barczuk-Falęcka, M.; Werys, K.; Czajkowska, A.; Mróz, A.; Witek, K.; Burrage, M.; Bakalarski, W.; Nowicki, D.; Roik, D.; et al. Cardiovascular magnetic resonance with parametric mapping in long-term ultra-marathon runners. *Eur. J. Radiol.* **2019**, *117*, 89–94. [CrossRef] [PubMed]
48. Gyöngyösi, M.; Winkler, J.; Ramos, I.; Do, Q.; Firat, H.; McDonald, K.; González, A.; Thum, T.; Díez, J.; Jaisser, F.; et al. Myocardial fibrosis: Biomedical research from bench to bedside. *Eur. J. Heart Fail.* **2017**, *19*, 177–191. [CrossRef]
49. Nguyen, M.N.; Kiriazis, H.; Gao, X.M.; Du, X.J. Cardiac Fibrosis and Arrhythmogenesis. *Compr. Physiol.* **2017**, *7*, 1009–1049. [CrossRef]
50. Creemers, E.E.; van Rooij, E. Function and Therapeutic Potential of Noncoding RNAs in Cardiac Fibrosis. *Circ. Res.* **2016**, *118*, 108–118. [CrossRef]
51. Thum, T. Noncoding RNAs and myocardial fibrosis. *Nat. Rev. Cardiol.* **2014**, *11*, 655–663. [CrossRef]
52. Clauss, S.; Wakili, R.; Hildebrand, B.; Kaab, S.; Hoster, E.; Klier, I.; Martens, E.; Hanley, A.; Hanssen, H.; Halle, M.; et al. MicroRNAs as Biomarkers for Acute Atrial Remodeling in Marathon Runners (The miRathon Study—A Sub-Study of the Munich Marathon Study). *PLoS ONE* **2016**, *11*, e148599. [CrossRef] [PubMed]
53. Sanchis-Gomar, F.; Lucía, A. Pathophysiology of atrial fibrillation in endurance athletes: An overview of recent findings. *CMAJ* **2016**, *188*, E433–E435. [CrossRef] [PubMed]
54. Schmitz, B.; Rolfes, F.; Schelleckes, K.; Mewes, M.; Thorwesten, L.; Krüger, M.; Klose, A.; Brand, S.-M. Longer Work/Rest Intervals During High-Intensity Interval Training (HIIT) Lead to Elevated Levels of miR-222 and miR-29c. *Front. Physiol.* **2018**, *9*, 395. [CrossRef] [PubMed]
55. Zhang, Y.; Huang, X.R.; Wei, L.H.; Chung, A.C.; Yu, C.M.; Lan, H.Y. miR-29b as a Therapeutic Agent for Angiotensin II-induced Cardiac Fibrosis by Targeting TGF-β/Smad3 signaling. *Mol. Ther.* **2014**, *22*, 974–985. [CrossRef] [PubMed]
56. Katsiari, C.G.; Bogdanos, D.P.; Sakkas, L. Inflammation and cardiovascular disease. *World J. Transl. Med.* **2019**, *8*, 1–8. [CrossRef]
57. Barros, E.S.; Nascimento, D.C.; Prestes, J.; Nóbrega, O.T.; Córdova, C.; Sousa, F.; Boullosa, D.A. Acute and Chronic Effects of Endurance Running on Inflammatory Markers: A Systematic Review. *Front. Physiol.* **2017**, *8*, 779. [CrossRef]
58. Tahamtan, A.; Teymoori-Rad, M.; Nakstad, B.; Salimi, V. Anti-Inflammatory MicroRNAs and Their Potential for Inflammatory Diseases Treatment. *Front. Immunol.* **2018**, *9*, 1377. [CrossRef]
59. Grabarek, B.O.; Wcisło-Dziadecka, D.; Gola, J. In silico analysis of CpG islands and miRNAs potentially regulating the JAK-STAT signalling pathway. *Adv. Dermatol. Allergol.* **2020**, *37*, 513–519. [CrossRef]
60. Helgerud, J.; Høydal, K.; Wang, E.; Karlsen, T.; Berg, P.; Bjerkaas, M.; Simonsen, T.; Helgesen, C.; Hjorth, N.; Bach, R.; et al. Aerobic High-Intensity Intervals Improve VO_{2max} More Than Moderate Training. *Med. Sci. Sports Exerc.* **2007**, *39*, 665–671. [CrossRef]
61. Keteyian, S.J.; Brawner, C.A.; Savage, P.D.; Ehrman, J.K.; Schairer, J.; Divine, G.; Aldred, H.; Ophaug, K.; Ades, P.A. Peak aerobic capacity predicts prognosis in patients with coronary heart disease. *Am. Heart J.* **2008**, *156*, 292–300. [CrossRef]

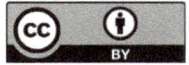

© 2020 by the authors. Licensee MDPI, Basel, Switzerland. This article is an open access article distributed under the terms and conditions of the Creative Commons Attribution (CC BY) license (http://creativecommons.org/licenses/by/4.0/).